RENEWALS 458-4574

WI[.]

UTS

D

O'

Addiction

Addiction

From Biology to Drug Policy

SECOND EDITION

Avram Goldstein

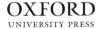

OXFORD
UNIVERSITY PRESS

2001

OXFORD

UNIVERSITY PRESS

Oxford   New York

Athens   Auckland   Bangkok   Bogotá   Buenos Aires
Cape Town   Chennai   Dar es Salaam   Delhi   Florence   Hong Kong   Istanbul
Karachi   Kolkata   Kuala Lumpur   Madrid   Melbourne   Mexico City   Mumbai
Nairobi   Paris   São Paulo   Shanghai   Singapore   Taipei   Tokyo   Toronto   Warsaw

and associated companies in
Berlin   Ibadan

Published by Oxford University Press, Inc.
198 Madison Avenue, New York, New York 10016
http://www.oup-usa.org

Library of Congress Cataloging-in-Publication Data
Goldstein, Avram.
   Addiction : from biology to drug policy / Avram Goldstein.—2nd ed.
      p.   cm.
   Includes bibliographical references and index.
   ISBN 0-19-514663-8 (alk. paper)—ISBN 0-19-514664-6 (pbk. : alk. paper)
      1. Drug abuse—Physiological aspects. 2. Drug abuse—Social aspects. I. Title.
RC564 .G66 2001
616.86—dc21   00-140048

9 8 7 6 5 4 3 2 1

Printed in the United States of America
on acid-free paper

Contents

Preface to the First Edition, 1993   vii

Preface to the Second Edition, 2000   xi

1. Introduction   3

PART ONE: DRUGS AND THE BRAIN   17

  2. Neurotransmitters: The Brain's Own Drugs   19

  3. Receptors: Locks for the Addictive Keys   37

  4. Addictive Behavior   53

  5. Pain and Pleasure   71

  6. The Seesaw Brain: "Highs" and Adaptations   83

  7. Are Addicts Born or Made?   99

PART TWO: THE DRUGS AND THE ADDICTS   115

  8. Nicotine   117

  9. Alcohol and Related Drugs   135

  10. Heroin, Morphine, and Other Opiates   157

  11. Cocaine and Amphetamines   179

  12. Cannabis (Marijuana)   195

  13. Caffeine   207

  14. Hallucinogens   219

PART THREE: DRUGS AND SOCIETY   233

  15. Prevention: Just Say No?   235

16. Treating Addiction, Preventing Relapse 249

17. Three Lessons from the Street 261

18. Three Lessons from Abroad 273

19. Prohibition vs. Legalization—A False Dichotomy 293

20. New Strategies for Rational Drug Policy 307

Suggestions for Further Reading 329

Index 341

Preface to the First Edition (1993)

This book grew out of my experiences during 25 years of laboratory and clinical research and teaching about the addictive drugs. The more I learned, and the more drug addiction became a subject of national concern, the more I realized how great was the gap between our growing scientific knowledge and the ever more heated debates about drug policy. A book directed primarily at intelligent non-experts might close this gap by translating what scientists have discovered about drug addiction into easily understood concepts. I believe it will be of interest, too, to students and practitioners of medicine, psychiatry, nursing, pharmacy, and other health professions, who deal with addicts as part of their daily work. Finally, it will provide teachers with solid factual information to help educate a new generation about this much-neglected societal problem.

The subject of drug addiction can be divided into three broad areas—how the drugs act on the brain, how each drug causes the medical disorder we call addiction, and what impact the addictive drugs have on society. Accordingly, the book is divided into three parts. I attempt to explain what we know about drug addiction in each of these three areas, how we know what we know, and what we can (and cannot) do about the drug problem.

I present the uncertainties of our present knowledge as well as the surely established facts. I avoid technical jargon; but where a technical term is essential, I define it at first use and also provide a reference to that definition in the index. I try to make the biomedical science interesting to the nonexpert by speaking whenever possible from my own point of view as experimenter and by attempting to convey the spirit of adventure as the scientist experiences it. When I write autobiographically, therefore, it is not to claim undue credit for research advances to which so many others, the world over, have contributed. And when I describe how the experiments are actually done, it is to help the reader follow the logic of the conclusions.

Many people and institutions contributed to this book. Stipend support for the writing was provided by the former Board of Directors of the Addiction Research Foundation of Palo Alto: Jean Kuhn Doyle, Herbert Dwight, Henry Organ, Martin Packard, Charles Schulz, and Brooks Walker, Jr.; I am deeply indebted to them all. With the help of Robert J. Glaser a grant was obtained from the Henry J. Kaiser Family Foundation to defray research expenses. The Albuquerque heroin addiction follow-up study described in chapter 11 was made possible through the generosity of the Carnegie Corporation of New York and its president, David A. Hamburg.

I owe a special debt of gratitude to Harold Kalant, who has been a valuable colleague over the years, who contributed much to my ideas on the pharmacology and sociology of the addictive drugs, and who offered helpful advice about the manuscript. Robert L. Campos has been an important source of information and assistance from the days of my first involvement in the treatment of heroin addicts. And for lively disagreements that helped sharpen my thinking about drug policy issues I am indebted to Ethan Nadelmann.

My scientific associates at the Addiction Research Foundation in Palo Alto who participated in most of my own investigations described here include Brian M. Cox, Priscilla Grevert, Barbara Judson, and Louise I. Lowney. Abbie Freiley was the skillful administrator of all the Foundation's efforts.

I am indebted to many people in Albuquerque. At the University of New Mexico are James Herrera, David Broudy, Marcia Starr, Walter Winslow, Al Vogel, Philip J. May, and Patricia McFeeley. Indispensable help in tracking subjects at the clinics and in the community was provided by Angie Barchus, Abigail Brooks, Steven R. Campos, Frank Fernandez, the late Paul Garcia, Ted Hicks, Marion Saxton, and Joseph Tartaglia. Special thanks are due to Robert Kahn for arranging access to the Monroe Clinic.

For their generous assistance and hospitality during my study visit in the U.K. I thank especially Griffith Edwards, Martin Mitcheson, Michael Russell, and John Shanks; for similar help in the Netherlands, Eddy Engelsman (who also commented on a draft of chapter 17), Charles Kaplan, and Govert van de Wijngaart; and in Zurich,

Aurelio Pasi. Several others who were helpful are mentioned by name in chapter 17.

Finally, I thank my colleagues Dora B. Goldstein, Mary Jeanne Kreek, and Roger E. Meyer for their helpful comments on an earlier draft of the manuscript; and my publishers, W. H. Freeman and Company, especially senior editor Jonathan Cobb, project editor Janet Tannenbaum, and copy editor Denis Cullinan, for criticism, suggestions, and expert assistance in bringing the book to publication.

AVRAM GOLDSTEIN, M.D.
Stanford, California
August 1993

Preface to the Second Edition

Scientific progress is so rapid nowadays that books about biology and medicine become obsolete in a few years. Revisiting a book about addiction seven years after its initial publication raises two questions. First, how much of it is still pertinent, how much just plain wrong? And second, are there new research findings or new political developments that in some fundamental way modify our understanding of addiction or of drug policies?

The answer to the first question is that nothing in the book has been proved wrong by time; the basics are the same, and my moderate views on drug policy also remain the same. The answer to the second question, however, is that these seven years have brought vast progress in our scientific understanding of addiction. The 1990s were fittingly dubbed "the decade of the brain" because brain research has moved forward at such an incredible pace. And because addiction is a brain disease, almost every advance in brain research impinges directly or indirectly on the study of addiction. I have retained the general organization of the book, but new developments are included in every chapter.

I had a difficult decision to make about citing individual scientists and clinicians by name. If I mentioned any, there would always be the question why not some others whose work was just as important. I took the easy way out. With very rare exceptions, I have not mentioned the names of any living researchers, even when their important contributions are described extensively.

In addition to those acknowledged in the preface to the first edition for having contributed to the genesis of the book, I am now indebted to other colleagues for recent discussions about the addictions. These include—among many others—Huda Akil, Gabriele

Bammer, Luca Cavalli-Sforza, Griffith Edwards, Zach Hall, Simon Hewett, Reese Jones, Alan Leshner, Barry McCaffrey, John Strang, Roy Wise, John Witton, Harold Kalant, and especially Alejandro Zaffaroni. Robert Kahn provided access to the Western Clinical Health Services methadone clinic in Albuquerque, where Lillian Gonzales and Wayne Brown facilitated my research. Of course, none of the above is responsible for my errors or misplaced emphases, nor do they necessarily share my opinions about addiction.

Finally, before launching into the substance of the book, I can do no better than quote General Barry McCaffrey, the "drug czar" in the Clinton administration, director of the federal Office of National Drug Control Policy (ONDCP):

> Facts, based in science and data collection, rather than ideology or anecdote, must provide the basis for rational drug policy.

Amen! This book is about the science of drug addiction—how we know what we know, what we still need to learn, and how what we learn must inform rational policies. Reader, you will find no ideology here and no sermons about morality, but only honest evaluations of the present state of addiction science by an addiction scientist.

AVRAM GOLDSTEIN, M.D.
Stanford, California
April 2000

For Dody

Addiction

Introduction

A 50-year-old man lies in a hospital bed, desperately ill. Emphysema has destroyed his lungs, and the pitiful sound of his labored breathing fills the room. Watch him! Incredible as it seems, he begs his wife to bring him a cigarette. Cigarettes put him here, cigarettes will surely finish him off. Why doesn't he quit? Why didn't he quit years ago when the first Surgeon General's report on smoking, widely publicized, had already made it clear what his future would be if he continued his pack-a-day habit?

This introduction could have started differently.

A 50-year-old man gets off the bus in a seedy downtown neighborhood. Just hours before, he was released after serving a two-year sentence for burglary, his third time in prison. His regular income as a grocery clerk had barely been enough to support his wife and child, so burglary seemed the only way to raise the large sums he needed for his heroin habit. Watch him! Only a block from the bus terminal he makes his "connection," buys a syringe and needle and some white powder. Heroin put him in prison three times, heroin will surely finish him off. Why doesn't he quit? Why didn't he quit years ago, when he could see clearly enough what his future would be if he continued using heroin?

Truths and Falsehoods about Addiction

Why did I choose to begin with an opening paragraph about nicotine addiction? Our society makes artificial distinctions among addictive drugs. We foster the false impression that because nicotine and alcohol are legal, they must be less dangerous and less addictive than the illicit drugs. Even the way we use (or don't use) the term "addiction" compounds this error. Addicts, we are accustomed to thinking, belong to an underclass; the word brings to mind street people, "junkies," ethnic minorities in the inner cities. For white middle-class folk in the suburbs, we use softer words to describe their "habits." We call them "heavy smokers," not nicotine addicts; "heavy drinkers" or perhaps even "alcoholics," but not alcohol addicts; "heavy coffee drinkers," not caffeine addicts. And even though many heroin and cocaine users are middle-class students or professionals, people like that seldom come to mind when we think about heroin or cocaine addiction.

Curiously, nicotine and alcohol and caffeine, in common parlance and political rhetoric, are often not even called "drugs," and they are rarely mentioned in our perennial "war on drugs." The frequent use of phrases like "alcohol and drugs" or "tobacco and drugs" reinforces this false idea. The objection to these phrases is not a matter of mere semantics; incorrect use of language shapes incorrect ways of thinking. So let me make it clear: there is no basis whatsoever in medical science for setting aside the legal addictive drugs as different from the illicit ones. As a matter of fact, the legal drugs are by far our greatest addiction problem—in part just because they are legal and readily available.

A drug is any chemical agent that affects biologic function. Drugs are typically used to treat or prevent disease. Some drugs act in the brain, some in other organs, and some in several parts of the body at the same time. A psychoactive drug is one that acts in the brain to alter mood, thought processes, or behavior. Nothing about drugs as such, even psychoactive ones, makes people like them or try to secure them. On the contrary, when physicians prescribe drugs, a major difficulty is getting patients to take them regularly. And this "compliance problem" is just as troublesome with many psychoactive drugs (such as those used to treat mental illnesses) as it is with drugs of other kinds. Among all the psychoactive drugs, however, there is something special about a very few. These addictive drugs are defined by the fact that they are self-administered without medical prescription—repeatedly, compulsively, even self-destructively. Once regarded with sympathy as an unfortunate disease, drug addiction in the United States was seen increasingly, during the twentieth century, as a morally reprehensible behavior, which addicts could control if only they made the effort. This book argues that drug addiction—although addiction to some drugs is often associated with crime—is primarily a public-health problem.

Dr. Alan Leshner, director of the National Institute on Drug Abuse, explains: "Drug addiction is a complex illness. It is characterized by compulsive, at times uncontrollable drug craving, seeking, and use that persist even in the face of extremely negative consequences . . . with relapses possible even after long periods of abstinence."

Addictive drugs pose dangers to the health of users, and they threaten nonusers as well. Like most public-health problems, addiction has multiple causes, many prevention strategies, and many approaches to treatment.

The Seven Drug Families

To speak of "the drug problem" is to oversimplify. The addictive drugs fall into seven families, which differ from one another in chemistry, effects on behavior, long-term harm, and the likelihood of a compulsive use pattern developing. Some addictive drugs— alcohol is a good example—disturb behavior in a way that threatens the safety of others even when used occasionally and not compulsively. Others—for instance, nicotine—are powerfully addictive but do not disturb behavior significantly. Still others—cocaine and methamphetamine are examples—cause excitation, sometimes an actual manic paranoid psychosis, and an extraordinary compulsion to go on using. Different drugs are taken into the body by different routes—injection into a vein or muscle or under the skin; intranasal (snorting); inhalation (as by smoking); or by mouth. Each drug is handled in its own way by the body, so that some are rapidly destroyed, while others persist for a long time. Moreover, rates of drug metabolism differ greatly among people, for both genetic and environmental reasons, resulting in individual variations in a drug's effect.

The features that distinguish the seven drug families have obvious implications for prevention, treatment, and social policy. To think rationally about drugs, we need to understand how each one modifies brain function, and how each one affects the user's health and the public health. In Part Two, I shall discuss the seven families of addictive drugs, one by one, at length; here I merely identify them:

1. Nicotine. The active principle in the tobacco leaf, this drug may be taken into the body not only by smoking (typically cigarettes) but also by absorption through the membranes of the mouth or nose when tobacco is chewed or used as snuff.

2. Alcohol and related drugs. In addition to beer, wine, and the distilled liquors, the alcohol family also includes the barbiturates and benzodiazepines (e.g., Valium). This family has legitimate uses in medicine, such as barbiturates for surgical anesthesia and the treatment of epilepsy and benzodiazepines for relief of anxiety and sometimes of insomnia. In the alcohol family, too, because their pharmacology is similar, are the volatile solvents, which are taken by inhalation, as in glue sniffing.

3. Opiates. This family contains the products of opium poppies, which are principally crude opium, morphine, and codeine. Heroin is prepared from morphine by chemical treatment. Codeine and several synthetic opiate painkillers (e.g., oxycodone, Dilaudid, Demerol), taken by mouth, are used by some opiate addicts. Heroin is typically administered by vein; but like crude opium it may also be smoked. If heroin is pure enough, it can be absorbed through the mucous membranes of the nose (snorted); and recent years have seen both increasing purity of street heroin and increasing numbers of smokers and snorters, especially among young people. Opiates other than heroin are usually taken by mouth. Many—especially morphine and codeine—are legitimately prescribed as pain-relieving medications, but heroin is not approved for this purpose in the United States. Methadone, LAAM, and buprenorphine are synthetic opiates used for treating heroin addicts.

4. Cocaine and amphetamines. Cocaine is the active principle of the coca leaf. There are two chemical forms of cocaine called hydrochloride salt and free base. The hydrochloride salt dissolves in water and can be injected or snorted. The free base ("crack") is smoked. In parts of South America where the coca plant grows, chewing the leaf is a long-established part of the native culture. Amphetamines are made in the laboratory. Their salts, like cocaine hydrochloride, dissolve readily and can be taken by vein or by mouth.

A pure form of one amphetamine (methamphetamine, "ice") is not readily destroyed by heat, so it can be smoked. The biologic effects of cocaine and the amphetamines are very similar. Both have certain approved uses in medicine—cocaine, for example, is a local anesthetic for the eyes, nasal passages, mouth, or throat.

5. Cannabis (marijuana, hashish, THC). Marijuana is the leaf of the hemp (cannabis) plant, hashish is a concentrated cannabis resin. Tetrahydrocannabinol (THC) is the pure psychoactive principle in cannabis, and is responsible for the psychoactive effects of marijuana and hashish. Marijuana is smoked, sometimes taken by mouth. THC has been a valuable research tool and it is now also available as an approved medication (dronabinol, Marinol) for a few conditions. Cannabis is otherwise illicit, but research into various possible medicinal uses continues.

6. Caffeine. Caffeine is the psychoactive principle in coffee beans and tea leaves, extracted into hot water, and taken by mouth as a beverage. It is also found as an additive in soft drinks and some over-the-counter medications. This is the only addictive drug that is completely legal, even for children.

7. Hallucinogens. This is a diverse family that includes many naturally occurring and synthetic compounds with mind-altering effects. Among the natural products are "magic mushrooms" (containing psilocybin and other active principles), cactus (containing mescaline), and a variety of exotic substances taken ceremonially by mouth, snorting, or smoking in native cultures throughout the world. Among the synthetics are LSD (lysergic acid diethylamide), MDMA ("ecstasy"), and PCP (phencyclidine, "angel dust"). There was a time in the sixties when hallucinogens were used therapeutically by some psychiatrists, but they are no longer used medically today.

Addiction as a Public Health Problem

How widely used are the various addictive drugs? That sounds like a simple enough question, but getting close to a true answer is a terribly complicated business. In the National Household Survey on Drug Abuse, a random sample of nearly 25,000 persons living in households is surveyed by skilled interviewers. But surveying householders is not the same as counting everyone in the population. People in prison, in the hospital, or homeless will not be surveyed, yet we know that the use of certain drugs is disproportionately high in just those groups.

Furthermore, it is doubtful how many people—no matter how skilled the interviewers—are likely to give accurate answers, especially about their use of illicit drugs. Much research has been done to estimate the "self-report bias," the tendency for people to under-estimate their own drug use. This applies not only to illicit drugs; if heavy use of any drug is disapproved of, people will tend to minimize what they say about their consumption of it. In an attempt to reduce self-report bias in the Household Survey, subjects are asked to answer some questions anonymously on a form that is then sealed and mailed in.

There is also the question of how to describe intensity of use. Categories typically used in surveys are "ever in lifetime," "at least once in previous year," and "at least once in previous month." These are rough attempts to distinguish between casual users who contribute only insignificantly (if at all) to the addiction problem, and true addicts. But the significance of such categories is different for different drugs—an important fact not considered in most surveys. With nicotine or caffeine, many users take small amounts but are not addicts; so the proper measure of intensity is the amount used each day. With cocaine, which is often taken in a weekend binge pattern, a weekly measure may be most relevant. With heroin, at least once daily characterizes the addict. With alcohol, most daily users present no problem to themselves or society even though they may have one or two beers or glasses of wine in a social context; here the best criterion is how much is taken in a day or at a single sitting, or whether drinking to the point of intoxication occurs.

With those reservations in mind, let us consider—in Figure 1.1—the latest information available (1997) for the United States. These estimates are for current users—defined as the number of people who used each drug at least once in the previous month. The data are estimates for a total population of 216 million over the age of 11. Caffeine use is nearly universal; it is a mild stimulant, and moderate use is probably not harmful to adults. Some medical authorities, however, are concerned that we do not know enough about possible effects of prolonged high caffeine intake on brain development and behavior in children.

Alcohol and nicotine (in tobacco) are the next most widely used addictive substances. Unlike caffeine, these two cause enormous

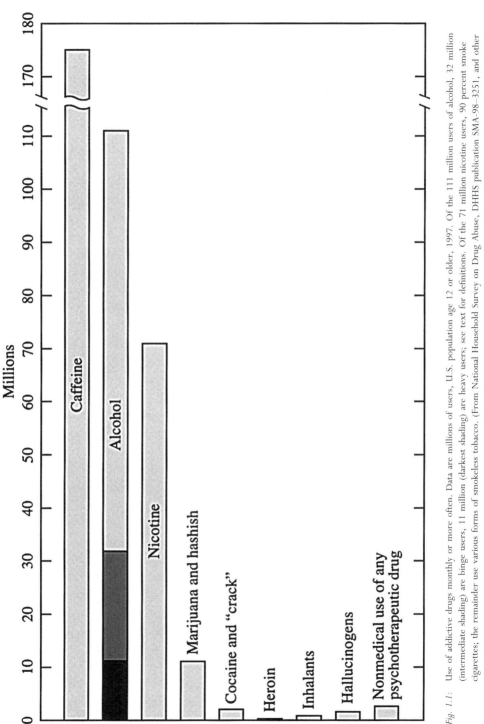

Fig. 1.1: Use of addictive drugs monthly or more often. Data are millions of users, U.S. population age 12 or older, 1997. Of the 111 million users of alcohol, 32 million (intermediate shading) are binge users, 11 million (darkest shading) are heavy users; see text for definitions. Of the 71 million nicotine users, 90 percent smoke cigarettes; the remainder use various forms of smokeless tobacco. (From National Household Survey on Drug Abuse, DHHS publication SMA-98–3251, and other sources.)

harm as measured by death and disability. Even casual users of alcohol can cause serious problems for society because of intoxication (e.g., highway fatalities, homicides). Of the 111 million current users, 32 million are "binge drinkers," defined as taking five or more drinks on the same occasion at least once during the previous month. Eleven million meet the criterion of "heavy drinking," engaging in binge drinking on five or more days during the previous month. C. Everett Koop, as Surgeon General, gave an even higher estimate—that 18 million have serious medical, social, and personal problems directly related to the use of alcohol.

The nature of nicotine addiction is such that as with caffeine, a person who uses tobacco at all takes it several times daily. As all the health damage of smoking is dose-related, the relevant measure of intensity is the number of cigarettes smoked daily. An insidious aspect of nicotine addiction is the absence of negative behavioral effects that might signal danger. The health impact (chronic lung damage, cancer of the lung and other organs, heart disease) is not due to nicotine itself but rather to products of the burning tobacco leaf. Carcinogens and irritants in tobacco smoke take many years to produce their cumulative damage, so—especially in the thinking of adolescents—the harm seems safely far into the future, while the satisfaction is immediate.

For reasons noted earlier, the figure for heroin (325,000 current users) is certainly a gross underestimate. The number of homeless people not counted in the Household Survey is estimated to be more than 800,000; and many of these transients are known to be users of heroin, cocaine, marijuana, and alcohol. Suppose there were actually a million homeless people, and suppose that every one of them used alcohol heavily; their contribution to the total number of alcohol users would be relatively small. Thus, their omission from surveys concerning alcohol makes little difference. In contrast, since there are so few heroin users in the population as a whole, omission of a group like this, with a high rate of heroin use, will result in a serious underestimate of the total.

About 14 million people used an illicit drug during the previous week, and for nine million of these, cannabis was the sole illicit drug. The principal illicit drugs—cannabis, heroin, cocaine, amphetamines, and hallucinogens—have a major impact on the user's health and on society. Addicts to these drugs may place their uncontrollable desire for the drug above all other needs and obligations. Thus, they may neglect nutrition and gainful employment while they devote inordinate amounts of time to drug-seeking behavior and associated criminal activities.

The total number who use nicotine or alcohol regularly far exceeds the number who use marijuana, cocaine, amphetamines, heroin, and "all others" (a category that includes volatile solvents and hallucinogens) combined. To state this fact is not to minimize the importance of the illicit drugs, but to set all drugs, licit as well as illicit, in a public-health context according to the aggregate harm done to users and to society.

To understand fully the public-health implications, one needs to know more than just the number of users. How many are directly and immediately harmed by the drugs? One way to obtain such information is from hospital emergency room records through the Drug Abuse Warning Network (DAWN). But as with the Household Survey, there are problems. Systematic reexamination of the DAWN records has cast doubt on their reliability; and remarkably, alcohol is not included at all, unless used together with another drug in an emergency room episode. Yet alcohol, used alone, causes emergency room admissions six times as often as when used in combination with another drug.

Keeping in mind, then, that the data are only very approximate, we can nevertheless get some useful information from DAWN. To get a rough indication of how dangerous each drug is to its user, we can compute the ratio of emergency room visits to the number of current users—in other words, how likely is the user of each drug to be brought to the emergency room? By this measure heroin is worst; in any given year as many as one in every three users is brought to an emergency room, often because of overdose due to uncertain and variable purity of the drug. Cocaine is next, with about one in 13 experiencing a serious adverse reaction; this is often a severe and life-threatening heart problem. Marijuana and the hallucinogens present far less immediate health hazards, affecting only one user in 200; and when adverse reactions do occur they usually take the form of psychiatric disturbances that are not life-threatening.

The term "comorbidity" describes the fact that drug abuse so often accompanies other mental illnesses. The National Institute of Mental Health (NIMH) established so-called Epidemiologic Catchment Areas to gather information about mental health in five representative communities. Data were collected in random face-to-face interviews by skilled personnel concerning a broad range of psychiatric disorders. Included were not only alcoholism but also "substance abuse disorder," a diagnostic category for any drug use that causes significant harm to the user. Current use of alcohol was found to cause serious problems for more than five million adults; why this estimate is lower than those cited above is unclear, but it is certainly high enough to command our attention. For addictive drugs other than alcohol, the number exceeded two million. Co-morbidity compounded the problems. Of those diagnosed with any mental illness, nearly one in three had an accompanying substance abuse disorder. Of those with an alcohol disorder, more than one-third also had another mental illness. And of those with a drug abuse disorder other than alcoholism, over half had another psychiatric diagnosis as well.

Addiction as an Infectious Disease

Drug addictions are in many ways like infectious diseases. A virus or bacterium infects some people but not everyone; there are differing degrees of relative immunity. Susceptibility (as for instance to tuberculosis) depends typically on a complex set of genetic and environmental factors. These include individual genetic vulnerability, ethnicity, degree of crowding, lack of sanitation, status of the immune system, and adequacy of nutrition. People carrying an infectious agent can transmit the disease to susceptible uninfected people. An infectious disease is spread most readily by people who have just caught it, and so it is with drug addiction; it is primarily new users who transmit the behavior to their peers.

Through public-health measures enforced by law, we try to eradicate infectious agents; this is analogous to attempts to control drug supply. At the same time, we provide for education about the kinds of behavior and lifestyles that expose people to infection or that reduce their immunity. We try to improve people's resistance in many ways, for example by vaccination. Finally, we offer treatment to all who are infected, not only to alleviate the illness (or cure it, if possible) but also to reduce the total pool of infection in order to limit the spread of the epidemic.

Some will object that the analogy to infectious disease is false because infected people are passive victims, whereas addicts actively seek out addictive drugs. But this distinction breaks down when one looks more closely; in both situations human behavior is partly or wholly responsible. Risk takers recklessly drink unsterilized water in areas where hepatitis or cholera or waterborne parasites are present. Careless people may not bother to use mosquito netting where malaria or encephalitis is prevalent. Heedless of the danger, some contribute to the AIDS epidemic through promiscuous sexual contacts without taking elementary precautions. Are those behaviors, which contribute to the spread of infectious diseases, really different in principle from that of cigarette smokers or alcoholics or cocaine addicts who start using a drug despite all the evidence of harm it will cause themselves and their families?

The unique characteristics of each specific infectious disease have to be understood before methods of prevention or treatment can be implemented. Likewise with the addictions—in every case policy must rest on a firm basis in medical science. Each addictive drug has its own characteristics, its own mode of action in the brain and its own pattern of biologic effects—severity of the addiction, disruption of behavior affecting the user and others, harmfulness to health, and long-term toxicity.

Many simplistic solutions to our drug addiction problem have been put forward. Some people want to step up the "war on drugs." They argue for stronger law enforcement to try to eliminate all the illicit drugs. Some people take a libertarian position. They would legalize all drugs, arguing that our drug problems are due primarily to the prohibitions, rather than to the drugs themselves. A moderate position seeks policies that try to balance the harm caused by the drugs against the harm caused by their regulation. To formulate that moderate position in specific detail, with its scientific basis, is the ultimate purpose of this book.

The misery suffered by addicts and their families is enormous. The costs to society—to all of us—are measured as loss of productivity, additional needs for medical care, dangers of drug-induced behaviors, destruction of family life, corruption of children, and burden on the criminal justice system. If we set aside political bombast, media sensationalism, and ill-informed calls for quick fixes, we can try—calmly and dispassionately—to examine what science can teach us about addictive drugs and addictive behavior. That requires a thorough analysis, drug by drug, of how each one acts and what harm each one does to users and to society.

What Does the Author Know and How Does He Know It?

The reader of a book that claims to impart authoritative information is entitled to know something about the author's qualifications. I am a pharmacologist, a neurobiologist, and a physician. Pharmacology is the scientific study of drugs and their uses in medicine; it should not be confused with pharmacy, the preparation and dispensing of drugs. In an academic career spanning more than 50 years, mostly at Stanford University, I studied and carried out experimental research on drugs, and I taught about addiction. My focus was on the opiates (morphine, heroin, methadone) and on nicotine and caffeine. My interest in opiate addiction led me to fundamental laboratory research on the brain receptors that are responsible for the drug effects. In the course of that research my colleagues and I discovered the dynorphins—one of the three families of endorphins, the morphinelike substances made in our own brains.

To learn more about heroin addiction and its treatment, I organized the first major methadone program in California. There I supervised the treatment of more than a thousand heroin addicts in San Jose and other communities of Santa Clara County. By means of rigorously controlled clinical trials, my colleagues and I were able to learn and publish a great deal about the most effective methods of treating and rehabilitating heroin addicts. I invented the first instantaneous method of urine testing for the presence of morphine, which would indicate heroin use; and this method was applied immediately to detect heroin users among our troops in Vietnam, in order to detoxify them before sending them home. I founded and directed the Addiction Research Foundation in Palo Alto, where I gathered a staff of talented investigators for basic neurobiology research at the laboratory bench, for research using normal human volunteers, and for clinical treatment research with heroin addicts.

After retiring from the university I kept in close touch with developments in drug addiction and its treatment as a member of the board of directors of the College on Problems of Drug Dependence, the principal organization of drug abuse researchers. I also served as a director of Drug Strategies, a national "think-tank" concerned with drug abuse research and policy. I have been a frequent advisor to the "drug czar," General Barry McCaffrey, who directs the Office of National Drug Control Policy (ONDCP). I served on the National Institute of Health Expert Panel on Medical Marijuana and was a reviewer of the 1999 Institute of Medicine report, "Marijuana and Medicine." Over the years, I have served as scientific advisor to several drug discovery companies.

What's Ahead in This Book

In Part One (Drugs and the Brain), I explain what we know about the biology of the drug addictions, and how we know it. How do the addictive drugs act on the brain and how do they affect behavior? What is there about this particular group of drugs that makes them so powerfully seductive? Why are some people much more vulnerable than others to becoming addicted? What long-term changes in brain chemistry are caused by heavy use of an addictive drug? What causes relapse after an addict has quit using?

In Part Two (Drugs and the Addicts), I discuss the medical and psychological features of each drug addiction. How do people fall into the addiction trap in the first place? What effects, positive as well as harmful, does each family of addictive drugs have on the people who use them, and what dangers do they pose for society? What special hazards (such as the transmission of AIDS and other infections) arise from intravenous drug use? What are the special dangers to the unborn if a pregnant woman uses drugs? What preventive measures and treatments are available, and how successful are they? Can addicts ever really put their addiction behind them?

In Part Three (Drugs and Society) I consider some of the history, sociology, and politics of the drug problem. The use of drugs to alter mood and behavior is not unique to our times; it may be as old as human civilization. But is it more widespread or more severe today than in the past? Is there really a "drug epidemic," or are politicians and the news media exaggerating? With what success have some other countries dealt with their drug problems? What methods of prevention education have been tried, and how effective have they been? How do harsh control measures (as have been employed often in some countries and occasionally in our own) compare with gentler ones? Finally, I present my own thoughts about drug policy for our nation—how to reduce the bad effects of addictive drugs on users and society while at the same time keeping to a minimum the harm caused by governmental intrusions and punitive sanctions.

Drug addiction starts with exposure of the brain to a substance belonging to one of the seven families of addictive drugs. To understand how that exposure affects behavior and why it leads to compulsive use, we first need to learn something about brain chemistry. That is the subject of the next two chapters.

Part One

Drugs and the Brain

2

Neurotransmitters:
The Brain's Own Drugs

Parts of this chapter and the next are rather technical. They explain how neurobiologists study addictive drugs by the modern techniques of molecular biology. The reader who is not deeply interested in the neurobiology may wish to skip those sections now, and return later for basic science information about aspects of addiction covered in other chapters.

Roger Whitcomb is absent from the office this afternoon. Unable to wait until evening, the craving nagging at him relentlessly, he quit work and rushed home. He is missing important business, but no business is as important as what he is about to do. Sitting on a soft easy chair, he places a pellet of crack cocaine in the bowl of a little pipe. He trembles with anticipation as he lights it and inhales deeply. A few seconds later he feels it "hit." An overwhelming sense of alertness, power, deep satisfaction, almost-orgasmic pleasure sweeps over him. A few hours later, he is still at it, using up his entire $200 supply of crack cocaine, needing more and more of it to sustain the euphoria.

How can a chemical in smoke transform a person's behavior so dramatically? How can it become so important to Roger and people like him? What does the cocaine do to his brain? As we shall see, not only cocaine but every addictive drug works by mimicking or blocking one of the substances that neurons (nerve cells) in the brain use to communicate with each other. These substances are called neurotransmitters. Each one locks onto its own special receptor in a process described by the famous lock-and-key analogy. By learning about the neurotransmitters and their receptors, we can begin to understand how addictive drugs produce such powerful effects.

Recall from chapter 1 that a drug is any chemical agent that affects biologic function. Then, we may rightly say that our bodies make drugs of their own. A familiar example is insulin, which is produced by the pancreas, and stimulates cell metabolism in other tissues; it can also be administered as a medication if the natural supply fails. In this same category are other hormones such as growth hormone, thyroid hormone, sex steroids, and the interleukins that regulate the immune system. The neurotransmitters are drugs that are made in neurons, and then are released from neurons to act on other neurons or on muscles or glands. When you walk, nerves in your leg tell each muscle when to contract by releasing a neurotransmitter, acetylcholine, directly onto that muscle. The acetylcholine is a chemical trigger that activates the machinery that causes the muscle fibers to shorten, thus exerting the force that moves your leg. When you are frightened, your adrenal gland releases a hormone, epinephrine (adrenaline), which circulates in the blood and acts on your heart to make it beat faster. When you salivate in anticipation of tasty food, it is because nerves are releasing their neurotransmitters onto your salivary glands.

Addiction is a behavior, and all human behavior has a biologic basis in the workings of the brain. The "hardware" of the brain consists of a thousand billion neurons with their complex network of interconnections, the neurotransmitters they manufacture, and the specialized receptors on which the neurotransmitters act. All this hardware develops initially according to the blueprints in the DNA of our genes, but it is also modified by experience. The "software" consists of the memories, learning, and conditioning that reflect inputs from the environment. Behavior is the traditional field of psychologists and psychiatrists. But because the brain is a chemical organ, brain chemistry is responsible for the finely regulated and coordinated functioning of both the hardware and the software. Thus, even psychologic disorders must arise ultimately through chemical changes. It is not a question of psychology versus biology; on the contrary, in the final analysis psychology *is* biology.

Chemical Transmission

The origins of our modern understanding of chemical transmission in the brain can be traced to the middle 1800s, in France. Explorers, long before, had brought back from South America an arrow poison called curare, which natives smeared on their blowgun darts to paralyze prey. Claude Bernard, the founder of the science of pharmacology, used frogs to study how curare paralyzes. When he applied a mild electric shock to a nerve in the frog's leg, the leg muscle contracted; but if he had first injected the frog with curare, it did not. Either the electrical stimulus was not reaching the muscle, or the muscle itself was not responding to it. Which alternative was true? Bernard soaked the nerve in a curare solution without exposing the muscle to the poison. No paralysis resulted; so it seemed that curare must paralyze the muscle directly. To his great surprise, however, when he soaked the muscle (but not the nerve) in curare and then shocked the muscle directly (not through the nerve), it contracted normally, even though it would not respond to nerve stimulation (Figure 2.1A). Bernard was forced to conclude that curare acted neither on nerve nor on muscle but somehow between the nerve endings and the muscle tissue. He was right; today we know

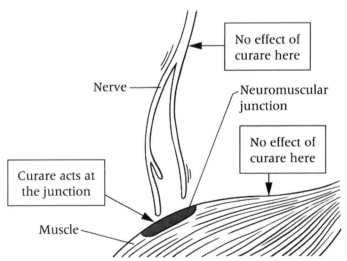

Fig. 2.1A: Historic experiments on neurotransmitters and receptors. Bernard's experiment.

there is a specialized structure there, the neuromuscular junction, on which curare acts.

In 1909 in England, at the University of Cambridge, J. N. Langley discovered that nicotine, applied directly to the neuromuscular junction, made the muscle contract; and remarkably, this action of nicotine could be prevented by curare (Figure 2.1B). No nerves were needed; even if they were destroyed, nicotine made the muscle contract, and curare prevented the nicotine action. The fact that curare could also block nerve impulses, as Bernard had shown years before, suggested to Langley that a nerve might normally stimulate muscle by releasing a chemical like nicotine, which would act on the neuromuscular junction and make the muscle contract (Figure 2.1C). Since various other substances did not do this, he also had to sup-

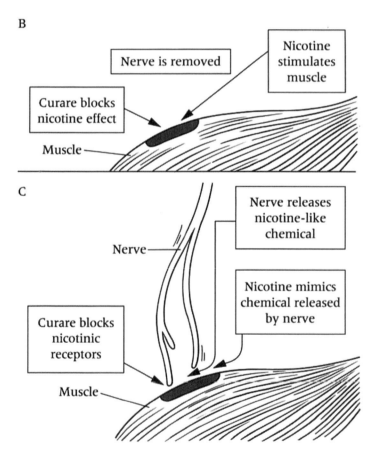

Fig. 2.1B,C: Historic experiments on neurotransmitters and receptors. Langley's experiment (B, above), Langley's conclusion (C, below).

pose that the neuromuscular junction contained some kind of specialized material upon which nicotine, as well as the postulated substance released by nerves, would act. Langley called this hypothetical material receptive substance, a name later shortened to receptor. So nicotine was said to act on a nicotinic receptor.

Shortly thereafter, in London, H. H. Dale discovered that visceral smooth muscles (as in the intestine, bladder, or pupil of the eye) behaved very differently from the skeletal muscles studied by Bernard and Langley. Nicotine did not stimulate them to contract, but a mushroom poison called muscarine did. Curare did not prevent the action of muscarine, but a plant poison called atropine did. Thus, the receptors on smooth muscle, which responded to muscarine and were blocked by atropine, were called muscarinic receptors. Dale's experiments first showed clearly that receptors were specific; nicotine and curare acted only on nicotinic receptors, muscarine and atropine only on muscarinic receptors.

What were the hypothetical substances released from nerve endings by nerve impulses, which caused these different types of muscle to contract? Not until the 1930s was it proved, in a famous experiment conducted by the Austrian pharmacologist Otto Loewi, that nerves actually did transmit their messages by means of neurotransmitters released from nerve endings. How was this shown? A frog heart, with its nerve intact, was placed in a small container of salt solution; it continued to beat. In another container was a second heart. Fluid from the first container, transferred to the second, had no effect on the heart there. Loewi slowed the beating of the first heart by stimulating its nerve electrically, then transferred the bath fluid to the second container. Remarkably, the second heart slowed, even though its nerve had not been stimulated. This proved conclusively that some substance released by the nerve onto the first heart had slowed it; and that the same substance, transferred with the bath fluid to the second heart, had slowed it, too. Dale and Loewi shared a Nobel Prize in 1936 for their fundamental discoveries about chemical transmission.

A few years later, the substance released by nerves in these experiments was found to be acetylcholine, the first of many neurotransmitters to be recognized. Langley's nicotinic receptors and Dale's muscarinic receptors were actually two types of acetylcholine receptor—the nicotinic one on skeletal muscle, the muscarinic one on visceral smooth muscle and heart.

Acetylcholine turned out to be responsible not only for neuro-transmission from nerve to muscle, but also from nerve to nerve, as in the brain (Figure 2.2). The junction (called a synapse) where the ending of one nerve contacts another is—like the neuromuscular junction—a microscopically tiny gap. A neurotransmitter released into this gap from the ending of one neuron can cross over to one of the nearby processes (called dendrites) on another neuron, and there it can stimulate a specific receptor. In this way, a "message" is transmitted across the synapse to the second neuron. Sometimes, if the right receptor is present on the nerve ending, a neurotransmitter can act back on the same nerve cell from which it was released, in a kind of feedback loop.

Nicotinic and muscarinic acetylcholine receptors are found in many regions of the brain, and acetylcholine is one of the brain's most abundant neurotransmitters. Nicotine, when delivered to the brain in a smoker's blood, combines with certain nicotinic receptors, mimicking the actions of acetylcholine.

The Neurotransmitters

The first neurotransmitters to be identified were, like acetylcholine, compact molecules composed of only 25 or so atoms. Called bio-genic amines, most of them—though not acetylcholine itself—are related to one or another of the 20 amino acids that serve as build-

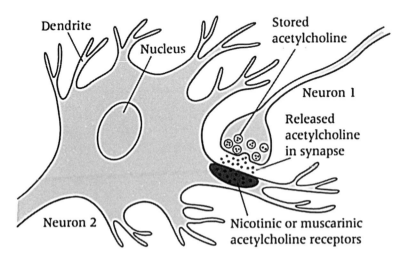

Fig. 2.2: Acetylcholine receptors in brain.

ing blocks for all the proteins in the body. The most important for addiction seems to be dopamine, derived from the amino acid tyrosine, and itself giving rise to two other biogenic amines, norepinephrine and epinephrine (adrenaline). Dopamine itself plays a key role in the midbrain "reward system" (see chapter 4). Serotonin (5-HT), derived from the amino acid tryptophan, is much involved in the regulation of mood and other behaviors. The amino acid glycine is itself a neurotransmitter (see below). The amino acid glutamate is an important excitatory neurotransmitter, which is converted in the brain to gamma-aminobutyrate (GABA), an inhibitory one. Another compact neurotransmitter of importance is adenosine, which is not related to the amino acids but to one of the four building blocks of DNA and RNA. These complex interrelationships illustrate how Nature ingeniously uses the same chemicals for quite different purposes.

Neurotransmitters of another kind are peptides, linear strings of amino acids, like a string of different colored beads. Peptides typically consist of between two and about 30 amino acids. Proteins are longer strings; insulin, for instance, is a small protein containing 51 amino acids. Dozens of peptide neurotransmitters are already known, and there could be many more. The number of possible arrangements of the 20 naturally occurring amino acids in a string (i.e., the number of different sequences) is incredibly large. Consider a peptide only five amino acids long. For each of the 20 possibilities at the first position, there are 20 possibilities at the second, thus 20 times 20. With five positions, we have 20 raised to the fifth power, or 3.2 million possible peptides, all different. For a protein several hundred amino acids long, the number of possibilities is truly astronomical. The enormous diversity of peptides and proteins that actually exist in the body represents only a small fraction of what is possible; and this small fraction has been selected by evolution over billions of years to serve all biologic needs.

Although the peptide neurotransmitters are bigger than the compact ones, they usually do not lie stretched out like a string of beads but fold into a more compact shape. Thus, many of them are able to fit into receptor pockets very much like those that accommodate the compact neurotransmitters. Likewise, compact molecules—ncluding all the addictive drugs—can fit into receptor pockets that ordinarily accommodate peptides. Many addictive drugs can bind selectively to a particular neurotransmitter receptor. The result is either to mimic the effect of whatever neurotransmitter would normally occupy that receptor, or to block that neurotransmitter by interfering (competing) with its binding to the receptor. Two examples: Nicotine mimics acetylcholine by acting on the nicotinic acetylcholine receptor; caffeine blocks the effect of adenosine neurotransmission by binding in an inert fashion to the adenosine receptor.

One neurotransmitter belongs to none of the groups just described; it is a long-chain fatty acid—a lipid—called anandamide. It—and a close relative also found in brain—is related to the naturally occurring prostaglandins. These lipids are of special interest because their receptors also accommodate tetrahydrocannabinol (THC), the active principle of marijuana.

An excitatory neurotransmitter stimulates neurons, exciting them electrically so that they release—onto yet another neuron—whatever neurotransmitter they contain. An inhibitory neurotransmitter quiets neurons, making them less likely to become excited. A modulatory neurotransmitter modifies the sensitivity of neurons to other neurotransmitters. Once we identify a certain neurotransmitter and its receptor, we still cannot predict what its effect will be on the brain. The reason is that the brain operates by such amazingly complex circuitry. Every circuit is switched on or off or modulated by one or more neurotransmitters, each with its associated specific receptor. Acetylcholine neurons (called cholinergic) and nicotinic acetylcholine receptors are found throughout the brain, acting in numerous circuits. As we shall see, the circuit primarily involved in the addictive effects of nicotine is located in the midbrain, where cholinergic neurons activate other neurons, which in turn release dopamine. Nicotinic receptors in many other brain areas, stimulated naturally by acetylcholine (or artificially by nicotine), are responsible for a variety of effects that are not related to addiction.

Endogenous Opioids (Endorphins)

The early discoveries that the plant products curare, nicotine, muscarine, and atropine bind to acetylcholine receptors should have raised this question: Does every substance of plant origin that acts on the brain mimic or block some neurotransmitter? And that question should have led to a deliberate search for unknown neurotransmitters that are counterparts of the known psychoactive plant products.

The ground has to be fertile, however, before an idea can sprout. As long ago as 1903 a French researcher, M. Mavrojannis, noted that when rats were given high doses of morphine, they became immobile, and they would hold any bizarre position into which they were placed. This strange kind of plastic immobility reminded Mavrojannis of similar states—catatonia, catalepsy—seen sometimes in schizophrenic patients. Making an intuitive leap of creative imagination he wrote:

> If one supposes that the organism normally produces narcotic substances, one can imagine that in certain cases at least, cataleptic phenomena are due either to an excessive production of these narcotic substances or to a defect in their elimination.

This remarkable insight had no effect whatsoever. It did not stimulate a search for "narcotic substances" in the brain. Conditions were not ripe, technology was not adequate, peptides (as the morphine-like substances in the brain turned out to be) were not even known—indeed, the amino acids themselves had not yet been discovered. When, three-quarters of a century later, the substances postulated by Mavrojannis were finally identified, his paper had been lost in the obscurity of forgotten archives.

The eventual discovery of the endogenous (i.e., made by the organism) opioid peptides had a great influence on the way scientists view drug addiction. They are called opioid (meaning "like opiates") because their biologic actions resemble those of morphine and other opiates. The family of opioids includes true opiates like morphine from the opium poppy, synthetic compounds related to morphine, and the opioid peptides. By the 1960s a very large number of compounds related to morphine had been synthesized in the search for a painkiller as strong as morphine but not addictive. These included both agonists (biologically active compounds) and antagonists (compounds that block the effects of agonists). It was evident from the way tiny chemical changes made big differences in the potency of the agonists, that a highly specific receptor had to be responsible for the pain relief. So the following question arose: Was it sensible to believe that highly specific receptors developed in the brain in order to combine with morphine—a substance apparently foreign to the body, a product of the opium poppy? Was it not more likely that there were natural morphinelike neurotransmitters in the brain and that these receptors had evolved to accommodate them?

Among the synthetic opiates was one that turned out, in the early 1970s, to be the key to searching for an endogenous opioid in the brain. This compound was an antagonist, naloxone. Apparently without biologic activity of its own, it nevertheless blocked the many actions of morphine. Because of this powerful antagonist effect, it came into clinical use for reviving victims of heroin or morphine overdose. Nothing in medical practice is quite so dramatic as a naloxone injection in the emergency room. A person is carried in, barely breathing, blue, and moribund; instantly after naloxone, the patient takes a deep breath, sits up, and wants to go home. Not only is naloxone highly effective in blocking the opioid receptors (see chapter 3), it does so in a specific manner, it fits those receptors and no others. Consequently it has a diagnostic value; if naloxone fails to revive a comatose victim, the problem must be other than an opiate overdose.

In 1972, the logic of using naloxone diagnostically was applied in laboratory experiments. It had been found that electrically stimulating the brainstem of a rat would abolish pain caused by—for instance—applying heat to the tail. The stimulation was evidently activating some kind of analgesic circuitry in the brainstem or spinal cord. Naloxone restored the pain, abolished the stimulation-produced analgesia. This key experiment suggested that neurons in the circuits mediating the analgesia were releasing a morphinelike substance. A handful of researchers (including my own laboratory group) began a search for that hypothetical substance. Naloxone would continue to play the key role in this work.

What was needed to find an unknown morphinelike substance in the brain? It would be easy enough to make extracts of animal brains. But how, on the laboratory bench, to detect the biologic action of a morphinelike substance in such extracts? The time-honored method of testing painkillers was to administer the drug to a live rat, rabbit, or monkey in a pain test. This was laborious and costly, and because individual animals vary so much in their sensitivity to drugs, even to obtain a single reliable result would have required repeated trials with many animals. Fortunately, Hans W. Kosterlitz, in Aberdeen, Scotland, developed the simple and practical method that was needed.

A tiny strip of muscle about an inch long, from the guinea pig small intestine, is fastened at one end to a hook in the bottom of a little tissue bath filled with salt solution. The other end of the muscle strip is attached by a thread to an electrical strain gauge, which signals the strength of the muscle pull. Electric shocks, one every ten seconds, make the muscle contract, pulling on the thread and writing a record on a moving strip of paper. Anything that changes the strength of the muscle pull writes a clear record of its effect.

The electric shocks activate nerves in the muscle, making them release acetylcholine. The released acetylcholine, as in Bernard's frog experiments, activates the muscle and makes it contract (Figure 2.3). Morphine blocks the muscle contraction by preventing the release of acetylcholine. But many other compounds block the muscle contraction in various ways. Since the strip is a typical visceral muscle, it contains several kinds of receptor, including the muscarinic type of acetylcholine receptor. So various poisons (such as atropine) also block the contraction. It follows that the method, as described so far, would be nearly useless for identifying a morphinelike substance. Something more was needed.

That "something more" was naloxone. If naloxone itself is added to the tissue bath it does not disturb the electrically stimulated muscle contraction. But in the presence of naloxone, morphine is totally ineffective. Moreover, if morphine is added first, and has already reduced the strength of the contraction, adding naloxone will promptly reverse the morphine effect, as illustrated in the figure.

The characteristic and specific naloxone blockade made possible the search for a morphinelike substance. In 1975, Kosterlitz and his team in Aberdeen, after laboriously purifying and testing material from thousands of pig brains, were able to isolate two active

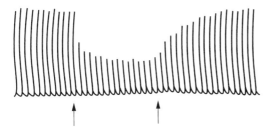

Fig. 2.3: Bioassay of an opioid. Actual record of electrically stimulated contractions (every 10 seconds) of guinea pig intestinal muscle. Morphine added at first arrow, naloxone at second arrow. (Experiment from the author's laboratory.)

substances that behaved like morphine. The big surprise was that the chemical structure of these substances turned out to be nothing like that of the compact morphine molecule. Named methionine-enkephalin and leucine-enkephalin, they were peptides, five amino acids long. The first four amino acids were the same in both—Tyr-Gly-Gly-Phe (these are the standard abbreviations for tyrosine, glycine, and phenylalanine). The fifth amino acid was methionine or leucine.

By searching through a database of all known amino-acid sequences, the Aberdeen scientists found a much longer peptide that contained the five amino acids of methionine-enkephalin, arranged in the same sequence indicated above. This peptide, 31 amino acids long (now called beta-endorphin), had actually been discovered years earlier in the pituitary gland, but its opioid character had not been suspected. Interestingly, this opioid peptide is made in the brain and other tissues as part of an even longer peptide that includes the pituitary hormone ACTH (corticotropin), which stimulates the adrenal gland in response to stress.

We know now that there are at least three families of opioid peptides, each encoded by its own gene. The enkephalins and beta-endorphin were followed by the dynorphins (described below). Because of their strong similarities, all three genes are thought to have evolved from a common ancestral opioid peptide gene. Opioid peptides are found throughout the animal kingdom and not only in the brain, but also in other tissues throughout the body. Dynorphins, for example, are present in the brain, spinal cord, intestinal tract, heart, and testes, as well as in the pituitary gland where we first discovered them.

An endogenous peptide, orphanin-FQ (also called nociceptin), is very closely related to dynorphin in its sequence, but does not bind to any of the opioid receptors; it has its own specific receptor (see chapter 3).

Two other compounds found in the brain have opioid actions through selective binding to one of the opioid receptors, the mu subtype (see chapter 3). To prove conclusively that a compound found in the brain is actually made there (or elsewhere in the body), it is necessary to demonstrate its biosynthesis in order to rule out laboratory contamination or an external source such as animal feed. In the case of a peptide, one needs to identify both the gene and the long precursor peptide, as with the endorphins. Endomorphins are two small peptides—Tyr-Pro-Trp-Phe amide and Tyr-Pro-Phe-Phe amide—that activate the mu opioid receptor, although they do not share the Tyr-Gly-Gly-Phe motif with the other opioid peptides. They appear to be present chiefly in the nerves that carry sensation and pain into and within the spinal cord and brain. Furthermore, as it is the mu receptor that mediates the addictive effects of the opiates, these peptides could be important for the addictions. At the present writing, however, neither the gene nor a precursor peptide has been identified, so we have to suspend judgment.

Curiously, morphine itself and two opiates containing the morphine structure have actually been found in beef brains. It is clear that these opiates, thought to occur only in plants, were really present in the brain rather than being laboratory contaminants. But as with the endomorphins, there is as yet no proof that they are actually made in the brain and have a function there. They could possibly originate in the animals' feed, be made by bacteria in the intestines, or even be introduced somehow in the slaughterhouse.

Discovering Dynorphin

To convey a feeling for the process of discovery, I can do no better than describe my own experience, which culminated in the discovery of the third family of opioid peptides. The reader will appreciate that far from being unique, my adventure has been repeated by the many investigators who discovered numerous neurotransmitters and their receptors during the past two decades.

My story illustrates how even a wrong idea in science can lead, by experiment, to a correct result. My colleagues and I wondered if one of the known hormones might be the sought-after endogenous morphinelike compound; after all, no hormone had been examined for such a possibility. Systematically, therefore, we tested many hormones on the muscle strip, as described above, but without success. Then one day in March 1975, there was a great commotion in the laboratory. I hurried over to one of the little tissue baths, where my colleagues were watching with excitement as the pen wrote its record. A crude sample of the pituitary hormone ACTH was being tested. The record showed clearly that the muscle contraction was reduced by the ACTH preparation, and that naloxone brought it back to normal. Obviously, either ACTH itself was morphinelike in its action, or else the impure ACTH sample contained a morphinelike impurity. Which alternative was true?

We were able to obtain a bit of chemically pure ACTH from a generous colleague; it had no effect at all on the muscle strip. The conclusion: Our ACTH sample, made commercially from pig pituitary glands, evidently contained a morphinelike impurity. When we exposed our crude ACTH to an enzyme that destroys peptides, the biological activity was lost, indicating that the morphinelike impurity was a peptide. So our task was cut out for us—to isolate that peptide from the crude ACTH and find out what it was. We turned to the Armour Company, which makes huge amounts of pituitary hormones as a sideline of their meat packing business. Fortunately a biochemist there had the foresight to realize that by-products, which would ordinarily be thrown away, might contain valuable substances as yet undiscovered. He had saved all such materials, and thus we were able to obtain many pounds of crude pig pituitary powder, the leftovers after preparing ACTH for the pharmaceutical market. We found right away that a soup made from this powder had typical naloxone-reversible morphinelike activity on the muscle strip.

Purification of a peptide is truly a laborious business. The crude soup had to be separated into its components (a process called fractionation), and each fraction had to be tested. We threw away whatever had no activity, and then we further purified the active fractions. We separated molecules according to size, obtaining dozens of fractions, from the size of small peptides containing only a few amino acids, to the size of large proteins containing hundreds. Testing revealed that all the biological activity was in a fraction corresponding to a length of around 15–20 amino acids. Then that active fraction was further fractionated according to a different criterion, electric charge. With a dozen or so fractions in hand, all of about the same size now but having different electric charges, we could again identify the active fraction (it turned out to have a strong positive charge) and discard the rest. We knew we were onto something novel because we found some important differences between the biological effects of our material and those of the enkephalins or beta-endorphin. It took us four years to obtain two micrograms (less than a millionth of an ounce) of a pure peptide with morphinelike activity.

Which amino acids did our peptide contain, and what was their sequence in the chain? A leading center for peptide sequence determination at that time was at Caltech in Pasadena. There, the nearly invisible speck of material went for analysis. I shall never forget the telephone call a few days later: "Here's the sequence: Tyr, Gly, Gly, Phe, Leu, Arg, Arg, Ile, Arg. . . ." I knew at once that we had discovered a completely novel opioid peptide. The first five amino acids were the familiar ones in leucine-enkephalin but everything after that was different from any known sequence.

The thrill of discovery is the main reward of scientific research. Knowing something about nature that no else in the world has ever known before is a wondrous experience, hard to convey in words. Here was this peptide, 17 amino acids long, the blueprint for which had been hidden in the genes for countless millions of years—and my colleagues and I had cracked the secret! Moreover, we had not only discovered a new opioid peptide neurotransmitter; as we soon realized, we had found one that was hundreds of times more potent than morphine or any opioid peptide then known. I named it dynorphin from the Greek prefix meaning power (as in dynamic) and the suffix-orphin (as in beta-endorphin).

Where in the Brain?

When a neurotransmitter is discovered and its chemical structure identified, one wants to know how it is distributed in the brain. Often, as with acetylcholine, neurons in every part of the brain contain it, so that no function can be assigned on the basis of distribution alone. Sometimes, however, the neurotransmitter is a prominent component of a known circuit with well established function. Its presence in the hippocampus, for instance, would suggest a role in memory processing; in brainstem and spinal cord, a role in pain regulation; in the visual, auditory, and olfactory systems a role in their well defined functions; in the cerebellum, a role in coordinating voluntary movements. Of greatest interest for addiction would be the presence of a neurotransmitter in the midbrain reward pathway (see chapter 4), where dopamine neurons are thought to play a key role in mediating pleasurable (hedonic) effects.

To discover where a neurotransmitter is localized one could, in principle, extract bits of brain tissue and measure directly with a biological assay, as described for the discovery process. In principle, yes, but not practical; the method is too laborious, and purifying the substance in question from each of hundreds of tissue samples would be out of the question. The efficient and universally employed technique is immunoassay, first invented in 1958 to measure tiny amounts of insulin. An animal (typically a rabbit) is injected with the substance we wish to detect—here a certain neurotransmitter, modified slightly to make it seem foreign to the animal's body. Within a few weeks, the animal's immune system reacts by making antibodies. These can be harvested from the animal's blood or directly from its antibody-producing cells.

An antibody is usually quite specific in recognizing and binding the same compound used to produce it. Specificity makes antibodies useful for localizing neurotransmitters by immunocytochemistry. Applied to a thin slice of brain tissue, an antibody will adhere only where it finds the substance against which it was made. All that is needed is a way to label the antibody, in order to make it visible under the microscope. Labeling is accomplished by attaching a fluorescent chemical or a radioactive atom, or by using a labeled secondary antibody directed against the primary one. Ultraviolet light makes the fluorescent chemical glow, radioactivity produces a photographic image on a film. By this method one can actually see the packages of a particular neurotransmitter stored in the nerve endings.

Summary

Neurotransmitters have many important functions, and they play a significant role in addiction, because every addictive drug mimics or blocks some neurotransmitter. According to the currently accepted hypothesis, dopamine is the key to "reward" (reinforcement), which underlies addiction (see chapter 4).

The story of the endogenous opioids has wider implications. The presence of an addictive substance in opium poppies led to the discovery of neurotransmitters with morphinelike actions in the brain. This encouraged scientists to look for other novel neurotransmitters in the brain, which might be related to known plant substances with psychoactive effects. One stunning success of this strategy was the discovery of endogenous substances that act like THC (the active principle in marijuana, see chapter 12).

Finding a neurotransmitter that is mimicked or blocked by an addictive drug is always a necessary first step in understanding the biological basis of an addiction. The next step is to learn about the brain circuits that contain that neurotransmitter. Finally, in the next chapter, we shall learn about the receptors on which the addictive drugs and their endogenous counterparts act in the brain, and how those receptors modify brain function when they are activated or blocked.

3

Receptors: Locks for the Addictive Keys

As in chapter 2, the reader who is not deeply interested in the basic molecular neuroscience may skip some of the technical matters covered here. It should, nevertheless, prove useful to return to this chapter for technical explanations of some aspects of addiction covered in later chapters.

For Bernard, Langley, Dale, and Loewi, receptors were more a concept than a physical reality. Whatever the postulated receptors might actually be, they were obviously highly specific. The lock-and-key analogy served to describe this specificity very early. The nicotine "key," as we have seen, activated the nicotinic receptor "lock" but did not fit the muscarinic receptor. Similarly the muscarine "key" did not fit the nicotinic receptor. If not for the variety of brain receptors with their amazing specificity, the brain could not function at all. It is largely the different receptors and their special locations in the brain that account for the differences among the addictive drugs—one a stimulant, another a depressant, one causing vivid hallucinations, another paranoid psychosis, yet another producing mutiple effects, one powerfully addictive at the outset, another only weakly so. All the receptors are proteins, so it is the properties of proteins that determine how receptors differ from one another and how neurotransmitters or addictive drugs interact with them.

Ligand Binding

A compound that binds to a receptor is called a ligand. A ligand molecule that is labeled (tagged) by a radioactive atom is called a radioligand. If a radioligand binds to its receptor, that binding is readily measured by an instrument that counts radioactive disintegrations. Ligand binding makes it possible to study receptors as physical realities, no longer just conceptual inferences (Figure 3.1).

The brain receptors of interest are embedded in the cell membranes that compose the outer sheath of the neurons. The brain of

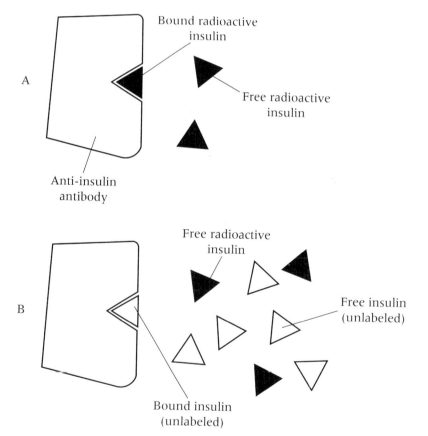

Fig. 3.1: The principle of competition at a binding site. Here the binding site is on an anti-insulin antibody, and radiolabeled insulin binding is measured by its radioactivity. (A) Radiolabeled insulin alone (black triangles); (B) competition by unlabeled insulin (white triangles).

a rat, mouse, or guinea pig (or of a human, obtained at autopsy) is removed and homogenized, as in a food blender, to break open all the neurons. Test tubes containing the homogenized material are rotated at high speed in a centrifuge to pack down the cell membranes with their receptors. After pouring off the watery soup, we stir up the membranes in salt water to wash them, then pack them down again. They are washed repeatedly, to get rid of all traces of everything but the membranes with their receptors. Finally, we divide the membranes into many test tubes, and to each tube we add— for example—an opioid ligand like morphine, which has been labeled with a radioactive atom. Of course the membranes contain receptors of many kinds, but our specific opioid radioligand will only bind to its own receptors. After allowing a little time for the binding to occur, we harvest the membranes with the bound radioligand on a small piece of filter paper to get rid of all ligand that is not bound.

The more radioligand we add, the more is bound to the receptors, until the binding sites are all filled. If ordinary nonradioactive morphine is added first, less radioligand can be bound, because the unlabeled morphine competes with the labeled morphine for the same sites. This competition step proves that the labeled morphine attaches to a limited number of specific binding sites, that it is not merely stuck to the surface of the membranes or the walls of the tubes. Substances that are not opioids fail to compete at all, proving that the binding is specific.

The most striking feature of specificity concerns chemically identical molecules of different "handedness." Our own two hands have exactly the same structure (thumb and four fingers, palm side and knuckle side), yet they are not actually identical in three-dimensional space. A glove can fit one hand but not the other. In the same way molecules can be "right-handed" or "left-handed." A left-handed molecule might be highly potent biologically, while its right-handed twin, containing exactly the same atoms, is entirely inert. This fact tells us that the receptor itself has an irregular, asymmetric, glovelike pocket, which accommodates only molecules with the correct three-dimensional shape. And although left-handed opiates compete for the binding sites, right-handed opiates do not, showing that the binding is stereospecific; this is consistent with the fact that only left-handed opiates produce the typical biological effects such as relief of pain.

With a brain slice, with membrane fragments from ground-up

nerve cells, or with cells grown in culture dishes, we can measure how many receptors there are (by the maximum amount of ligand that can bind) and also how tightly a ligand binds (its affinity). The more avidly a ligand is bound (the higher its affinity) the lower the concentration that is needed to fill the receptors. A high-affinity ligand would typically occupy the sites at a concentration of 1 nanomole per liter or less. This corresponds to a single grain of salt dissolved in a 250-gallon tank of water! Differences in binding affinity are largely responsible for the fact that LSD—as an example—is psychoactive in remarkably tiny amounts, whereas the biologic activity of a drug like caffeine requires hundreds of times higher dosage.

Sex-hormone receptors and insulin receptors were the first to be studied in this way, about 30 years ago. Shortly thereafter, a ligand binding technique was developed for detecting brain opioid receptors. Ligand binding is key to understanding the drug addictions because by labeling an addictive drug, we can learn which receptor is its target. Then we can study how that receptor is made in the body, how its production is regulated, how it is affected by chronic exposure to the drug. Finally, ligand binding helps us to learn the structure of the receptors (as discussed below) and how they mediate the biological effects of drugs. I have illustrated the methods by reference to the opioid receptors, but a very similar description would apply to receptors for other addictive drugs.

The ligand binding assay lets us characterize a receptor according to what ligands it will or will not bind and with what relative affinities. We say that a receptor is selective for a particular ligand if it binds that ligand with substantially higher affinity than other ligands. Binding assays give direct information about ligand affinities, but cannot distinguish readily between agonists and antagonists, since both bind. An antagonist binds without activating a receptor—like a wrong key that fits a keyhole but fails to turn the lock mechanism. To distinguish an agonist from an antagonist, we have to look at receptor function by measuring some biological consequence of the binding. For example, we might measure the response of the electrically stimulated muscle strip to an opioid, as described in chapter 2. Such functional assays give information about the biological potency of an agonist or antagonist. Potency is a measure of the agonist concentration needed to produce the biological effect, or the antagonist concentration needed to block it. Potency is usually related to binding affinity, but it is not the same thing; sometimes a full biological effect results from occupancy of only a small fraction of the receptors.

The nicotinic and muscarinic acetylcholine receptors in brain exemplify a general principle—that virtually all receptors come in families, with subtypes having strong similarities but also important differences. An apt analogy might be the breeds of dogs, all easily recognized as dogs, but with characteristic differences among them. Typically, subtypes of a receptor can bind several ligands in a set of closely related chemical structures, but with different relative affinities. In the case of the opioid receptors, one subtype (designated by Greek letter mu) is selective for morphine and beta-endorphin, another (delta) prefers enkephalins, and yet another (kappa) has greatest affinity for dynorphins. With most receptors, there are even subtypes of subtypes, and probably more subtypes yet to be discovered. The evolutionary purpose of receptor subtypes is probably to allow fine-tuning of biological processes by closely related but different endogenous ligands.

Where Are the Receptors in Brain?

To learn where an addictive drug acts in the brain and to get further information about how it acts there, we need to know in what parts of the brain the specific receptors for that drug are located. We can, of course, cut the brain into small pieces according to the known anatomy—cortex, cerebellum, hippocampus, brainstem, and so on—and apply the homogenization procedure to each piece. This method is useful, but the information it gives is not detailed enough. What we really want is a high-resolution map that shows which neurons contain a receptor of interest and where on those neurons that receptor is deployed. Instead of homogenizing, we can carry out the radioligand binding procedure with thin tissue slices, which are then pressed against photographic film—a technique known as receptor autoradiography. The radioactivity bound selectively to the receptor sites in each tissue sample makes a pretty map of the receptor distribution on neurons throughout the brain.

A powerful technique for locating receptors in the living human brain is positron emission tomography (PET scan). In a ligand PET scan, the radioactivity of a bound radioligand can be detected through the skull. Thus, a computerized three-dimensional image is obtained, showing the receptor distribution. A glucose PET scan measures the uptake of radiolabeled sugar by neurons. Sugar is taken up most rapidly by neurons that are most active (as they need sugar for energy) and that have an abundant blood supply. If an addictive drug stimulates a particular group of neurons, the local blood flow will increase, and radiolabeled sugar will rush into the cells, marking that region in the PET scan. A related method for identifying nerve activity in the living brain is functional magnetic resonance imaging (fMRI). The glucose PET scan and fMRI have shown, for example, that nicotine stimulates certain highly localized areas in the brain; and the ligand PET scan, using labeled nicotine, confirms that these are indeed areas dense in nicotinic acetylcholine receptors.

Regulation by Feedback

As every synapse has at least one input neuron and one output neuron, the nerve endings that release a neurotransmitter into the synapse are called presynaptic, while sites on another neuron, which receives the neurotransmitter, are called postsynaptic. Nicotinic or muscarinic acetylcholine receptors are usually postsynaptic, positioned strategically just across the synapses from the endings of acetylcholine neurons. Presynaptic receptors control the release of neurotransmitters into the synapse. For instance, when activated by an opioid agonist, the presynaptic opioid receptors on the endings of acetylcholine neurons suppress acetylcholine release from those neurons.

Both presynaptic and postsynaptic receptors form parts of regulatory feedback circuits. Excessive stimulation by agonists—as seen with several addictive drugs—generally leads to a reduction in the number of receptors, whereas insufficient stimulation results in an increase. Thus, receptor up-regulation and down-regulation are important mechanisms by which the brain maintains its chemical equilibrium. One way these adaptive changes are brought about is by altering the balance between receptors on the cell surface and those inside the cell, where ligands cannot reach them. By a slower process, the expression of receptor genes—their transcription into messenger RNA (mRNA)—can be increased or decreased, so that more or fewer receptors are made.

Just as receptors are regulated by the activity of neurotransmitters, so are the production and release of neurotransmitters regulated by the degree of stimulation of the receptors. Too much stimulation of a receptor calls for less ligand to be made and released, too little stimulation calls for more. With respect to the regulation of both receptors and neurotransmitters, the brain behaves as though trying to maintain all its operating systems on an even keel. The addictive drugs upset this normal balance.

A special example of synaptic adaptation is called long-term potentiation (LTP), in which repeated stimulation at a synapse makes subsequent stimulation at the same synapse more effective—thus, a kind of synaptic memory, which is thought to underlie memory in general. Little is yet known about how addictive drugs affect this process, but (as later chapters describe) memory plays a key role in the craving that triggers relapse to addiction.

Receptor Structure

A receptor is a complicated miniature molecular machine. The binding site for the ligand is like the ignition lock in a car; the key activates the engine, but taking apart the lock would not tell us anything about how the car runs. We want to know not only how the receptors are constructed and how they bind ligands, but more important, how their machinery works. Revolutionary advances of the last decade are a major leap forward toward that goal.

When a ligand binds to its receptor, that binding is only the first step. If the ligand is an antagonist, it merely occupies the binding site passively, and thus excludes agonist ligands. However, if it is an agonist, the binding event transmits some kind of signal to the cell's machinery, to bring about an effect—for example, to make a neuron fire electrically or stop firing. The mechanism whereby the receptor controls biochemical events inside a cell is called signal transduction. When an agonist ligand binds, it causes a change in the conformation (shape) of the receptor and/or (in some receptors, like the acetylcholine receptor) by movement of receptor subunits relative to each other. Such a change may cause parts of the receptor that protrude into the cell to interact with other parts of the cell machinery. The three-dimensional structure of an unoccupied receptor can be studied by physical means, and the change induced by ligand binding can be discovered. The Holy Grail of receptor research is a complete understanding of the molecular steps between agonist binding and the signal transduction events within the cell.

Receptors are large proteins, chains of several hundred amino acids. Which amino acids are present in the chain, and the order in which they are strung together, determine how the chain is folded and therefore account for the distinctive three-dimensional structure. One method of finding the sequence of amino acids starts by purifying exhaustively, in order to obtain a tiny amount of the absolutely pure receptor protein. The method is much like that described for our little dynorphin peptide in chapter 2. The numerous proteins in brain tissue can be fractionated according to size, electric charge, and so on, while the receptor protein we want to purify is traced by its ability to bind a ligand. When purification is complete, so that the only protein present is the receptor, it can be sequenced—if there is enough of it. Because the protein chain is so long, it first has to be cut into overlapping fragments; then each fragment can be sequenced by starting at one end, and removing and identifying each amino acid in turn.

Alternative and far more efficient methods take advantage of the fact that every receptor—like every other protein in the body—is specified by a gene. The DNA of a gene (and of its working copy, mRNA) is composed of four different building blocks (called nucleotides) in a linear sequence. In DNA, these building blocks are designated by the abbreviations of their bases—A, T, C, and G (adenine, thymine, cytosine, guanine). The chemical properties are such that A can bind tightly and specifically to T, and C to G. Such pairs of bases (A:T and G:C) are the glue that holds together the two complementary strands of DNA—"complementary" because all the way along the gene, every A is opposite a T, every C is opposite a G. The same bases make up the long single strands of mRNA, except that instead of T, a closely related molecule called U (uracil) is present, which binds to A just as T would (i.e., A:U).

One important advance made possible by the complementary pairing principle is the mapping of specific mRNA molecules in brain tissue. This method, called in situ hybridization, requires that we know at least a portion of the sequence of the mRNA that encodes a certain receptor or peptide neurotransmitter. In practice, a labeled probe is synthesized, complementary to the known part of the mRNA we wish to map in the brain. Wherever that mRNA is present in a thin brain slice, it will bind the probe, be visible under the microscope, and take its own picture on a photographic film. The specific mRNA is present only where the neuropeptide or receptor of interest is in the process of being assembled—not necessarily the same place it is stored and released. One would expect a neurotransmitter and its receptor to be in very close contact, as with acetylcholine receptors in the neuromuscular junction. But that is not always true. Proteins are made in the cell body of the neuron, and then are transported to sites (sometimes quite distant) in the same neuron, where they will function. Furthermore, some neurotransmitters diffuse a considerable distance before contacting their receptors. These complexities often make interpretation difficult and lead to lively controversies among neuroscientists.

Determining directly how much neurotransmitter or how many receptors are present paints a valuable but static picture. Measuring the mRNA by in situ hybridization provides a dynamic picture of what is being made at the moment. That can give insight into how addictive drugs disturb regulatory processes in the brain. Regulatory mechanisms enable an organism to adapt when a drug or hormone upsets the normal equilibrium. For example, if a person is treated for a long time with cortisol (a hormone product of the adrenal cortex), the normal production of ACTH (a necessary stimulant of the adrenal cortex) by the pituitary gland is suppressed, as though to compensate for the high cortisol level. Sometimes thyroid hormone is administered medically in order to shut down the normal stimulation of the thyroid by thyroid-stimulating hormone from the pituitary. With neurotransmitters and their receptors, too, addictive drugs can cause suppression or stimulation of gene expression. As an illustration, studying specific mRNA by in situ hybridization can tell us whether chronic exposure to an opiate shuts down the production of the endogenous opioid peptides, the opioid receptors, or related proteins—effects that might lead to a state of tolerance and dependence (see chapter 6).

Expression Cloning

Modern biotechnology has provided alternative ways to learn the sequence of amino acids in a receptor. Let us examine the powerful method called expression cloning. Since every protein is built according to the blueprint in the DNA of the genes, it is often possible to analyze the gene sequence directly or—what amounts to the same thing—the sequence of the mRNA. A gene is said to be expressed when it is copied into mRNA, which will then serve as the template on which the protein is assembled from its constituent amino acids. Genes are expressed only when and where they are needed; otherwise, since every body cell contains our entire genome, we would have the ridiculous situation that all proteins would be made all the time in every tissue.

Gene expression is like reading out the linear information on a magnetic tape. Here the linear sequence of bases on one strand of the DNA (called the coding strand) directs the assembly of a complementary strand of mRNA. The base sequence in mRNA then directs the assembly of amino acids into a growing protein chain according to the rules known as the genetic code. Each triplet of bases directs the entry of one particular amino acid, so it follows that if the base sequence of DNA or mRNA is known, one can deduce the amino acid sequence of the expressed protein—receptor or neurotransmitter or whatever.

Typically we have a ligand in hand, and we know from biological activity and ligand binding that there must be a specific receptor for that ligand in the brain. We start with a tissue that is known to be making the receptor of interest. This means that the mixture of mRNA molecules in that tissue (e.g., brain), or in a population of cells, will contain the mRNA that specifies the receptor of interest. From this mixture of mRNA molecules, using the appropriate enzymes, we prepare a corresponding mixture of complementary DNA (cDNA). This step reverses the original copying of the gene's DNA into mRNA, and therefore it is called reverse transcription. The cDNA is then incorporated into a molecular structure known as a plasmid. A plasmid is a kind of artificial gene, which contains all the instructions for multiplying inside cells. Each plasmid incorporates just one of the thousands of cDNA molecules in the mixture. So, among all the plasmids will be just one or a few that contain the cDNA encoding the receptor we are seeking. The plasmids are put into bacteria, and the bacteria multiply, so the plasmids multiply too.

Next, the plasmid DNA is transferred into mammalian cells. These cells are allowed to grow on a gelatin surface in dishes, so that each cell, as it multiplies, gives rise to a discrete colony containing thousands of cells. Of course, as each colony arose from a single cell, and as that single cell contained only one kind of plasmid, the colony will now express just a single foreign protein. Every cell, following the instructions of its plasmid DNA, produces proteins just as though the instructions were in its own genes. Now the question is: Which ones of all these colonies (if any) express the receptor of interest? The answer is provided by ligand binding as described above.

Once we have identified a colony that does bind our ligand, we have only to retrieve that plasmid DNA and amplify it (make more of it) by the polymerase chain reaction (PCR)—the same method used with tiny amounts of DNA to identify or exonerate criminal suspects. Then all that remains is to sequence that DNA—a procedure that is now automated and rapid, as used typically in the Human Genome Project. Thus, we obtain the full sequence of base triplets that specifies the receptor, and the sequence of amino acids in the receptor can be deduced, even though the receptor itself was previously unknown. This is how, in 1992, the first sequence of an opioid receptor gene (the one encoding the delta receptor) was identified.

Cloning by Homology

The principle that receptors come in families has led to a remarkable development. The conditions of DNA hybridization can be varied at will. With a probe in hand (as described above) we can find only an exactly complementary strand, or we can be less demanding. Low-stringency hybridization can yield genes with sequences that are similar, but not identical, to the one represented by our probe. This is a powerful way to find previously unknown receptors that are related to those we know about already. Once the sequence of the delta opioid receptor was known, for example, cloning by homology yielded the mu and kappa opioid receptors very quickly.

A curious outcome of this technique is the discovery of orphan receptors, entirely unknown before, and presenting the question— what are these for, and what are their endogenous ligands? Here the usual procedure is stood on its head. Ordinarily we start with a drug effect, ask what receptor mediates it, then obtain the receptor and its gene by one of the methods described above. Here, on the other hand we start with a receptor gene, obtain a related (homologous) receptor, and then seek the endogenous ligand and its function.

A good example is the discovery of the orphanin receptor and its endogenous ligand. Cloning by homology, starting with an opioid receptor probe, led to a completely unknown receptor, closely related in structure (as expected), but without the ability to bind any opioid ligand. Then the search for an endogenous ligand led, surprisingly, to a previously unknown peptide very much like dynorphin, but with several differences among its 17 amino acids. This peptide, christened orphanin-FQ, binds to the orphanin receptor but not to any opioid receptor. Clearly, evolution had selected a mutated form of some primitive opioid receptor to serve a new purpose, or a mutated form of a primitive orphanin receptor to accommodate opioid ligands (we are not sure which came first). Apparently, orphanin-FQ acts on orphanin receptors on dopamine neurons in the mesolimbic reward pathway (see chapter 4) to suppress the release of dopamine. This effect, which is opposite to the action of endogenous opioids, is a continuing subject of active research. Orphanin-FQ is also called nociceptin because in certain circumstances it intensifies pain, opposing the analgesic actions of the endogenous opioid peptides. Its wide distribution in the brain and elsewhere suggests it has many other functions.

Finally, a new and powerful technique is being widely applied for deleting a gene of known sequence in an animal, producing what is called a gene knockout. Provided that absence of the gene is not lethal, what happens when it is knocked out may let us infer its normal role. In some respects this is an improvement over using an antagonist to infer a normal function, because here one specific receptor (the product of a single gene) is deleted, whereas no antagonist is totally selective for a single receptor. Knockout mice lacking the mu opioid receptor are born and develop normally, and their behavior is not grossly aberrant, but they do not respond to morphine. It is not analgesic for them, and it does not affect any of their body systems in the way morphine normally does. Most relevant to opiate addiction, they neither self-administer morphine nor become dependent on it (see chapter 4).

Some Receptors That Are Targets of Addictive Drugs

With sequence information in hand, knowing something about the structure of a receptor and its signal transduction mechanism, knowing the locations of the receptor and its endogenous ligands, we can begin to understand how an addictive drug affects the brain.

The first receptor to be sequenced, in 1982, was the nicotinic acetylcholine receptor at the neuromuscular junction, the same one that Claude Bernard first identified by means of curare, the same one activated by nicotine. It is a channel composed of five different proteins. Each protein chain crosses the cell membrane four times, and thus the whole structure is an array of 20 parallel segments forming a cylinder that traverses the membrane, with a pore that runs down the middle (Figure 3.2). This kind of receptor is called a ligand-gated ion channel because it is designed so that when a ligand binds at the mouth of the channel, the pore widens. Then certain ions (electrically charged atoms) can pass, which previously could not. Positively charged sodium ions rush into the cell, reducing its internal negative electric charge, and thus they initiate an electric signal. In muscle, this sudden reduction in electric charge is propagated along the fibers, causing them to contract. In the brain, when acetylcholine is released from the ending of one neuron, crosses a synapse, and binds to the receptor on a second neuron, an electric signal is propagated down that second neuron. Nicotine mimics this process. Muscarinic acetylcholine receptors belong to an entirely different family (see below).

The GABA receptor in the brain is also a ligand-gated ion channel. When the neurotransmitter GABA is released from a nearby nerve ending, it opens the channel of the GABA receptor to allow passage of negatively charged chloride ions. This increases the total negative charge inside the cell, making the neuron less responsive to the neurotransmitters that ordinarily excite it. Thus GABA is an inhibitory neurotransmitter, whereas acetylcholine is an excitatory neurotransmitter. The GABA receptor has a special binding site for the psychoactive and addictive benzodiazepine drugs (like Valium),

Open channel entrance

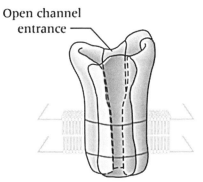

Fig. 3.2: Typical structure of a ligand-gated ion channel, the nicotinic acetylcholine receptor. Here 20 parallel protein chains delimit the outer channel boundary. The two solid parallel lines near the bottom represent the cell membrane of the neuron. (Adapted from J.P.Changeux et al., *Quarterly Review of Biophysics* 25:395,1992.)

and a different binding site for the psychoactive and addictive barbiturates. It is also one of several receptors where alcohol and inhalant solvents exert their main effects. All these drugs, when they bind, loosen the channel structure, make it easier to open, and thus enhance the inhibitory effects of GABA on neuron function.

Another ligand-gated ion channel in the brain is the NMDA receptor, a subtype of glutamate receptors, which respond to the abundant excitatory neurotransmitter glutamate. Glutamate opens the channel, allowing sodium, potassium, and calcium ions to flow into the neuron, thus exciting it. Alcohol—directly or indirectly—interferes with the opening of this ion channel. As the GABA and NMDA receptors have opposite effects on ion channels, one inhibitory, the other excitatory—alcohol produces a similar end result by enhancing GABA inhibition and opposing glutamate activation. Phencyclidine (PCP) has its own unique binding site on one of the NMDA receptor subunits (see chapter 14).

An entirely different architectural motif is represented by a very large group of receptors—the seven-helix family (Figure 3.3). These include muscarinic acetylcholine receptors and the receptors for dopamine, THC, adenosine, serotonin, and many neuropeptides including the opioids. A seven-helix receptor is a single protein chain of about 350 amino acids that threads back and forth across the cell membrane seven times, forming a cylindrical barrel something like

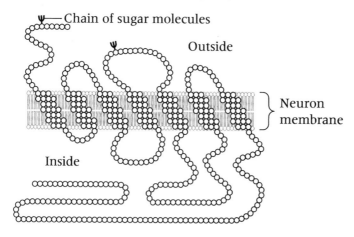

Fig. 3.3: Dopamine D1 receptor, typical of the seven-helix family. Unlike Fig. 3.2, in which only the gross structure is portrayed, here each amino acid is shown as a small circle. Each point of attachment of two chains of sugar molecules is depicted by a special symbol attached to one specific amino acid in the protein chain. (From D. R. Sibley and F. J. Monsma Jr., *Trends in Pharmacological Sciences* 13:64,1992.)

the ion-channel receptors, but without a central pore. The mouth of the barrel is a pocket, exposed on the outer surface of the cell membrane, into which a ligand molecule can fit. A compact ligand fits snugly into the pocket; a compacted segment of a long peptide ligand can also fit into the pocket, while the rest of it interacts with portions of the receptor that protrude out of the membrane.

For all receptors in this family, we are beginning to understand how an agonist binds differently from an antagonist, making different contacts with the amino acid residues that line the ligand-binding pocket. Inside the neuron, a special protein (called G-protein) interacts with parts of the receptor that extend through the cell membrane. When an agonist binds in the outer pocket of the receptor, the helixes move; this causes the G-protein to be released and to activate other functional proteins within the cell. Often, such a released G-protein interacts with some ion channel inside the same cell, thereby regulating its open or closed state and thus controlling the activity of the neuron. Agonist binding also causes two receptors of this family to interact, forming twins (dimers); and dimers may even contain different subtypes (e.g., mu and delta), and some properties of the dimers differ from those of the single receptor units. Finally, agonist binding promotes internalization of receptors—a regulatory feedback that makes fewer receptors available at the cell surface.

A third family of receptors relevant to addiction are the transporters, which are embedded in the nerve cell membrane and are specialized for carrying specific ligands across into the cell. Many essential molecules—for instance sugars and amino acids—are unable to penetrate the oily cell membranes because they are too soluble in water, and "oil and water don't mix." Without transporters, cells could not survive, for they require many water-soluble nutrients. Transporters remove some neurotransmitters from synapses after their release; this process of reuptake into the same neurons from which they were released not only terminates the action of neurotransmitters, but also conserves them to be used again. The transporters for several neurotransmitters such as GABA, serotonin, and dopamine share a similar architecture. Typically, a transporter protein chain crosses the cell membrane 12 times, leaving two long tails inside the cell and loops of different sizes outside. Just how such a structure actually moves a neurotransmitter like dopamine across the neuronal cell membrane and into the inside of the neuron is the subject of active research. Cocaine and amphetamines bind to the dopamine and serotonin transporters, and block their function. Then dopamine and serotonin accumulate to very high levels in the synapses, instead of being taken up by the neurons; and the effects of these neurotransmitters—especially of dopamine—are enhanced (see chapter 4). Knockout mice that specifically lack the dopamine transporter have synaptic dopamine levels many times higher than normal, and they are extremely hyperactive and excitable.

Summary

The preceding account will have made it apparent that scientific knowledge about brain receptors is still a work in progress. Nevertheless, the knowledge gained already has helped pinpoint sites of action of addictive drugs in the brain, and has implicated specific receptors and neurotransmitters. The molecular structure of the receptors has been revealed, and the signal transduction mechanisms have been elucidated. This research has opened the way for understanding how addictive drugs alter brain chemistry, and how the brain adapts to those chemical changes. The adaptations result in altered sensitivity to the drugs, as in the processes of sensitization, tolerance, and dependence (see chapter 6). Especially important is ongoing research on how each addictive drug affects the neurotransmitters and their receptors that regulate the natural reward systems of the brain, to be described in the next chapter. The complexity of neurobiology is awe-inspiring and rather daunting; but the good news about complexity is that it reveals ever more entry points for specific interventions in the addictions, by novel drugs not yet invented or even imagined.

4

Addictive Behavior

As we have seen in previous chapters, neurotransmitters and receptors are the neurochemical units on which the addictive drugs act.
Our ultimate aim is to understand how the neurochemical effects of
the drugs cause changes of mood and behavior—changes that lead
to compulsive drug use. This chapter describes three different experimental approaches to studying the behavioral effects of addictive
drugs. It presents evidence from animal and human experiments
that bears on the following three questions:

> How is a drug recognized by the distinctive feeling it produces,
> so it can be discriminated from other drugs, and be preferred for
> self-administration?
> What are the principles and patterns underlying compulsive
> drug-seeking and drug-using behavior?
> What are the brain circuits and mechanisms that are respon-
> sible for the addictive properties of the seven drug families?

Answering these questions requires direct experiments because simple observation, anecdotes, and historical study of human societies
can never prove or disprove any interpretation decisively. Controlled
experiments are needed if unambiguous conclusions are to be

reached. Although human research is difficult, it is necessary, feasible, and informative; but there are problems. The most relevant experiments would require administering addictive drugs to people (even children or adolescents) who have had no prior drug experience; but that would be totally unethical. Ethical research—always with the informed consent of the subject—can be carried out with addicts, especially in testing alternative treatments for addiction. Studies involving administration of addictive drugs to ex-addicts can be useful, but raise serious ethical questions if the subjects are trying to remain abstinent.

Drug Discrimination: How Rats Tell One Drug From Another

People who seek out a particular drug will know when they have found it because they will recognize how it feels, provided they have had it before. This subjective recognition is called drug discrimination. It is that certain feeling, different for each kind of psychoactive drug, that users seek. Without it there would be no possibility of repeatedly seeking out and using a particular drug, and therefore there could be no drug addiction. An experienced drug user knows very well the difference between feeling drunk on alcohol, "stoned" on marijuana, or "high" on cocaine.

Drug discrimination can be demonstrated in animals as well as in humans. I illustrate with experiments carried out in my own laboratory. Our aim was to see if rats could discriminate the subjective feelings caused by nicotine from those caused by other drugs or by an inert placebo. It might seem ridiculous to expect a rat to tell us what it feels when we give it nicotine; but there is a way. A device called a T-maze (Figure 4.1) has a central alleyway (the stem of the T) with a grid floor that is constantly electrified. A rat placed on the stem of the T will receive a continuous mild but unpleasant foot shock. It looks desperately for a way to escape and finds that it can run forward and then go into the right or left cross-arm of the T. At the end of each cross-arm is a safe haven with a gate that can be open or closed according to the experimenter's design. Neither gate can be seen by the rat from a distance. So in trying to escape the foot shock, the animal runs up the stem of the T and then the whole length of either cross-arm. Then, if that gate is closed, it has to retrace its steps and try the other cross-arm.

To train a rat in this apparatus, we first take the animal out of its

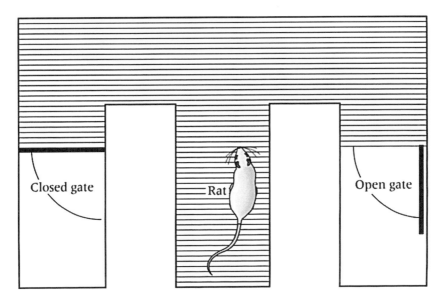

Fig. 4.1: Overton T-maze. Electrified grid floor is shown, with controlled access to safe haven on either side.

home cage and give it an injection of an inert salt solution, a placebo. A few minutes later we place the rat in the stem of the T, leaving the right gate open, the left gate closed. Either by good luck or after trying the wrong cross-arm, the rat finds the safe haven, escapes the shock, and is then removed and replaced in its home cage. The same procedure is repeated day after day. The rat learns that as soon as it is placed on the stem of the T, it must run straight ahead, make a fast turn to the right, run to the end of that cross-arm, and scurry through the open gate into the safe haven.

Once the rat has learned this lesson, we inject a dose of nicotine instead of placebo, and this time we close the right gate and open the left one. Of course the rat applies what it has learned; it turns to the right. When it finds the gate closed it is astonished and confused (if we may impute human emotions). It desperately seeks another way to escape the foot shock, and sooner or later discovers the safe haven on the left.

We make an injection every day, sometimes placebo, sometimes nicotine. Whenever it is placebo, we open the gate on the right; whenever it is nicotine, we open the one on the left. Sooner or later the rat begins to adopt a strategy that works. It behaves as though it were reasoning, "Aha! When I feel my normal self, I can escape to the right but when I have that peculiar feeling, I have to turn to the left." After about a month of daily trials, most rats learn the lesson perfectly.

The procedure has now trained the rats to "tell us" if they have had nicotine or not and we are ready for a test session. We make an injection and see which way a rat turns. With placebo or with nicotine, we know what the correct behavior should be, and we find almost perfect discrimination. What happens, then, if we give a drug that is chemically related to nicotine, one that might or might not act like nicotine in the brain? Trained rats can classify such a drug for us as nicotinelike or not nicotinelike by simply turning one way or the other after a test injection.

We can train rats to distinguish other psychoactive drugs such as morphine, cocaine, or diazepam (Valium) from a placebo. Now, suppose a rat has been trained to recognize nicotine, and then at the test session it is given one of these other drugs. What does such a rat do? A reasonable guess would be that since the animal was trained to discriminate nicotine from placebo, it will recognize morphine or cocaine or diazepam as "not placebo." We would guess that the animal, feeling "drugged," will respond as it did to nicotine.

We would be wrong. Remarkably, what the rat does is to discriminate nicotine from not-nicotine; in other words the discrimination is highly drug-specific. Indeed, an animal can be trained easily to discriminate one drug from another, as long as the two drugs belong to different families, so they bind to different receptors. This drug-specific recognition is not really too surprising if we think about how readily humans distinguish between different addictive drugs.

The same method can be used to test antagonists. First, we give a drug that we think might be an antagonist to nicotine. Will it block nicotine discrimination? A few minutes after injecting such a drug, we give nicotine. If the rat was trained as described above, it can tell us "I feel nicotine" by turning to the left, or "I don't feel nicotine" by turning to the right. Trained rats are tested with different antagonist doses. If the dose is small enough, the rat will indicate nicotine. As the dose is increased, a point will be reached at which the rat no longer indicates nicotine. The dose at which the rat's behavior changes is a measure of the antagonist potency.

Experiments have shown that nicotine discrimination is highly specific, therefore that it depends on receptors in the brain. Very small changes in the chemical structure of nicotine made big differences in the dose required to make a rat say "Yes, it's nicotine." These differences in potency for drug discrimination are consistent with the potencies for pharmacological effects that are known to be mediated by brain nicotinic acetylcholine receptors.

Drug Discrimination: Can People Do As Well As Rats?

A fascinating human experiment in drug discrimination was carried out with volunteers who had a long history of heroin use, who knew exactly what they liked about heroin. They could even put a price on a heroin injection according to its strength. The aim of the experiment was to test the effectiveness of the heroin antagonist naltrexone, a drug that is closely related to naloxone. A dose was given by mouth, followed by a standard effective dose of heroin intravenously. The subject was then asked "How much would you have been willing to pay for that injection?" On different days and with different subjects, various doses of naltrexone were tested. The subjects were unaware of what doses, if any, they were getting. Drug discrimination worked as well as in the rat experiments; the results were remarkably clear, especially in view of the seemingly crude measurement technique. After a zero dose of naltrexone (i.e., a placebo) the standard heroin injection was rated, on the average, as worth 18 dollars. After a sufficient dose of naltrexone, the same dose of heroin was rated worthless. And there was a regular dose-response relationship, intermediate doses yielding intermediate dollar-value estimates. The theory behind the therapeutic use of naltrexone is that if people take this antagonist regularly, they will not continue buying heroin because heroin will be worthless to them. In chapter 10 we shall discuss how this works out in practice for preventing relapse to heroin use.

Most drug testing in humans requires double-blind design. This means that neither the subject nor the experimenters know whether a drug or a placebo is administered or—in studies of dosage—what dose is given. The purpose is to exclude subjective biases. But the very ability to discriminate psychoactive drugs can make double-blind design in human experiments difficult or even impossible. We could even find ourselves in the absurd situation that the subjects would have no trouble discriminating drug from placebo by the way it felt, while only the experimenters were left in the dark! This is not to say double-blind design should be abandoned, only that the investigator has to be aware of the problem and try to devise clever ways of getting around it. One such approach—but not very satisfactory—is to use an active placebo, an unrelated substance that has some psychoactive properties of its own.

Taking a Drug Again and Again

If a person self-administers a drug repeatedly without a medical reason, we conclude that there must be something satisfying about it, that the user is seeking a desirable sensation or pleasurable state (a hedonic effect) produced by the drug. Experimental animal psychology has taught us that behaviors are often determined by their consequences. This means that if a particular behavior results in a desirable outcome such as access to food or water for a hungry or thirsty animal, the probability will increase for that behavior to be repeated.

Suppose a pigeon, mouse, rat, monkey, or other animal can press a lever to obtain food. The animal does not know this at the outset, and merely explores its surroundings, eventually pressing the lever by accident. Food appears at once, and the animal eats it. If we keep a continuous record of the lever pressing activity we see that a pattern soon emerges, as the animal learns how to bring about the desirable consequence. We say that the food is a reinforcer because it strengthens (reinforces) the probability that the appropriate operant (active, self-initiated, working) behavior—in this case lever-pressing—will be repeated.

Human behavior is subject to many complex influences, but the same rules often apply. An apt analogy to the experiment just described is a person working one of those gambling machines called a "one-armed bandit." If it never paid out, people would soon stop putting in their coins. The money it delivers is the reinforcer; putting in coins and pulling the handle is the operant behavior that is being reinforced. In gambling devices, as in laboratory experiments, there can be many different payout schedules. Payout could occur every lever press, or every so many lever presses, or at the first lever press after a time-out period according to some entirely random schedule, and so on. It is interesting that for laboratory animals as for people at Las Vegas the strongest incentives are provided by variable schedules of reinforcement, in which the number of lever presses (or coins) needed to produce a reward is random and unpredictable.

In order to study self-administration of a drug by an animal, we implant a thin flexible tubing into the jugular vein, arranging matters so that the animal can move about freely in its cage. Now instead of food, a certain number of lever presses will deliver a small dose of an addictive drug like heroin or cocaine. The animal sooner or later discovers that pressing a lever repeatedly will eventually produce a drug injection, and soon it will be taking the drug on a regular schedule. Clearly, in this case the drug itself is the reinforcer. Which drugs act as reinforcers in animals? In general the same ones that are addictive in people, and that are recognized by their pleasurable effects in drug discrimination experiments.

Animals will sometimes work amazingly hard to get a drug. If every lever press results in the injection of a small but effective dose, an animal will press the lever only occasionally, evidently allowing one dose to wear off before taking another. But what if we change the rules and require 10 lever presses (or 100 or 1,000) to get a single injection? The animal will quickly adapt to the new arrangement, as though trying to take the same amount of drug as before, but now working many times harder to get it. How hard an animal is willing to work for a drug is one measure of the drug's addictiveness. By this criterion, cocaine is the most addictive drug of all; a monkey will self-administer it to exhaustion—not eating, not drinking, and ignoring opportunities for sexual activity. Eventually such a monkey will die taking cocaine—of starvation or dehydration or sudden heart stoppage caused by the drug excess in the body.

An interesting feature of self-administration behavior for many (but not all) drugs is the way an animal will tend to maintain a certain effective concentration in its bloodstream and brain. This is called self-titration. If the schedule is unaltered with respect to the number of lever presses required, but the dose delivered at each lever press is changed, the animal responds appropriately. Make each single dose bigger, the animal presses less frequently; decrease each single dose, the animal presses more frequently. If the dose is suddenly reduced to zero, there is usually a burst of pressing (as though expressing frustration?) before the animal gives up. Again the slot machine comes to mind; if the rules suddenly changed, and payouts inexplicably stopped, we can imagine the frustrated gambler furiously pumping more coins into the machine or shaking it in furious frustration.

An experiment in human self-administration was carried out to see if smokers titrate their intake of nicotine. Would they adjust their rate of smoking in order to obtain a certain desired amount of drug? Addicted cigarette smokers were gathered in a room, ostensibly to be tested on their problem-solving ability. Paper-and-pencil tasks kept them busy. Each subject was given an ashtray and told to feel free to smoke. Hospital-style intravenous drip systems were set up, into which injections could be made—out of a subject's sight. Some subjects were chosen randomly to receive nicotine injections, others to receive placebo. At completion of the experiment a few hours later, the ashtrays were collected, and the cigarette butts were counted and weighed. The result was clear. The more nicotine had been injected—without the subject's knowledge—the fewer cigarettes were smoked. Experiments like this one answered an old question—do smokers smoke primarily for oral gratification, for the visual pleasure of watching the smoke, or for the nicotine? Here it was evident that they smoked primarily for the nicotine, unconsciously adjusting their smoking behavior according to the nicotine level in their blood and brains.

However, as often happens with scientific hypotheses, the outcome was not perfectly unambiguous. Yes, the subjects did adjust their smoking as stated, but no, the titration was not perfect; some smoking continued even when nicotine levels were so high that one would have expected smoking to cease entirely. This result sheds light on an essential feature of drug self-administration in humans— that spiking drug levels in the brain are far more rewarding than steady-state levels, no matter how high. And spiking, over and above a high level, will still be reinforcing. We shall return to this issue of spiking versus steady-state in connection with methadone treatment of heroin addicts (see chapter 10).

The self-administration procedure lets us test various active drugs and antagonists, much as we did with drug discrimination. Suppose a rat is working on a regular schedule for heroin injections and is then given a small dose of naltrexone. The antagonist spreads through the body and reaches the brain. The rat discovers that the heroin injections produced by lever pressing seem suddenly to have become weaker, as in the discrimination experiment with human subjects that was described earlier. The rat responds accordingly by working harder, taking more heroin to overcome (if possible) the antagonist. Sooner or later, however, if lever pressing yields no reward at all, the animal quits, and the behavior is said to be extinguished. Thus an animal's self-administration record can give us information about whether a novel compound antagonizes the effect of a rewarding drug, and if so, how potent it is.

For drugs that are effective by mouth, the self-administration procedure can be as simple as presenting a choice between two water bottles, one of which contains the drug, and the other a placebo solution made to taste like the drug. This free access drinking choice arrangement is less artificial than lever pressing. Rats and mice can be housed socially, can have opportunities for exercise, can have places to explore and toys to play with. Then one can test how the choice between drug and placebo is affected by environmental influences. One such experiment showed that the preference of rats for morphine over plain water was greater under conditions of isolation than in a more normal social setting. With people too, the generally accepted wisdom (though not rigorously proved) is that the use of addictive drugs is influenced strongly by environment, by social circumstances, especially by the availability of alternative activities and sources of alternative satisfactions.

How Rats Learn Where to Get Their "Fix"

Another way to study the reinforcing properties of drugs, and to localize drug reinforcement in the brain, is called conditioned place preference (CPP). A special kind of two-compartment box is used, with the compartments designed to appear and feel very different, in order to help a rat distinguish one side of the box from the other. The animal can move freely within the box, shuttling as it wishes between the two sides. A rat is placed in the box every day, and the time it spends in each side is carefully recorded. Then, one day, the animal is placed in the nonpreferred side, injected with a drug (perhaps heroin or cocaine) or a placebo, prevented for a while from returning to its preferred side, and then returned to its home cage. The procedure is repeated daily for a week or two.

After this period of conditioning, the rat is simply placed in the box without any injection. What does it do? If the daily injections were placebo, or if they were drugs known not to be reinforcers in other tests, the animal's behavior is unaltered; it chooses to stay on the side of the box it preferred at the outset. On the other hand, if a reinforcing drug was injected during the conditioning period, the rat will have learned to associate the rewarding effect of the drug with the place where the injections were given (thus the name of the procedure), and it will linger on that side of the box as though waiting for its drug "fix."

This experiment shows plainly that CPP can distinguish drugs that are rewarding from drugs that are not. The procedure can also be used to find where in the brain a drug acts to produce reward. Under surgical anesthesia, a very fine injection needle is implanted into a selected site in a rat's brain. This microsurgery has no obvious effect on the animal's behavior; and we know from neurosurgical procedures in people, that such fine needle implantations are harmless. Then, place conditioning is carried out as before; but now the daily drug injections (of tiny amounts of drug) are made into the small area of brain surrounding the needle tip instead of into a vein. Different groups of rats are used for each brain site tested—a truly laborious experiment.

The results are dramatic. Drug injections into most parts of the brain do not modify the animal's behavior at all. But a certain few locations are effective in producing place preference. These are the same brain sites into which animals will self-administer addictive drugs. They are in a dopamine-containing nerve tract in the midbrain, which is described below.

Feels So Good!

A key experiment, nearly 50 years ago, first demonstrated reinforcement by electrical brain stimulation. A thin wire electrode was implanted into a rat's brain and hooked up so that by pressing a lever, the animal could give itself a mild electric shock. Most placements of the wire were ignored by the rat, but at certain specific brain sites it "liked" the electrical stimulation, and pressed the lever repeatedly. The method is called intracranial self-stimulation (ICSS). By trying all sorts of electrode placements it was possible to learn where in the brain stimulation is reinforcing.

With rats, we have to infer that ICSS is pleasurable because it is reinforcing, but people can report their subjective experience. ICSS has been carried out in human patients during attempts to find a surgical cure for epilepsy. Patients fully conscious on the operating table report that ICSS does indeed produce an intensely pleasurable and satisfying feeling, provided the electrode is positioned correctly.

Deep in the middle of the brain is a site especially favorable for ICSS—a nerve tract known as the mesolimbic dopaminergic pathway (Figure 4.2). Many of the neurons here originate in the ventral tegmental area (VTA) and extend forward in the brain to the nucleus accumbens (NAc) and frontal cortex. These long neurons contain the neurotransmitter dopamine. When stimulated at the VTA they deliver dopamine from their terminals at NAc and frontal cortex, where dopamine receptors are found. This nerve tract is called a reward pathway because animals will press a lever to stimulate it with electric shocks, just as they work to get a food reward if they are hungry or a water reward if they are thirsty—and just as they work to get an injection of a drug that is a reinforcer.

The generally accepted view—the dopamine hypothesis—is that this neurotransmitter, released from the nerve endings of the mesolimbic pathway, is a key link in the complex chain of events responsible for reinforcement. It supposes that dopamine causes the feeling of pleasure and satisfaction—the hedonic effect—that leads to self-initiated repetition of the stimulation. That dopamine is released at NAc by ICSS or by reinforcing addictive drugs is beyond doubt; dopamine release has actually been measured by special instruments placed deep in a rat's brain. Dopamine spikes at NAc are caused by morphine and other opiates microinjected into either end of the reward pathway—at VTA or directly at NAc. Cocaine is effective only at NAc (see below). Thus, these two reinforcing addictive drugs act in the same pathway that animals self-stimulate with electric shocks in the ICSS procedure. A strong piece of evidence supporting the dopamine hypothesis is that blocking dopamine receptors abolishes the effects of various reinforcing stimuli.

In one experiment, dopamine release at NAc was measured in a freely mobile rat. If the rat was food-deprived and then allowed to eat, the local dopamine level soared. Readers with a sweet tooth will be amused to learn that chocolate caused the greatest dopamine surges! If a male rat was placed in a cage with a receptive female but separated by a wire screen barrier, dopamine release increased. If the screen was removed and copulation was allowed, the dopamine level went higher. Experiments like this show that dopamine release at its receptors in NAc and frontal cortex is closely associated with rewarding events of the same kind that lead to repeated ICSS or

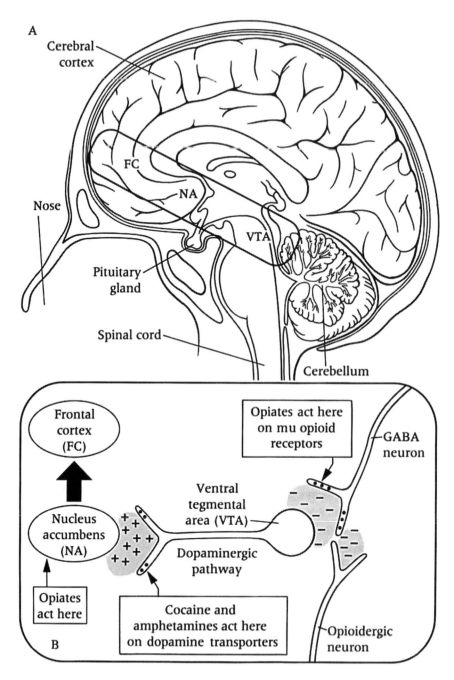

Fig. 4.2: Mesolimbic dopaminergic reward pathway. A. Human brain sliced open lengthwise, showing the relevant midbrain and forebrain area, outlined by an oval, with ventral tegmental area (VTA), nucleus accumbens (NA), and frontal cortex (FC) labeled. B. Cartoon diagram of the area outlined in A and described in text. Heavy dots represent stored neurotransmitter at nerve endings (+ = excitatory, − = inhibitory) and released into synapse.

drug self-administration. It appears that some action of dopamine on its receptors in NAc (and probably frontal cortex) may be the rewarding event in both cases. Consequently, anything that causes dopamine to be released there or that enhances its action there— whether by electrical stimulation or by drug stimulation—is rewarding.

How does cocaine or an amphetamine act at NAc? There, in the endings of the dopaminergic neurons, the stored neurotransmitter awaits the arrival of a nerve impulse. Immediately upon its release into the synapses, the dopamine combines with its receptor on another neuron. Then it is quickly taken up again (sponged up, one might say) by the dopamine transporter (see chapter 3) on the same neurons that released it, thus terminating its action. Cocaine and amphetamines block the transporter. Then dopamine accumulates in the synapses, and its effects are greatly enhanced. Amphetamines, in addition, act directly on dopaminergic nerve endings to cause excessive release of dopamine into the synapses. Both cocaine and amphetamines act at the nerve terminals that release dopamine at NAc, whereas opiates and other drugs also act elsewhere in the reward pathway—often at the origin of the pathway in VTA. A long-term effect of addictive drugs is to shut down dopamine production by a feedback mechanism, as the brain regulatory controls attempt to compensate for the excessive dopamine.

Mice without dopamine transporters ("knockouts," described in chapter 3) have synaptic dopamine levels 10 times higher than normal, and they are extraordinarily hyperactive, as one might expect. One might also expect cocaine not to be rewarding for them. But surprisingly, these animals still do self-administer cocaine, and they also show cocaine reward in the place conditioning (CPP) apparatus. This seeming paradox suggests that cocaine acts on other targets (perhaps other transporters) in addition to the dopamine transporter, and therefore that dopamine may not be the sole mediator of reward.

How do opiates produce their rewarding effects? We know that opioid receptors on a nerve ending are inhibitory, suppressing the release of whatever neurotransmitter that neuron contains. If the neuron in question releases an excitatory neurotransmitter, then morphine, by diminishing that release, will reduce the excitation. On the other hand if the neuron in question releases an inhibitory neurotransmitter, morphine will reduce the inhibition and thus cause increased excitation. This may seem a complicated regulatory system but it is effective for fine control, much as a car set to idle fast while in gear could be accelerated by releasing pressure on the brake pedal.

That stimulation can result from disinhibition is illustrated by the effect of morphine on a part of the brain known as the hippocampus. Here morphine provokes intense electrical activity, sometimes causing seizures. The principal neurons here are held continuously in check by the braking action of other neurons, which release the inhibitory neurotransmitter GABA. Presynaptic mu opioid receptors are deployed on the ends of these GABA neurons. When morphine (or an endogenous opioid) activates these receptors, GABA release is impeded, so the braking action of GABA is greatly diminished, and the principal hippocampal neurons become more active. As one might expect, the mu opioid receptors on the GABA nerve terminals are normally activated by nearby neurons that release opioid peptides as part of the normal regulation of hippocampal activity.

In the reward pathway, neurons originating in VTA are held in check by GABA. By inhibiting GABA release, opiates diminish the braking action on these dopaminergic neurons, so they fire more frequently and release more dopamine from the nerve terminals at NAc. A similar disinhibitory effect of opiates presumably accounts for their stimulatory action when applied directly at NAc.

Dopamine effects in the reward pathway are enhanced not only by cocaine, amphetamines, and opiates, but also by nicotine and alcohol. As the evidence accumulated, many researchers came to the view that this common mechanism of reinforcement is shared by all the addictive drugs—therefore that stimulation of a dopaminergic reward pathway is what makes a drug addictive. But we have no idea how dopamine stimulation in NAc actually produces the reinforcement. A crude way of putting this uncertainty is to ask: Where in the brain is the feeling of pleasure and satisfaction localized? Is NAc only a way station, a relay in a much more complex network of neurons? The question may not even make sense; perhaps a mood state is not localized at all but is spread over many parts of the brain.

Some scientists remain skeptical of the simple (perhaps simplistic) dopamine hypothesis, feeling that conclusive proof is still lacking—or at least that there is much more to the story than we have learned so far. Most unsettling is the fact that in real life, the various addictive drugs, although they all cause dopamine release from the mesolimbic pathway, are nevertheless not interchangeable; nicotine will not substitute for heroin or alcohol, nor marijuana for cocaine, nor morphine for amphetamine. Thus, it has been proposed that do-pamine may play a role in calling attention to any hedonically active addictive drug rather than itself providing the rewarding effect. The participation of dopamine in relapse after abstinence is discussed in chapter 6.

Despite all the uncertainties that remain, the studies described here are opening the way for deeper understanding. Most important, there seems to be no reason to think that the biological mechanisms of drug reward in the human brain are different in any fundamental way from those uncovered by experiments in rats.

Rewarding and Aversive Opioids

Opioidergic neurons containing enkephalins, beta-endorphin, and dynorphins are found in the VTA. Not surprisingly, an enkephalin or beta-endorphin, if injected directly into the VTA, acts like an addictive opiate, evidently activating mu opioid receptors there. But the dynorphin peptides, which act preferentially on kappa opioid receptors, have an opposite effect; they activate a system that me-diates aversion, that delivers punishment rather than reward. Ani-mals will not self-administer kappa (dynorphinlike) agonists. More-over, in the CPP procedure such drugs condition a rat to avoid rather than prefer the side of the shuttle box where they are administered.

What about people? A human volunteer was given a synthetic opiate agonist that is selective for kappa receptors. It was expected that the subject would find the drug unpleasant, as animals seemed to. What actually happened was dramatic and totally unexpected. The kappa agonist was more than just unpleasant—it produced a frightening psychotic state, with weird distortions of time and space, a terrifying feeling of impending death, and hallucinations. How could the experimenters be sure that these bizarre drug effects were due to activation of kappa opioid receptors and not to some non-specific toxic disturbance of brain function? First, the kappa agonist they used was available in both left- and right-handed forms, as de-scribed earlier for other opioid ligands; and only the left-handed one was active, signifying interaction with a specific opioid receptor. Sec-ond, and most convincing—and to the great relief of experimenters and subject alike—the subject's mental state reverted to normal instantly when the opiate antagonist naltrexone was injected.

Summary

A natural system exists in the brain for signaling both reward and punishment. Most of the evidence indicates that this reward pathway operates by releasing dopamine in the forward part of the brain, at the nucleus accumbens and frontal cortex. Reinforcing stimuli, including addictive drugs, cause dopamine release at those sites. Opioid peptides and their receptors seem to play a central role in reward, even when the primary reinforcing addictive drug belongs to a different family. For example, blocking mu opioid receptors with naltrexone suppresses relapse in alcohol addiction (see chapter 9). Also, as mu opioid agonists are reinforcing, while kappa opioid agonists are aversive, it may be that the balance of these two opioid activities regulates our normal mood and state of well-being.

Natural neurochemical mechanisms in brain signal "good" when food is found and eaten by a hungry animal, when water is found and drunk by a thirsty animal, when sexual activity is promised and consummated, or when a threatening situation is averted. They signal "bad" when harmful behavior is engaged in or when pain is experienced. These signals become associated with the situations in which they are generated—and they are remembered. Thus, the conditioning observed in the CPP procedure seems to represent the necessary process by which an animal learns to seek what is beneficial and avoid what is harmful.

That addictive drugs "feel good" must be understood in this evolutionary context, for in a sense they are not even foreign to the body; they merely mimic or block the neurotransmitters that function normally to signal reward. However, they activate the pathways artificially—short-circuiting the natural process, one might say—and thus they disturb the mechanisms that keep people on an even keel. This delicately regulated system was perfected by evolution over millions of years to serve the survival of all species, and to let us humans experience pleasure and satisfaction from the biologically appropriate and necessary behaviors of daily life. No prudent person would try to beef up the performance of a personal computer by jolting it with high voltage electric shocks. It always astonishes me, therefore, to hear users of addictive drugs and apologists for their use—some of whom are sensible people in other respects—defend what is really a reckless chemical attack on the human brain. The more we learn about addictive drugs and brain chemistry, the clearer it becomes that the brain is far too delicate to tamper with, too complex an organ to risk damaging its intricate regulatory controls.

5

Pain and Pleasure

In the Cornaro Chapel in Rome a brilliant shaft of sunlight illuminates the masterwork of the great seventeenth-century sculptor Bernini. A marble statue of Saint Teresa, it depicts the moment of her famous ecstasy, when an angel with a flaming golden arrow pierced her heart repeatedly. In her own words:

> The pain was so great that I screamed aloud but simultaneously felt such infinite sweetness that I wished the pain to last eternally. It was the sweetest caressing of the soul by God.

Saint Teresa's words express the familiar yet mysterious psychological relationship between pain and pleasure. Pain relieved leaves not merely a normal pain-free state but a special kind of pleasure and satisfaction in its absence. Pain unrelieved can activate endogenous mechanisms that not only suppress the pain but also can produce pleasure in their own right. And though it is considered pathological, some people derive masochistic pleasure from pain itself.

It is interesting, therefore that this pleasure-pain connection is grounded in neurochemistry. Not only the endogenous opioids but other neurochemical systems—for example the endogenous cannabinoids (chapter 12)—are responsible both for suppressing pain and for producing pleasure through the reward systems. The same duality applies to the behavior of opiate addicts—they use heroin for pleasure, certainly, but also for relief of physical and emotional pain. This chapter focuses on the endogenous opioids because we know most about their relationship to pain, pleasure, and addiction. It is likely, however, that a general principle is at work here—that suppression of pain and enhancement of pleasure are mediated by the same or closely related neural circuits. Indeed, addictive drugs other than opiates—for example caffeine, alcohol, and marijuana—have pain-relieving qualities too.

Pain Suppression by Endogenous Opioids

Opioid receptors and opioid peptides are found in the dopamine reward pathways of the midbrain, as described in chapter 4. They are also distributed widely elsewhere in the nervous system—throughout the brain and spinal cord and in the nerves that supply the extremities, the skin, the blood vessels, and most of the internal organs of the body. Opioid receptors are deployed all along the pain pathways, at successive levels of the sensory systems, starting at the skin or joints or internal organs and progressing up into the spinal cord and brain. Thus, morphine is effective locally in suppressing activation of the sensory nerves by pain—as when injected into the knee joint during arthroscopic surgery. When the sensory nerves reach the spinal cord, they release a special peptide neurotransmitter called a neurokinin, which stimulates the next neuron in the pain pathway at that synapse. Opioid receptors on the endings of the neurokinin neurons can suppress neurokinin release. When morphine is given as an injection for pain relief, it activates these receptors and thus interrupts the pain pathway at the spinal cord. The most dramatic effect of morphine, however, occurs in the higher centers of the brain, which handle emotional and intellectual functions. There, morphine disconnects the perception of pain from the usual emotional response; as some patients put it, "I know the pain is still there but I don't mind it any more."

Because the seemingly magical property of abolishing both emotional and physical pain underlies the addictive use of heroin (and of some other addictive drugs), we need to understand how our endogenous opioid system for suppressing pain works. Is it turned on by painful and stressful stimuli? How might we obtain direct experimental evidence about this? Suppose, for example, that the opioid peptide beta-endorphin were a neurotransmitter in such a system; then we would want to measure its release inside brain and spinal cord in response to pain. In humans, we can easily take a blood sample, but not a sample of brain or spinal cord. Consequently—especially before the development of ligand PET scans (see chapter 3)—many measurements were made on blood after painful and other stressful stimuli. The most popular version of this approach sought to relate the "runner's high" to increased beta-endorphin blood levels. Unfortunately, such measurements are based on radioimmunoassays, which cannot distinguish between opioid-active beta-endorphin itself and precursor peptides that are chemically related to beta-endorphin but have no opioid activity. Most of this blood "beta-endorphin" consists of these other peptides, which are released from the pituitary gland (not the brain) along with the stress hormone ACTH. Therefore, although this immuno-reactivity in blood does measure a stress response, it is misleading to suggest that it has anything to do with pain regulation or emotional states in the brain or spinal cord.

We can measure endogenous opioids in animal brains. However, even in animals, it is not too useful to know how much beta-endorphin or enkephalin or dynorphin is present, stored in nerve endings and waiting to be released. The real question is: Do painful or stressful stimuli provoke their release? After all, it is the dynamic release process that matters. If you wanted to analyze the operation of a water wheel on a river, you would have to measure the flow of water running down the river, not the height of water behind the dam in an upstream reservoir.

A method long in use for measuring neurotransmitter release in the central nervous system is to analyze small samples of cerebro-spinal fluid from the spinal canal or base of the brain. There is a major problem, however. It takes many minutes for a substance re-leased deep inside the brain to appear in the spinal fluid, and during that time, a peptide is very likely to be destroyed. One needs to measure release at the actual site of release. One successful method is by a push-pull cannula inserted deep into the spinal cord or brain of a live rat under anesthesia. This cannula is an extremely fine double-barreled glass tubing filled with a salt solution. A tiny stream of fluid is pushed into the tissue through one barrel of the cannula and withdrawn continuously through the other, thus bathing the synapses that surround the cannula tip. The amount of such substances as beta-endorphin in the withdrawn fluid is then measured by immunoassay. By this procedure it has been shown that extreme stress, pain, and electroacupuncture (see below) actually do release opioid peptides at several levels of the pain pathway, and not only within the spinal cord but also at higher levels of the brain.

Another method is based on the principle of competition for receptor binding. A thin slice of rat brain is maintained in a functional state in a shallow dish, under a microscope. It is exposed to a radiolabeled opioid ligand, yielding a picture showing the location of opioid receptors in the slice. One of the neural pathways that is known to contain endogenous opioids is stimulated electrically before the slice is exposed to the radioligand. Now the picture shows a reduction in radioactivity compared with unstimulated tissue. In other words, an opioid peptide released by the stimulation has occupied the receptors, excluding the radioligand, as described in chapter 3. This method can establish which opioid ligands are released, and with which opioid receptor subtypes they combine when known nerve pathways are stimulated. Similar methods are applied to the VTA, NAc, and other parts of the reward pathways implicated in the addictions.

A novel technique—also based on the competition principle— uses a fine needle coated with an antibody that is specific for a particular peptide neurotransmitter, for instance the neurokinin that transmits pain signals. The needle is inserted into a rat's spinal cord and the animal is subjected to pain by pinching a paw. After a suitable time the needle is removed and immersed in a solution of radiolabeled neurokinin. The radioactive neurokinin binds everywhere along the needle except where endogenous neurokinin (not radioactive, of course) was released in the spinal cord, and had bound to the needle, filling the antibody binding sites. Wherever the needle bound radioactive neurokinin, the photographic image of the needle is black; but where endogenous neurokinin was released, a clear band is seen, where the radiolabeled neurokinin was excluded. This experiment proved that painful stimulation released neurokinin at precisely the site in the spinal cord where the endings of the incoming pain neurons are known to be—the same site where opioids suppress neurokinin release.

How Antagonists Reveal Ongoing Opioid Activity

The opiate antagonists naloxone and naltrexone can shed light on which brain functions require participation of an endogenous opioid. The logic is simply that because these antagonists are so specific for opioid receptors, any function that is altered by them is probably mediated by an endogenous opioid. If low doses suffice, the mu receptor (for which naloxone and naltrexone have highest affinity) is most likely responsible.

A good illustration of this approach is the effect of naloxone on circulating testosterone in blood. A brain peptide called gonado-tropin-releasing hormone (GnRH) stimulates cells in the pituitary gland to secrete the sex hormone gonadotropin (also called LH) into the blood in sexually mature male rats. LH, in turn, stimulates the testicles to produce testosterone, which is responsible for many male sexual characteristics and behaviors. In sexually mature rats, naloxone causes a huge increase in circulating LH and testosterone because of greatly increased release of GnRH in the brain (Figure 5.1). From this result we conclude that some endogenous opioid acts as a continuous brake on GnRH release—a brake that is revealed

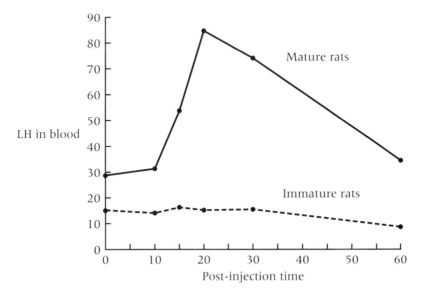

Fig. 5.1: An opioid antagonist reverses ongoing inhibition of luteinizing hormone release from rat pituitary. Blood levels of LH are shown at various times after naloxone injection. Lower record, immature rats; upper record, sexually mature rats. (From T. J. Cicero et al., *Journal of Pharmacology and Experimental Therapeutics* 246:14–20, 1988.)

when naloxone removes it by blocking the opioid receptors. Consistent with the rat experiment, morphine or heroin acts in an unregulated manner to shut down sexual function in men and to suppress the menstrual cycle in women—dysfunctions that characteristically afflict heroin addicts.

To test whether an endogenous opioid suppresses pain, we carried out a naloxone experiment. When a mouse is placed on a hot plate, warm enough to be uncomfortable but not hot enough to burn the feet, the mouse reacts by lifting a paw or jumping within a few seconds. The greater the discomfort, the sooner the mouse reacts, so the delay in jumping (called the latency) is a measure of the intensity of the pain, as experienced by the animal. If groups of mice are injected with morphine before being placed on the hot plate, the average latency is greatly prolonged; the animals experience less pain. If naloxone is given first and then morphine, the morphine effect is prevented. These preliminary tests tell us that the method works, that suppression of pain by an administered opiate can be measured as increased latency on the hot plate, and that naloxone blocks that opiate effect. Now, if pain is being suppressed to some extent by an endogenous opioid, we would expect naloxone itself to make it worse. Using fresh mice and without giving any morphine, we injected naloxone alone. The latency was reduced; the mice jumped sooner than normal, as though the pain had been intensified. We concluded that under the conditions of this experiment, an endogenous opioid system was, indeed, suppressing pain; and by blocking that system naloxone made the pain worse.

A useful feature of naloxone and naltrexone is that they are harmless enough to use in humans. We carried out experiments with many volunteers. Knowing the result of the mouse hot plate experiment, we expected naloxone to intensify pain. We produced pain by the following standard procedure: We shut off the circulation to the forearm by inflating a blood pressure cuff to a very high pressure. We had the subject exercise the hand for a few minutes, and then relax. I can say from my own experience as a subject, that without any blood flow to carry away the products of muscular activity, a severe throbbing pain develops—tolerable, but only barely so. The subject reported the increasing severity of pain on a numerical scale. The procedure could be terminated by the subject at any time, but otherwise was stopped after 10 minutes. To our great surprise we found that naloxone had no effect whatsoever on the pain, as rated by the subjects.

Surprising results are the best kind, because they point to something new, something that was misunderstood and needs further research. We soon realized that whereas in the mouse experiment the animals were severely stressed, the human volunteers—made comfortable and reassured by the investigators—remained calm and relaxed, despite their discomfort. Although painful, the procedure was not stressful. Other investigators have since shown that if pain is experienced while under stress, naloxone does indeed make it worse. For example, actual clinical pain (always stressful)—as after tooth extraction—is intensified by naloxone. Thus, stressful pain in humans can activate our endogenous opioid system. Moreover, we know now that severe stress alone, even without pain, activates the endogenous opioids so that noxious stimuli then become less painful than they would be otherwise.

In animal experiments, stressful procedures reveal this mechanism. We place a rat in cold water, so that it has to swim to a distant platform—a stressful task. Then we remove it and test for pain sensitivity by applying heat to the tail and measuring how many seconds pass before the animal reacts. Such an animal displays a much more sluggish reaction to the painful stimulus after the cold-water swim than before, and this suppression of pain is abolished by naloxone.

A common response of animals to an overwhelming threat or to extreme pain is total immobility ("freezing"), giving the impression of paralysis or indifference. This reaction may be mediated by endogenous opioid release, as in a few instances it has been shown to be prevented by naloxone. In the rat, morphine does cause an immobile state (described in chapter 2), which is reversed by naloxone. We do not know if such reactions in humans are also mediated by endogenous opioids, but it would not be surprising if they were. An extraordinary and possibly relevant case is the description by the famous explorer David Livingstone of being attacked by a lion:

> He caught my shoulder as he sprang . . . he shook me as a terrier does a rat. The shock produced a stupor similar to that which seems to be felt by a mouse after the first shake of the cat. It caused a sort of dreaminess in which there was no sense of pain nor feeling of terror, though [I was] quite conscious of all that

was happening. . . . This peculiar state is probably produced in all animals killed by the carnivora; and if so, is a merciful provision by our benevolent creator for lessening the pain of death.

Lawrence Durrell in his Alexandria Quartet describes something similar; but it is not clear whether this passage is based on fact or whether it is pure fiction:

> The camels of Narouz were being cut up for the feast. Poor things, they knelt there peacefully with their forelegs folded under them like cats while a horde of men attacked them with axes in the moonlight. . . . The animals made no move to avoid the blows, uttered no cries as they were dismembered. . . . Whole members were being hacked off, as painlessly, it seemed, as when a tree is pruned.

Speaking of camels brings to mind an amusing story that illustrates how a scientific myth can take hold, based on premises that may sound logical but turn out to be completely wrong. Chapter 2 recounted how beta-endorphin is produced in the pituitary gland and brain as part of a long precursor peptide. As long as it is part of the longer peptide, beta-endorphin has no biological activity, and it does not relieve pain; the long precursor peptide has to be cleaved first to release free beta-endorphin. Shortly after the long peptide from pig pituitary glands was isolated, a young foreign scientist who had worked on the project returned home from the laboratory where he had worked in San Francisco. He attempted to isolate the long peptide from camel pituitary glands to see how it differed from the pig peptide. Remarkably, he could find no precursor peptide at all—only free beta-endorphin in extraordinarily large amounts.

The renowned senior chemist who had been the project director explained at scientific meetings: "Now we know why camels are so insensitive to pain; they have a huge amount of free beta-endorphin." When other foreign scientists tried to isolate the camel peptide, they found the long precursor but almost no free beta-endorphin. Were there two kinds of camel? Not at all. The explanation lay very simply in a difference of refrigeration; without adequate freezing during storage, enzymes in the pituitary glands cleave the long precursor peptide after death, releasing free beta-endorphin. Live camels do not have an unusually large amount of beta-endorphin after all. An original false result had been attributed to an equally false "fact"—that camels are insensitive to pain. Despite

Durrell's account, there is no evidence whatsoever to suggest that camels are less sensitive to pain than are other species of mammals. In science, one has to establish the facts securely before interpreting them!

Pain Suppression by Acupuncture

The ancient Chinese procedure of acupuncture employs fine needles to stimulate local nerves under the skin. Largely because acupuncture had been claimed to cure every imaginable disease, Western medicine tended to discount the whole thing as superstition. Only in the late 1970s, when Western scientists could again visit China freely, did they see for themselves that acupuncture produces real pain relief—in surgical operations on animals, as well as on humans.

Experiments over many years at Beijing Medical University have demonstrated that electroacupuncture (stimulating nerves in the skin by a mild electric shock) reliably produces pain relief, not only in humans but in laboratory animals as well. I recall the first visit of a Chinese colleague to my laboratory, in 1978, just after the Cultural Revolution. "The problem for science," he told me, referring to acupuncture, "is to sort out the superstition from the reality." He himself had wisely decided to concentrate on pain relief by acupuncture, putting aside all the other supposed benefits of the technique. He used rats, applied electric shocks of known strength and frequency through the needles, used standardized pain stimuli, measured pain by response latency (as described above), and employed the whole toolbox of modern neurobiology to get at the mechanism. He established beyond doubt that pain relief by electroacupuncture is a reality, and he soon found that it is blocked by naloxone. As explained above, this indicates that electroacupuncture causes the release of endogenous opioids; and he could actually measure such release within the spinal cord and brain at several sites along the known pain pathways. These pioneering studies established acupuncture as a valid technique for relieving pain, and they have since been extended to humans.

Endogenous Opioids and the Emotions

The discovery of reward pathways, and the feelings of pleasure and satisfaction evoked by heroin or morphine, suggested that certain kinds of emotional pleasure might be caused by endogenous opioids, released onto opioid receptors within the brain, perhaps in the mesolimbic dopaminergic reward pathway.

I looked for a way to study an emotional response under experimental control in the laboratory. Emotionally arousing experiences produce a "thrill" in many people. This sensation is a pleasant tingling vibration that starts at the back of the neck and travels down the spine, often also sweeping over the arms and down the legs. It may be accompanied by tears, sighs, a "catch" in the throat, and even gooseflesh on the arms or chest. The word "thrill" is interesting for its double meaning, long established in our language; a thrill is both a vibratory sensation (the common meaning in medicine) and an emotionally arousing experience. Thrilling events are often described as "raising the hackles" (i.e., gooseflesh that causes hairs to rise at the back of the neck) or as "making chills run up and down the spine." Thrills are evoked by many kinds of moving experiences. Some people (I am one of them) get thrills from certain passages of music. Opera fans are familiar with the intensity of these emotional reactions, typically after a superb performance of one of the great operatic arias.

Musical thrills are easily studied in music-loving volunteers. I reasoned that if the thrills were mediated by the release of endogenous opioids in the brain, they should be blocked by naloxone. All of my volunteer subjects knew from experience which musical passages gave them thrills. One by one, they listened to their favorite music in the laboratory, and—by means of finger signals—they reported the occurrence and intensity of thrills. Then they were given an injection—double-blind, with all the injections coded, so neither I nor the subjects knew which was naloxone and which was placebo. After the injection, they listened again to the same passage, and rated the thrills once more. Altogether, there were 10 subjects and 10 sessions for each, spaced a week apart. Without any injections at all, or after placebo injection, repeating the same musical passage yielded the same pattern and intensity of thrills.

In some subjects, naloxone consistently blocked the thrills, suggesting that endogenous opioids do play a role in this purely emotional response, possibly through the dopaminergic reward pathway. This was a small-scale experiment, really only a pilot trial. It ought to be repeated by other investigators with more subjects and with higher doses of naloxone, as the doses I used are now known to be only marginally effective. But it is a difficult and expensive experiment, and unfortunately, even many years later, no one has attempted to replicate it.

Summary

The endogenous opioids constitute a natural protection against pain. The endogenous cannabinoids (chapter 12) may represent a parallel pain-suppressing system. Acupuncture produces analgesia by releasing endogenous opioids at several levels of the spinal cord and brain. The hallmark of opiate action is not only direct relief of pain, but also suppression of the anxiety and distress associated with pain. Moreover, opiates relieve emotional pain, even in the absence of physical pain. Finally, endogenous opioids seem to mediate emotional satisfaction and pleasure, as suggested by the "thrills" experiment. This unique mixture of psychoactive effects goes a long way toward explaining why powerful painkillers like morphine and heroin are also powerfully addictive. When emotional suffering is caused by intolerable conditions of life or by a pathological reaction to life's ordinary stresses, a quick "fix" offers immediate satisfaction, immediate pleasure, immediate escape from misery.

6

The Seesaw Brain:

"Highs" and Adaptations

The brain resists any disturbance in its neurochemical equilibrium. It recognizes a chemical change immediately, then adapts to it slowly. An addictive drug that mimics or blocks a neurotransmitter or receptor is like a weight thrown suddenly onto one side (let's call it the drug side) of a balanced seesaw. The sum of all the adaptations is like a counterweight added slowly to the opposite side (the adapting side) until the level state is reached again. If a drug floods the brain suddenly (a drug spike), an immediate change in brain function results. In the vernacular, if this effect is hedonic (pleasurable), it is called a drug "high;" the drug side of the seesaw drops. If the same drug is trickled slowly into the brain instead of spiking, adaptations can occur even while the drug level is increasing; the "high" is muted or nearly absent, while a plateau drug level is established.

The seesaw of an adapted brain is in balance despite the drug's presence. Now, to obtain a psychoactive effect again, the dose has to be raised to override the adaptation, to unbalance the seesaw again. And then, the dose has to be raised yet again, and so on. This is the phenomenon called tolerance, which is discussed at length later. An exception to this process of adaptation is seen with cocaine and other psychostimulants, which may initially have enhanced effects on rapidly repeated use (sensitization, see below).

Drug Spikes, Drug "Highs," and Drug Metabolism

The route of administration affects how quickly a drug will enter the brain and there have its hedonic effect. Suppose a drug is injected into an arm vein, a typical route for heroin or cocaine. The drug is carried in the blood to the right chamber of the heart, where it mixes with all the venous blood returning from the rest of the body, then is pumped through the circulation of the lungs, returns to the heart, and finally is delivered to the brain. This all takes about 16 seconds, and the drug arrives at the brain greatly diluted. Then, depending on how quickly it can pass through the brain capillaries into the spaces between the neurons, the drug will first exert its psychoactive effect.

Now suppose the same drug can be smoked. Some of it may pass directly into the venous blood through the membranes of the mouth or nose. Most of it, however, if deeply inhaled, will spread throughout the tiny alveolar sacs in the lungs. This network of fine lacy membranes can allow some drugs to pass directly into the blood. The inhalation route differs from the intravenous route in two important ways. First, the blood carrying drug molecules from the lungs to the left side of the heart is pumped directly to the brain without dilution, and it bypasses the liver's metabolic enzymes entirely. Second, the transit time from lungs to heart is very short— only about three seconds—minimizing the time of exposure to metabolic enzymes in the blood. Most important, each breath produces an immediate drug spike in the brain, and thus an immediate "high," more powerful than by the intravenous route.

Some recent research suggests that the lung tissue itself may buffer the intense drug spike by binding certain drugs like nicotine and possibly cocaine. In consequence, the brain spikes are not as high as would be expected if all the inhaled drug had passed directly to the brain. But although the spikes may be smaller than expected, the principle of spiking still applies. From the user's point of view, the sharpest spikes give the best "high." That is why the inhalation route is so popular; and conversely, it is why the oral route (with slow absorption from the stomach and intestine) is—with few exceptions—not favored. Important practical issues depend on the difference between spiking and plateau drug levels. In Part Two this question will be revisited with respect to each drug; it is especially significant in understanding why, in the treatment of heroin addicts, oral methadone maintenance cannot be considered a heroin substitute (chapter 10). It is also highly relevant to the differences between tobacco smoking and the nicotine patch (chapter 8), and between smoking "crack" cocaine and chewing coca leaves (chapter 11).

By whatever route a drug reaches the brain, when it leaves the brain and enters the general circulation it becomes vulnerable to destruction by enzymes in blood and liver. A few drugs—THC in marijuana is an example—are metabolized slowly or not at all but are stored for a very long time in body fat, trickling out into the bloodstream and being excreted in the urine for days or even weeks after a single dose.

To illustrate the diversity and complexity of drug metabolism, let us consider how three important drugs (alcohol, heroin, and cocaine) are handled by the body. Alcohol is converted by a liver enzyme to a very toxic product, acetaldehyde. Then a second liver enzyme destroys the acetaldehyde as fast as it is made, so that very little accumulates. Were it not for this second enzyme (acetaldehyde dehydrogenase), alcohol would be too poisonous to drink. In chapter 9 we shall see that one way of discouraging alcohol addicts from drinking is to preserve the acetaldehyde in their blood so that even a single drink will make them severely ill.

Heroin is actually a pro-drug, an inactive precursor; it is not biologically active in its own right because its two acetic acid groups, which confer the property of rapid passage from the blood into the brain, also prevent its binding to opioid receptors. In the brain, first one then the other acetic acid group is removed, yielding psychoactive morphine. That morphine is then acted on by liver enzymes that attach sugar molecules to it in two different ways. One such attachment inactivates the morphine, but the other (which also happens in the brain) makes it even more potent. So here we have one process that converts a pro-drug to an active drug, another that destroys the drug's biological activity, and a third that enhances its psychoactive effect. To make matters even more complicated, people differ in the proportions and activities of these three processes.

Cocaine is destroyed very fast—within minutes—both in blood and liver, by enzymes that cleave the molecule into two inert halves.

A major attraction of smoked "crack" cocaine is economic; by moving so rapidly and without dilution from lungs to brain, much of the cocaine escapes destruction by these enzymes, and thus each brain spike requires less cocaine than would be needed by the intravenous route.

In general, because people differ from one another in these complex patterns of metabolism, they differ widely in their sensitivity to any given drug, and therefore in the necessary dosage of that drug. The dose of any psychoactive drug is whatever is necessary to establish an effective concentration in the brain. That will depend on the affinity of the particular drug for its receptors, on the efficiency of signal transduction in the person's neurons, and also on drug metabolism and distribution. All these differ greatly among people, for both genetic and environmental reasons. Average doses at first use vary widely among different drugs. We express dosage in grams, milligrams, and micrograms; a gram is one twenty-eighth of an ounce, a milligram is one thousandth of a gram, and a microgram is one thousandth of a milligram. An average psychoactive dose of heroin or morphine, injected directly into a vein, is between 2 and 10 milligrams; of nicotine, a fraction of a milligram; of cocaine or amphetamine, about 20 milligrams; of LSD, about 20 micrograms; of caffeine, about 150 milligrams. Alcohol is least potent of all. About 10 grams by mouth is required; that is one-third of an ounce of 200-proof pure alcohol, whether taken undiluted or as beer or wine.

A psychoactive drug takes effect as soon as enough of it reaches the brain, where it acts on its receptors. The hedonic effect wears off as the drug concentration there declines. How long a single dose lasts is different for each drug and for each user, depending on how fast the drug is removed from the blood by the metabolic processes and by excretion in the urine, and how fast the brain adapts. As the drug level—whether spike or plateau—falls in the blood bathing the brain, the drug concentration at the receptors eventually drops below an effective level, the drug leaves the receptors and is carried away in the blood, and the psychoactive effects wear off.

Tolerance and Sensitization

With most addictive drugs, repeated administration over a long time, on a regular closely spaced schedule, leads to a loss of effect, so that more and more is needed to produce the same "high" as before.

That is the definition of tolerance. It reflects the neurochemical adaptations in the seesaw analogy. Addicts who have become tolerant to some drugs may have to self-administer many times their original dosage in order to get the same "high" as before, sometimes even a dose that would have been lethal at the outset.

With some drugs (especially psychostimulants like cocaine and amphetamines), certain patterns of repetition can lead to sensitization. This is a state in which the drug effect is enhanced rather than reduced. It is typical of what happens with binge administration of cocaine. (A binge is a rapidly repeating sequence of drug-taking.) Nevertheless, regular and continuous administration of cocaine leads to tolerance, as with other addictive drugs. We still understand sensitization poorly—and no more will be said about it here— whereas the classic seesaw description of tolerance is supported by many years of research results.

Metabolic tolerance means that the body (primarily the liver) adapts to a drug by developing an increased capacity to destroy it. Thus, each repetition of the initial dose provides less and less drug for shorter and shorter times at the sites of action in the brain; so progressively higher doses are needed to produce the desired effect. Metabolic tolerance develops if a drug causes increased production of the very enzyme that destroys it. A familiar example is pentobarbital, a short-acting barbiturate that was once widely prescribed as a sleeping pill. An initial dose sufficient to cause sleep remains in the blood for a few hours, but with repeated dosage the drug is destroyed more and more rapidly and thus becomes less effective.

Cellular tolerance results from changes within the brain itself. The neurons adapt to the drug, becoming less sensitive to it with continued exposure. Even at the moment the first dose wears off, repeating that same dose may produce a somewhat smaller effect than before; the dosage will have to be increased to obtain the full original intensity of drug action again. This pharmacological need contributes to the reckless compulsion that drives the addict's drug-seeking behavior. As the neurons continue to adapt to higher and higher drug doses, their function remains seemingly normal although they are bathed in the drug. The seesaw stays in balance. In this state, when the hedonic effect of a dose has just worn off, a considerable drug concentration remains—enough to have caused an extreme behavioral effect originally. The apparent normality of brain function masks the underlying neurochemical adaptation that only becomes manifest if the drug is withdrawn. The brain has become dependent on the drug, as explained later.

If naloxone is given just before every dose of an opiate, in order to prevent all the opiate effects, neither tolerance nor dependence will develop. Thus, the mere presence of an addictive drug is not sufficient for the development of tolerance and dependence; the drug must activate its receptors and produce its psychoactive effects. The seesaw model incorporates this fact—that the brain's adaptive mechanisms do not attack or block the drug directly, but rather in some manner oppose the drug's effects.

The development of cellular tolerance has a time course all its own, one that can be studied experimentally. For many drugs, there is a critical interval between doses—the shortest time that must elapse before repetition of the same dose will produce the same effect as the one before. With any shorter interval, tolerance (and dependence) will build up, so that successive doses have to be increased in order to obtain the original drug effect. The critical interval for heroin in humans can be recognized by the typical experience of novice users. They inject it into a vein and experience the "high." A week or two later they take another "fix" and again get the desired effect. If they continue using heroin at an interval of a week or so, the dose requirement does not escalate, and some people manage to control their use in this manner for months or even years. Most, however, once they have started, are unable to resist the temptation to experience the heroin "high" more often, and they start to use it more frequently. When the interval becomes shorter than a day or two, the dosage begins to be less effective. With use several times a day, the required dosage escalates sharply.

Years ago, before the development of modern ethical standards for human experiments, a study was conducted with ex-addict volunteers monitored closely in a locked hospital ward. When heroin or morphine was made freely available for self-administration, the maximum permissible doses were eventually taken—amounts that greatly exceeded what would have been an effective dose at the outset. In one famous instance a subject escalated his dose of morphine to ten thousand times what was initially effective—and still demanded more. In other experiments with heroin in human volunteers, it was found that allowing frequent access and dosage escalation ad lib did not satisfy the addicts' desire for heroin. On the contrary, it became increasingly difficult for them to obtain rewarding effects comparable to those produced by the initial lower dosages. Eventually a negative mood state developed, with increasing irritability, hostility, and paranoia. A similar picture is seen with escalating dosages of cocaine or amphetamines. These observations argue strongly against the simplistic notion, sometimes advanced, that if only we let addicts have all the heroin or cocaine they want, the problems associated with their addiction would be solved.

Cocaine has a shorter duration of action than heroin (measured in minutes instead of hours), and also a much shorter critical interval, so that the need for higher dosage develops very quickly, even during a single "run" of cocaine use. During a typical cocaine binge—and despite sensitization—the addict injects (or smokes) again and again, increasing the dosage, until the entire supply of drug is exhausted.

The ultimate degree of tolerance that can develop is different for each drug and also probably varies among users. Opiates represent one extreme: there seems to be virtually no ceiling on tolerance. With nicotine addicts, on the other hand, tolerance seems to have a ceiling; they rarely smoke more than three packs of cigarettes daily. This produces, in their blood and brain, nicotine spikes about ten times the nontolerant level—a nicotine concentration that would be lethal to the nonsmoker. Likewise, when tolerance develops to alcohol, quite large amounts may be consumed every day, but the amount taken at a single sitting (binge) is rarely more than four or five times the initially effective dosage. Caffeine intake by tolerant coffee drinkers may be as great as 10–20 times the usual single dose (one cup of coffee) in the course of a day.

Tolerance makes life difficult, especially for heroin and cocaine addicts, because as their dosage escalates, expenditures for the drug become ever more difficult to afford. Ordinary legitimate sources of income soon prove insufficient for all but the wealthiest addicts; then robbery, burglary, theft, embezzlement, other property crimes, and prostitution are seen as practical ways to obtain the necessary wherewithal. In addition, the danger of overdose becomes greater if the addict who has become accustomed to large doses of an impure street drug gains sudden access to a product of greater (but unknown) purity. As described fully in chapter 18, remarkably large doses of heroin are given to addicts in a large Swiss government program and also in Britain. Dosages 100 times the ordinary psychoactive dose of heroin (as used in Britain for analgesia) are used routinely in these highly tolerant addicts, protecting them from any effects of the much lower heroin doses they may acquire on the street. The same principle is standard practice in methadone maintenance programs (chapter 10).

Thus, tolerance is very important because of the problems it creates for the untreated addict and for society. However, from the standpoint of understanding the neurobiology of addiction, tolerance may not be fundamental; it is not a cause of addiction but a consequence of addiction. To be addictive, a psychoactive drug must be reinforcing, must stimulate a reward system in the brain; but it need not necessarily lead to tolerance. Finally, one might well ask: If addicts get into trouble because of the dosage escalation, why don't they just stop using the drug and let the tolerance (which is fully reversible) dissipate? We do not have a complete answer, but dependence undoubtedly plays a role in perpetuating an addiction.

Dependence

Accompanying tolerance, a state develops in which stopping the drug suddenly ("cold turkey") causes a withdrawal sickness, which is dramatically relieved by another dose of the same drug. That state is called dependence. If all the drug is suddenly removed—faster than the brain can de-adapt—the abrupt unmasking of the adaptation is manifested as a withdrawal syndrome. In the seesaw analogy, "cold turkey" causes the weight of all the adaptive mechanisms to tilt that side down when weight is suddenly removed from the drug side of the balanced seesaw.

The seesaw model describes the fact that the onset and termination of drug action are rapid compared with the much slower adaptation and de-adaptation. Furthermore, the model predicts that the signs and symptoms of withdrawal should be opposite to those of the drug itself; and this is in large measure true. Withdrawal from stimulants like cocaine and amphetamines causes depression, probably because of dopamine depletion due to repeated overstimulation. Withdrawal from depressant drugs like opiates or alcohol causes excitation. Loss of sensitivity to endogenous opioids could contribute to the severe aversive (unpleasant, dysphoric) reactions experienced during opiate withdrawal. In the intestine, for instance, where endogenous opioids normally inhibit bowel movement, and morphine causes constipation, diarrhea is a prominent effect of morphine withdrawal.

Dependence (originally called physical dependence) is not a drug effect in the usual sense, for it can only be observed in the absence of the drug that caused it. Only when repeated drug administration is suddenly stopped do brain disorders ensue, known collectively as a withdrawal syndrome (also called abstinence syndrome).

Remarkably, despite their dramatic features, the withdrawal syndromes seen after chronic use of opiates or alcohol were only first recognized as such during the 1930s and subsequent decades. Before that, physicians and law-enforcement personnel believed that the vociferous complaints of opiate addicts deprived of their drug were merely manipulative behaviors designed to secure an opiate. And many physicians thought that the alcohol withdrawal syndrome (especially delirium tremens) was actually due to a persistent direct toxic action of alcohol itself on the brain. The confusion was finally clarified by controlled clinical studies with human subjects.

In the 1930s, at the U.S. Public Health Service hospital for addicts at Lexington, Kentucky, C. K. Himmelsbach and his colleagues demonstrated unequivocally that the opiate withdrawal syndrome—nausea, vomiting, sweating, gooseflesh, diarrhea, tremor, chills, and fever—was caused predictably by discontinuing morphine administration in a person who had been maintained on a regular schedule of morphine injections with escalating dosage. The prime necessity in studying anything scientifically is to be able to make measurements—if at all possible—and collect the quantitative data needed to analyze what happens when this or that circumstance is changed. Himmelsbach's contribution was to develop a method of scoring the intensity of the withdrawal syndrome, placing emphasis on easily recognized objective disturbances of physiology rather than on subjective complaints. At the same time, he trained medical personnel in using the method, so that consistent results could be obtained. With the Himmelsbach scale one could accurately chart how long it took for the withdrawal disturbances to develop after the last dose of morphine (about 48 hours) and how long it took them to dissipate (about 10 days). The scores also showed that the intensity of withdrawal was directly related to the prior daily morphine dosage.

Proof that the alcohol withdrawal syndrome was due to discontinuing alcohol rather than to a toxic effect of alcohol itself was accomplished by the same group of medical scientists. Alcohol withdrawal, as was first recognized in these experiments, is much more severe and dangerous (potentially fatal) than that due to opiate withdrawal (rarely fatal). When alcohol leaves the body after a period of high intake, a state of agitation develops, with severe tremor, sometimes leading to major seizures like those of epilepsy. In some people, bizarre psychiatric disturbances also occur during alcohol with drawal, including vivid and lurid hallucinations (delirium tremens, "the D.T.s").

Proof that the dramatic opiate and alcohol withdrawal syndromes were consequences of drug dependence led to confusion about the psychoactive drugs that did not produce such an obvious constellation of physiologic abnormalities when withdrawn. Thus, it was long held that cocaine is not addictive, because stopping its use does not produce a withdrawal syndrome of the opiate or alcohol type. We know now, however, that cocaine is intensely addictive, in that an overpowering compulsion develops for the addict to continue using it. And not surprisingly, there is—after all—a cocaine withdrawal syndrome; it is manifested primarily by psychologic disturbances such as severe fatigue and even suicidal depression. Early doubts about the addictiveness of caffeine, nicotine, and marijuana had the same origin; with each of these drugs (as described in later chapters), sudden withdrawal mainly affects mental functions and mood state rather than causing gross abnormalities of physiology in the body's organ systems.

Each drug has its own characteristic rate of development of dependence, determined by how fast the brain brings into play the mechanisms that counteract the drug effect. Once the dependent state has been established, stopping the drug will lead to a gradual onset of the withdrawal syndrome, depending on how quickly the drug leaves the body and how quickly the brain de-adapts.

Researchers can study opiate dependence easily in laboratory animals because the opiate withdrawal syndrome can be brought on quickly and intensely (precipitated withdrawal) by the opioid antagonist naloxone, which abruptly abolishes all the effects of opioid agonists on their receptors. This is equivalent to removing everything at one swoop from the drug side of the seesaw. Mice in precipitated withdrawal jump in a bizarre manner reminiscent of popcorn. The "popcorn jumping" can be scored (how many in a group jump, how frequently they jump) in order to establish quantitatively how drug dosage and dosing interval determine the intensity of dependence and withdrawal. The greater the dependence on an opiate (as from higher dosages or more frequent injections), the easier it is to precipitate withdrawal with naloxone—in other words, the lower the naloxone dose that is needed.

Using this standard procedure, we measured the average dose of naloxone required to make a group of mice jump. If mice were not exposed to an opiate, even a very large dose of naloxone did not provoke jumping. The very first dose of an opiate produced a small but measurable degree of dependence, indicated by the fact that a large dose of naloxone could now make the mice jump. Testing a few animals at a time with fairly large doses of naloxone, hour by hour after a single injection of an opiate, we found that jumping behavior developed, reached a maximum after about 8 hours, and had disappeared entirely in 16 hours. This indicated that the mouse brain adapted to the opiate in about eight hours (balancing the seesaw), then de-adapted in another eight. We predicted that repeated opiate injections within the eight-hour critical interval would lead to a buildup of dependence, because the previous brain adaptation would not have had a chance to wear off. That is exactly what happened; the dependence became increasingly severe (smaller doses of naloxone sufficed to precipitate jumping), the shorter the interval; and this process paralleled the development of tolerance (as described above).

In people who are not users of opiates, as in normal animals, naloxone is virtually without effect. Therefore, naloxone can be used as a diagnostic test for opiate dependence in addicts. A tiny dose, administered with care, precipitates a very mild set of incipient withdrawal signs, revealing the opiate-dependent state.

Accompanying every withdrawal syndrome is an intense craving for the drug that was withdrawn. The opiate withdrawal syndrome can be terminated instantly by an injection of opiate. The alcohol withdrawal syndrome can be terminated by a drink or by sedative hypnotic drugs like benzodiazepines or barbiturates, which act like alcohol. The seemingly magical ability of an addictive drug to relieve its own withdrawal syndrome makes it hard for addicts to abstain; they know that the drug will bring immediate relief. With alcohol, a "hangover" is the beginning of a withdrawal syndrome, and alcohol addicts know that the easiest way to suppress it is to take "a hair of the dog that bit you"—namely, another drink. Early-morning headache is the first sign of caffeine withdrawal, and caffeine addicts know how to cure it with that first morning cup of coffee. Nicotine addicts typically awake in the morning in withdrawal, and light the first cigarette of the day as soon as they can.

Brain Mechanisms of Adaptation

Dependence, like tolerance, is a consequence of addiction, but it also drives the addiction. Even a single dose of an addictive drug produces a tiny amount of dependence, so that during the critical interval after an initial dose there is evidently a mild and subtle but real withdrawal syndrome. In my experiments, I only demonstrated this with opiates in mice; but it is probably true of other addictive drugs, and also in people. The incipient disequilibrium in the brain, as a single dose wears off, could produce just enough discomfort to motivate the user to repeat the dose. If we understood fully the brain's biochemical, cellular, and molecular adaptations in tolerance and dependence, and if we could then develop pharmacological means of preventing them, we might be able to reduce the tendency for one dose to lead to another.

Unfortunately, the present state of knowledge concerning the brain chemistry underlying tolerance and dependence is rather confusing. Numerous biochemical changes have been demonstrated in specific brain regions (like the nucleus accumbens) of rats made tolerant and dependent with morphine or cocaine. These include, for example, alterations in the way phosphate groups are added to certain proteins—a mechanism for making enzymes and receptors more or less active. Changes also occur in other systems (like the G-protein mechanism described in chapter 3), through which the drugs act. Finally, opiates switch on or off the transcription (the copying of a gene into mRNA) of certain genes—again, in some brain regions but not others. During withdrawal from opiates, most of these biochemical effects are reversed; but much research interest attaches to the question whether some of the changes may be irreversible. All these diverse modifications of brain chemistry are interesting and significant; but a coherent picture has not yet emerged to explain fully—for any addictive drug—either the immediate rewarding effects (the "high") or the long-term tolerance and dependence.

What kinds of neurochemical change could account for the adaptation that underlies the state of dependence? We do not yet have a complete answer, but we have partial answers.

There are well-known mechanisms for regulating the number of receptors according to need. If a hormone or neurotransmitter is present in excess, the brain may turn off production of the relevant receptor by shutting down transcription of the receptor gene. Then, fewer receptors means reduced sensitivity to a drug—in other words, tolerance. Fewer receptors also means dependence, because when the drug is suddenly withdrawn, an abnormal state of receptor deficiency will be unmasked. Another biological mechanism for reducing the number of receptors is to stop their transport from inside the cell, where they are made, to the cell membrane in the synapse where they normally function.

The production and release of neurotransmitters are also regulated precisely in order to ensure normal brain function under changing conditions. Artificial continuous activation of receptors, as by repeated administration of an agonist drug, would have the same significance for the regulatory systems as a grossly excessive release of endogenous ligands. The brain would "think" too much ligand was present, and in response would suppress production. When the drug is withdrawn, the unmasked neurotransmitter deficiency would then be functionally equivalent to a receptor deficiency. This mechanism is illustrated by the dopamine deficiency that results when cocaine or amphetamine (which raise dopamine levels) is withdrawn.

Even without any change in the receptors or neurotransmitters, the signal transduction mechanisms could undergo an adaptive change. It will be recalled from chapter 3 that signal transduction is the process that mediates the biochemical events inside a neuron when an agonist binds to a receptor. On repeated opiate administration, the G-protein that is coupled to the receptors and mediates their biologic action becomes less efficient, making the receptor less sensitive (i.e., tolerant) to endogenous as well as administered opioid agonists. Again, the result would be functionally equivalent to a receptor deficiency.

Finally, we have to acknowledge our profound ignorance of the brain mechanisms that drive relapse. Even after prolonged abstinence, an ex-addict may inexplicably revert to drug use. This behavior is often accompanied by conscious craving, so that the craving seems to drive the relapse; but a cause-and-effect relationship has not been proved conclusively. One can even imagine that conscious craving is simply a state that accompanies an independent and automatic unconscious compulsion, which is directly provoked by stored memories of hedonic satisfaction. In experiments with former cocaine addicts, craving has been provoked by conditioned cues— for example, video scenes associated with former drug use. Brain imaging reveals that specific areas known to process emotional memories "light up" with such provoked craving.

That conditioned cues provoke relapse after a period of abstinence has been shown in rats as well as in people. Very recently, what seems to be the neurochemical basis of relapse has been demonstrated in rats. The animals were allowed to self-administer cocaine by pressing a lever, as described in chapter 4. An associated signal, such as a light or tone, tells the animal that the lever is active, that pressing it always provides cocaine intravenously. After this association is well established, cocaine is no longer delivered, and the conditioned behavior (i.e., pressing the lever) is extinguished. Then, as long as eight days later, the signal alone not only causes relapse to lever pressing (no cocaine reward) but remarkably, caused a massive release of dopamine from neurons at both the nucleus accumbens and the amygdala (see chapter 4).

Summary

The important differences between spiking drug levels and plateau drug levels in the brain have been discussed, and how drug metabolism and the route of administration influence the addictive process for each drug.

Although I have spoken frequently here about opiates (chiefly because we know so much about them), many of the same considerations apply to all the addictive drugs. The possible kinds of adaptive change described here have been demonstrated experimentally in one system or another, with one addictive drug or another, yielding a confusing abundance of results. We can say that many biochemical changes do occur in response to drug administration. Some of these are immediate, presumably related to the drug "high," and possibly also reflecting the early changes that lead to tolerance, sensitization, and dependence. For each addictive drug it will be necessary to learn much more about which specific changes account most satisfactorily for the observed acute and chronic behavioral effects. At the moment we seem to have a surfeit of data coupled to a deficit of understanding; but future research will surely change that.

A major problem in addictions is the tendency of abstinent ex-addicts to relapse. One can make the case that relapse is the single most important issue in addiction. We can easily detoxify addicts—routinely, humanely, and effectively—and bring them to a state of abstinence. Therefore, if we had a way to prevent relapse, the addiction problem would largely be solved. The difficulty is that we still know almost nothing about the brain mechanisms that drive relapse, except for the obvious inference that memory—conscious or unconscious—plays a role. Making a formerly rewarding drug aversive seems, in principle, to be a useful approach to preventing relapse; but putting that principle into practice has not been highly successful (see chapter 9).

7

Are Addicts Born
or Made?

Of all the people who try an addictive drug, some will never use it again; they just don't like it. Some are willing to use it occasionally, to enjoy it socially with friends; but it is not important to them and they can happily do without it. Some become regular users and integrate the drug into their lives, but nevertheless are able to give it up without much trouble if they decide to. Finally, there are those who use a drug frequently and regularly and find themselves unable to quit, or at least can quit only with the greatest difficulty, and even then are likely to relapse. This last group—the addicts—represents the greatest problem for society and the greatest challenge for medical science.

Who Is Vulnerable to Addiction?

The same pattern of vulnerability applies to all the addictive drugs. Consider caffeine. Except for a small group who abstain on religious grounds, almost everyone, even in childhood, uses this drug—primarily in coffee, tea, and soft drinks. Studies on caffeine consumption in children reveal the classic pattern. Some kids don't like it and don't use it. Many drink caffeinated beverages in moderation.

A few have a very heavy intake, and these few experience unpleasant symptoms (withdrawal effects) if they quit abruptly.

Or consider alcohol. Some people just don't like this drug, especially the light-headed dizziness and loss of control it produces, and they abstain or limit their intake to an occasional sip for sociability or as part of a ceremonial ritual. Many people drink regularly—one or two drinks daily—and have no problem; indeed, there may even be health benefits in moderate drinking. But for some, alcohol takes over their lives and their decision-making powers. These alcohol addicts appear to be slaves to the drug; they have great difficulty quitting or cutting down, even though the effects on their mental and physical health are obvious. And once abstinent, they tend to relapse.

The pattern described here has nothing to do with whether a drug is legal or illicit, but illicit drugs (especially marijuana, heroin, and cocaine) are special in two ways. First, a person's willingness to try and then go on using an illicit drug depends very much on their life circumstances, alternative sources of pleasure and satisfaction, attitude toward the law and society, and whether they like to take risks. Second, the consequences of being addicted are much more devastating if obtaining and using a drug entails criminal activity.

Whichever drug we consider, who becomes an addict? Might some people have it in their nature—be especially vulnerable—to becoming addicted? And if that were so, would a person's vulnerability be restricted to a single addictive drug or would it apply to addictive drugs as a class? Data are still sparse, while speculation is abundant; but new epidemiological and molecular genetic approaches are yielding solid information. Genetic predisposition is emerging as a serious research topic in our attempt to understand drug addiction.

Addiction as Self-medication?

Much that is said about a possible genetic basis of vulnerability to addiction is pure speculation. But as we are concerned here with neurotransmitters and receptors in the human brain, making actual measurements presents great difficulty. Nevertheless, scientists have begun to tackle the problem with promising new methods such as brain imaging and actual studies of candidate genes in connection with the Human Genome Project. Some of these exciting new developments are described later in this chapter.

First, some speculation. Might some addicts have a defective reward system for which they try to compensate by using drugs that stimulate that system? Our genes determine the structure, production, and regulation of every protein in our bodies, and therefore, a gene defect (a mutation) can result in an abnormal or missing protein. Thus, mutated genes could be responsible for defective production or regulation of those hormones, neurotransmitters, and receptors that are essential for reward, pleasure, and satisfaction.

Think of the days before 1889, when the role of the pancreas and of insulin deficiency in juvenile diabetes had not yet been discovered. A young person with diabetes would be ill, and medicine could offer a diagnosis but no remedy. Now imagine a "pusher" offering an illicit drug for injection, prepared from pig pancreas and (as we now know) containing insulin. Most people, if persuaded to try this substance, would experience a drastic fall in their blood sugar; they would feel dizzy and weak after an injection and would refuse to try it again. But diabetic youngsters would feel right and normal for the first time; thereafter they would pay any price, take any risk, for the opportunity to secure and inject that substance. This youth would surely become "addicted." Fanciful as this allegory may be, it reminds us that once a condition has been diagnosed as a medical one, lifetime dependence on a therapeutic drug is not stigmatized as an addiction.

Suppose, for the sake of argument, that some people are born with a deficient reward system. They might be unable to achieve normal satisfactions from social interactions and other pleasant life pursuits. Unlike a person with sickle cell anemia or cystic fibrosis, who would have been diagnosed as suffering from a known genetic disease, they and their families and friends would be unaware of the genetic deficit. They might display emotional flatness, have difficulty in social relationships, lack enthusiasm for anything—a classic picture of depression. Then, one day during adolescence, an acquaintance offers some heroin. Suddenly a feeling of normalcy would be experienced: "Now for the first time I feel the way a person should feel. Now I realize what I have been missing all my life."

I have asked many heroin addicts to recall their first experience with heroin. All of them say it was pleasurable; many also say it made them feel "right" for the first time. Unfortunately, this kind of fuzzy information based on romanticized memory, self-justification, and a desire to tell what the doctor wants to hear is neither dependable nor decisive; we can hardly take it seriously as an argument for genetic predisposition.

Genes and Environment

The idea that vulnerability to drug addiction can be inherited has been widely misunderstood. It is obvious—indeed it is a trivial statement—that if a drug were totally unavailable, no one could become addicted to it, regardless of their heredity. In that sense, drug addiction differs from clearcut genetic diseases that do not depend on external factors. The position may be closer to that of diseases with strong hereditary influences like the common kinds of heart disease, or like cancers of the breast or colon, in which environmental factors play a major role.

The strong influence of environmental factors is nowhere more obvious than in nicotine addiction. Forty-five years ago, a large majority of young Americans began smoking as they entered adolescence, but today only a small minority (around one-fifth) become smokers. Moreover, of all the people who ever smoked, two-thirds have been able to quit. Obviously the genes have not changed in 45 years; the change must be due to other factors such as intensive education about the health consequences of smoking. Unlike the genes, these other factors can be modified to reduce addictive behaviors—by prevention education and by laws restricting where and when smoking is allowed. Despite such efforts, however, one-third who ever smoked have been unable to quit. These are the hard-core addicts, who go on smoking despite full knowledge of the harm to their health. And if they do manage to quit, they tend to relapse—again and again.

Societal attitudes are important in determining the likelihood of a young person's starting to smoke cigarettes. Among a circle of friends we call this peer pressure; in the wider society it may be described as social custom or social acceptability. As an addiction becomes less popular, it becomes less acceptable. This sounds like a meaningless tautology but it expresses an important fact—that a positive feedback operates. As information about the health dangers of smoking takes hold, fewer people smoke; and as fewer people smoke, the attitudinal change is reinforced throughout society. Restrictions on smoking become increasingly acceptable and more willingly complied with. For some people, none of this matters because they have always observed total abstinence, either on religious grounds (for example, Mormons) or because of strong family tradition. Such people never become addicted, regardless of the drug or of their genetic makeup. At the other extreme are a minority who reject the societal consensus and violate the prohibitions, whatever the drug; some of that group become addicted, and they constitute a persistent problem.

Socioeconomic class influences social acceptability of addictive behavior because people are generally more influenced by what their own group does than by the wider culture. Thus, the decline in smoking has been much greater in affluent middle-class circles than in blue-collar society, probably reflecting a difference in educational level as well as in self-confidence about being able to change the circumstances of one's own life. Very likely this class difference in smoking behavior will disappear with time, but change in societal norms is typically slow.

The tobacco industry argues that their advertising is not intended to recruit smokers, but only to promote one brand over another. Regardless of what is intended, however, advertising unquestionably contributes to the climate of social acceptance of this lethal addiction. That is especially important when athlete heroes and popular music groups—role models for so many young people—are deliberately associated with cigarettes in advertising and product promotions.

The same environmental influences and the same social patterns apply to illicit drugs, except that the relative importance of the various factors is different. The Vietnam experience sheds light on how social acceptance by a peer group, coupled with easy availability, can influence drug use. American young men were wrenched from their families and home environment. Placed in a situation that was alternately terrifying and boring, with cheap heroin of high purity readily available, they used it in remarkable numbers. At the height of the epidemic, some 15 percent of U.S. ground forces were actually using enough heroin to have become dependent on it. However, follow-up studies have shown that the great majority of them, after returning home, put their heroin use behind them and did not seek it out again.

In civilian life, on the other hand, to use an illicit drug in the first place requires a decisive rejection of societal standards. Experts believe that a rather special psychologic temperament often plays a role, described sometimes by psychiatrists as "antisocial personality disorder." One kind of addict is a risk-taker, a sensation seeker, a nonconformist, and readily influenced by nonconforming peers. But again we see, as with the legal drugs, that of all those who have this predisposing psychological makeup and actually do try an illicit drug, only a small fraction become addicts. Does genetic predisposition also play a role, then, in determining who will belong to that small fraction?

Some would deny a role for genetics, arguing that only psychological factors are operative. But this only begs the question, because genetic factors contribute strongly to psychological makeup—personality, responses to stress, rational thinking, decision making, and other patterns of behavior. Thus, a genetic predisposition to a drug addiction might be caused by changes in genes that are responsible for the production and regulation of the neurotransmitters and receptors in brain that influence those personality characteristics. Among these could be abnormalities in a reward pathway, causing a functional deficit in the feelings that are normally associated with pleasure and satisfaction. The abnormal state would be present before the individual is ever exposed to a drug. Interestingly, the simultaneous presence (comorbidity) of a mental illness (often major depression) is seen in about half of all who are dependent on an addictive drug.

Unfortunately, detailed information about the psychological status of addicts is rarely available before they become addicted. Therefore, after they are addicted there is no way to determine whether abnormal psychological traits are consequences of chronic drug use, or whether they predated the first exposure to the drug. To gain such understanding, it is necessary to study children, and then years later to assess their drug use in adulthood. In one such investigation the personality and behavioral traits of several hundred Swedish 11-year-olds were recorded. Then the same subjects were evaluated 16 years later, to see which had become alcoholics. Children who displayed character traits of impulsivity, novelty-seeking, and readiness to take risks were far more likely than their classmates to use alcohol excessively as adults. Similar long-term studies in the United States have suggested that attention disorders and aggressive behavior, manifested as early as first grade, may be associated with addictive drug use at later ages, especially among males.

Not genes alone, then, nor environment alone, but the interactions of environmental with genetic factors are keys to understanding predisposition to addiction.

Genetics of Predisposition to Addiction in Animals

Addiction is a behavior. Anyone who doubts that genes can control behavior has only to look at dogs. More than 100,000 years ago, some wolves with a particular genetic makeup found it useful to attach themselves to human habitations. Those animals with the characteristics we value in modern dogs—friendliness, loyalty, protective instinct, and so on—were bred selectively. What is of greatest interest is how modern breeds differ in their instinctive behaviors—behaviors that are determined entirely by the genes. A nice illustration in my own family is Rudy, an Australian Shepherd. This animal never saw a sheep or a cow, and his mother never taught him how to herd. Yet when our family goes for a walk, Rudy herds us as though we were sheep or cattle. He tries to bring a straying grandchild back to the group. He becomes agitated if someone is missing, as though he keeps count of the members of our family, for whom he feels responsible. Similar genetically determined behavior is familiar to all dog owners, each different breed doing what its genes prescribe and have been selected for over many dog generations—shepherds, terriers, bloodhounds, retrievers, sled dogs, lap dogs, guard dogs, and so on.

Of course, addiction cannot be determined exclusively by genes in the same manner as instinctive behaviors; an addictive drug has to be available. Given that availability, however, and the cultural milieu in which initial use is acceptable, a person might then use the drug or avoid it, and that choice could be influenced strongly by genetic factors. That is what we mean when we speak of predisposition (or vulnerability) to addiction. In animal experiments we can study predisposition in a more rigorous manner than is possible with humans. By selective breeding, scientists have obtained strains of laboratory animals that will choose to take an addictive drug, and others that will avoid that same drug. Mice, for instance, can be offered a free choice of water bottles, one of which contains a drug. By repeatedly selecting and inbreeding animals that prefer a drug and others that avoid the drug, high-preferring and low-preferring lines have been obtained. This inbreeding has been done successfully with rats as well as mice, and with several addictive drugs, showing that genetic factors are, indeed, able to influence the predisposition to use a drug.

Numerous studies have shown that genes influence sensitivity to the effects of drugs, and much effort has been devoted to understanding the neural and molecular mechanisms. This research is certainly interesting, but most of the effects of any drug are on pathways in the brain that have nothing to do with addiction. For example, alcohol makes mice (like humans) lose their balance and even become unconscious, seeming to be asleep. Selective breeding has produced "long-sleep" and "short-sleep" strains, proving that sensitivity to this alcohol effect is genetically controlled. There is even evidence that certain brain receptors, upon which alcohol is known to act, are more resistant to alcohol in short-sleep than in long-sleep mice. But such effects of an addictive drug may have nothing to do with an animal's tendency to self-administer that drug and become addicted. From the standpoint of addictive behavior, most actions of a drug in the brain should be thought of as side effects not germane to the hedonic reinforcing action that drives addiction. Therefore, vulnerability to addiction must be studied directly by the self-administration or place conditioning techniques described in chapter 4.

Genetics of Predisposition to Addiction in Humans

The pioneering studies on predisposition to addiction in humans dealt with alcohol. The data were from identical and fraternal (nonidentical) twins. Identical twins have identical genes; fraternal twins share only half their genes, like any siblings. For any disease, if environment has no influence, identical twins will be concordant (alike) with respect to that disease; both twins of a pair will have it or neither twin will have it. To the extent that environmental factors contribute, the concordance rate among pairs of identical twins will be less than 100 percent. A lower concordance rate among fraternal than among identical twins would reflect the contributions of both genetic and environmental factors. Thus the heritability of a disease can be computed from the differences in concordance rates for sets of fraternal and identical twin pairs. Data from several countries show that identical twins do (or do not) become alcoholics with a significantly higher concordance rate than fraternal twins, suggesting a significant heritability of a predisposition to alcohol addiction. In one large study, for instance, 54 percent of identical twin pairs were concordant but only 28 percent of nonidentical pairs were.

Other studies have revealed a similar difference between identical and fraternal twins with respect to nicotine, cocaine, marijuana, and heroin. The genetic effect is most striking in the progression from moderate use to heavy use and dependence. A striking example: For cocaine dependence, in a recent study of nearly 2,000 twins, concordance was 35 percent for identical twins but zero for fraternal twins. Genetic factors are more important in males than in females. All the studies point to some predispositions that make a person vulnerable to addiction in general, others that are drug-specific.

Unfortunately, this standard twin-pair approach suffers from a serious defect. Identical twins tend to be more alike than fraternal twins in many ways that have nothing to do with genetics. During childhood, their parents tend to dress them alike and treat them alike. Growing up to be alike in many respects, they tend to copy each other's behaviors, and this could also apply to the development of drug likes and dislikes. This problem—that identical twins share many environmental factors to a greater extent than do fraternal twins—plagues all twin studies concerning behavior, making it very difficult to sort out the influences of genetics from those of environment. Therefore, the most persuasive data come from studies of identical twins raised from birth by different families in distant locations.

Convincing evidence comes from cross-adoption studies, not necessarily with twins. Sons of alcoholics adopted at birth and raised in a nonalcoholic family were found to have a fourfold greater probability of becoming alcohol addicts than did their stepbrothers. Conversely, sons of nonalcoholic parents adopted and raised by alcoholic families did not tend to become alcohol addicts, even when their stepbrothers did. This result speaks strongly in favor of some kind of inheritance of a predisposition to alcohol addiction. It also tends to discredit the idea that family environment plays the predominant role in the genesis of alcoholism, although it does not rule out a contributory role for environmental factors.

Direct evidence of inherited differences in a response to alcohol has been sought in various studies with sons of alcoholic fathers.

The subjects, who were young enough not to have developed immoderate drinking habits, were compared with control subjects from nonalcoholic family backgrounds. All subjects were evaluated on standardized paper-and-pencil tests of mental abilities, memory, and vigilance, after being given a placebo and after receiving a low and a high dose of alcohol. On some of the tests, the sons of alcoholic fathers showed significantly less disruption of performance by alcohol than did the matched controls. As none of the subjects had yet become problem drinkers, this insensitivity to alcohol could not be attributed to acquired tolerance, but appeared to be an intrinsic characteristic of the men with alcoholic parentage. Brain wave patterns have also been found, in some studies, to be different and less affected by alcohol in sons of alcoholic fathers. As noted earlier, however, sensitivity or resistance to some effect of alcohol might have nothing to do with vulnerability to alcohol addiction.

Finding the Genes that Predispose to Addiction

Predisposition to a drug addiction is probably never due to a single defective gene. In this respect it differs from the hemoglobin gene in sickle-cell anemia (see below) or the ion-channel gene in cystic fibrosis. Nevertheless, the amazingly rapid advances in gene technology are making it possible to search for predisposing genes even in complex conditions caused by multiple gene defects. The Human Genome Project, which is mapping all the bases of all the nucleotides on all the genes of our 22 pairs of chromosomes and two sex chromosomes (X and Y), is opening the way to understanding vulnerability to each of the drug addictions in molecular genetic terms.

The genotype is the whole set of genes carried by an individual in every cell of the body. The phenotype is what we are—the expression of all our genes. Phenotype includes physical features, mental capacities, and behavior. If we could accurately describe an addictive phenotype (whether in relation to one drug or to many) we might then try to find the responsible genotype. As we shall see, however, there are problems identifying an "addictive phenotype" and problems of a different kind identifying a relevant genotype.

Small differences in DNA sequences (called polymorphisms) occur throughout an animal or human population. One common kind is called a single nucleotide polymorphism (SNP for short) in which mutation of a base at a particular position in the DNA sequence has changed it to another, such as A to G. We humans have a total of about three billion bases in our DNA, encoding 70,000 or more different proteins; and each of us carries a SNP in every few hundred bases.

Most of these SNPs are without consequence for us. Many occur in the large parts of the genome that do not encode any protein. Even a SNP in a coding region of the gene is harmless if the altered DNA encodes the same protein as before, or if the slightly altered protein functions just as well as the original. For example, the same amino acid may be encoded by more than one triplet of bases; AAA and AAG (see chapter 3 for names of bases) both encode the amino acid lysine, so a mutation of A to G in the third position of AAA would have no consequence at all. The same A to G mutation in the second position, yielding AGA, would encode a different amino acid, arginine. But arginine is chemically quite similar to lysine, so the resulting protein might still function well. However, changing AAA to GAA would yield glutamate, which has entirely different chemical properties. Usually—but not necessarily—that kind of change would drastically alter the ability of the protein to function; but in some locations, the effect could be negligibly small. A certain few triplets, instead of encoding an amino acid, signal the machinery to stop making a protein altogether; so a SNP that yields such a "stop co-don" is likely to have a devastating effect. Finally, some polymor-phisms are not SNPs but rather involve deletions or rearrangements of parts of a gene; and these frequently result in major alterations of the gene product.

To understand how a SNP can cause a disease, we can do no better than to consider sickle-cell anemia, the first hereditary disease for which a molecular cause was discovered, by Linus Pauling about 50 years ago. Hemoglobin is made chiefly in the bone marrow, where it is packaged into the red blood cells, which carry oxygen to our tissues. The protein scaffold of the hemoglobin molecule consists of two chains of amino acids called alpha and beta. The gene that encodes the beta chain is on chromosome 11. The sixth amino acid in the beta chain is normally glutamate, encoded as GAG in the DNA. An A-to-T SNP in this triplet yields GTG, encoding the amino acid valine, the properties of which are very different from gluta-mate. As a result, the hemoglobin (now called sickle hemoglobin, hemoglobin S) behaves quite abnormally, forms fibers, and distorts the shape of the red cell. If a person inherits the mutated DNA from two parents (i.e., on both copies of chromosome 11) all their hemoglobin is of the S kind. Then their sickle-shaped red cells clog the smallest blood vessels and are destroyed, causing sickle-cell anemia. People who inherit only one copy of the SNP are carriers; they make enough normal hemoglobin to get by, but they can pass the mutated chromosome to their children.

One method of finding mutations looks for restriction fragment length polymorphisms (RFLPs). Certain enzymes (called restriction enzymes) are used to cut DNA into many fragments, each enzyme operating only at a particular sequence of six or so bases. If that key sequence is altered by a SNP, the enzyme will not cut (Figure 7.1). Consequently, the normal DNA fragment will be cut in two; but if a SNP is present, only the original uncut fragment will be seen. As DNA fragments are easily separated by size, the fragment containing a SNP can be distinguished readily. This method tells us where a mutation is, but it does not identify what base has mutated.

Remarkable new technologies allow us to find and identify SNPs. One method uses a "gene chip." Thousands of DNA fragments that

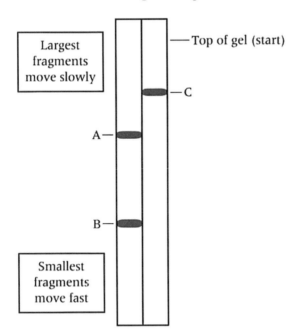

Fig. 7.1: Restriction fragment length polymorphism (RFLP). In this method, DNA fragments are driven downward on a gel slab by an electric current; the smaller the fragment, the faster it runs. Gel at left contains same DNA as at right, but first cleaved by a particular restriction enzyme, as explained in text.

include known SNPs are attached to a surface as a regular matrix of dots. Fragments of a genome to be tested are heated to separate the two strands of the DNA helixes, then added to the chip. Whenever a strand of a genome fragment is exactly complementary to one on the chip (because it includes the same SNP), it will adhere (hybridize) and can be identified. The method is like in situ hybridization, described in chapter 3. If we did this with the genome of a patient with sickle cell anemia, a fragment from his or her chromosome 11 would adhere to the tiny dot containing the known SNP that is responsible for this disease.

Now we can consider the two kinds of problem alluded to earlier—the phenotype problem and the genotype problem. The phenotype problem is this: People who are addicted to a certain drug may differ from one another in the mechanism of their addiction in ways we do not yet understand. In a disease like cystic fibrosis the diagnosis is clear, and seems to depend on a single mutated gene. But mental diseases of various kinds are ambiguous. Schizophrenia, for example, may well be a cluster of different conditions that we have not yet learned to separate diagnostically. Addictive behavior is at least as complex; this means, unfortunately, that not one but several genes may be involved. Behavioral abnormalities, in general, are probably polygenic. Different genes may underlie what seems superficially to be the same condition in different people. And more than one gene may contribute to the condition in a single person. The only possible (though partial) solution to the phenotype problem is more accurate diagnosis; for addictions this means trying to distinguish among addictive behaviors that may seem superficially to be the same.

The genotype problem is this: No two humans (except for identical twins) have exactly the same DNA sequence. As noted above, on average every person has a great number of SNPs and other kinds of mutation in his or her genome. Suppose we are seeking some mutation that might underlie nicotine addiction. Obviously we could try to analyze all the DNA, chromosome by chromosome, gene by gene, in a group of heavily addicted smokers, and compare with the DNA of people in the same environment as the smokers but who never smoked. Unfortunately, the polymorphism(s) associated with nicotine addiction would be swamped by all the many DNA differences between any two groups of people. The signal we are looking for would be lost in the noise.

The solution to the genotype problem is to reduce the noise—to compare addicts with nonaddicts in a population that is as genetically homogeneous as possible. In that comparison, the genetic difference between addicts and nonaddicts should stand out against a low background of random mutations. Fortunately, there are population isolates in many parts of the world—people descended from a very small group of founders—who have intermarried little or not at all with outsiders. A prime example is the population of Iceland, founded in the ninth century, with very little immigration since then. A major effort is being made to exploit this population's special advantage by sequencing the genome of all the country's inhabitants. Another example is provided by the 8,000 residents of the little island of San Pietro off the south coast of Sardinia, descended from a few founders—Genoese fishermen and their wives—in the sixteenth century. The Basques of northern Spain and southern France have been an isolated population since the stone age. Finally, about 1.5 million people living in the central valley of Costa Rica are descended from a small number of sixteenth-century Spanish founders. In this case, a history of admixing with the natives can be recognized, in males, by a distinctive Y chromosome found only in American Indians. The existence of these and other population isolates makes scientists optimistic about finding the genetic sources of complex polygenic diseases, including the drug addictions.

At the present writing, a few genetic traits have been found to be associated with addiction to one drug or another; but the number will surely have grown by the time this book is published. A few examples:

(1) Many people of Chinese or Japanese extraction are made ill by alcohol even in tiny doses (see chapter 9). The face flushes (the so-called "Oriental flush"), a severe headache develops, and other more serious reactions may occur. The cause is a mutation in the gene that encodes the acetaldehyde dehydrogenase enzyme. This enzyme, in its normal form, destroys acetaldehyde, the very toxic substance that is produced by the metabolism of alcohol in the body. The defective enzyme allows acetaldehyde to accumulate whenever alcohol is present, so it is obvious why people carrying the mutant gene would avoid alcohol. Epidemiologic studies show a low prevalence of alcoholism in China and Japan, but there is controversy about how great a protective role is played by the enzyme deficiency. Strong evidence for protection is the fact that only very rarely do

Japanese alcoholics have the altered enzyme, compared with about 50 percent in the Japanese population as a whole; in other words, those with the mutant enzyme avoid alcohol.

(2) A certain SNP in the gene that encodes the mu opioid receptor is more frequent among a group of heroin addicts than among people who never used heroin. This finding is provocative, but it is not obvious why the altered receptor should make a person more vulnerable to heroin addiction.

(3) A certain SNP in the gene encoding a dopamine receptor is more frequent in certain types of alcoholics than in nondrinkers. This finding was at first hailed as demonstrating the molecular basis of alcoholism. However, much controversy soon arose; it appears now that the altered receptor may play a role in various comorbid mental states that are associated with one kind of alcohol addiction.

(4) A SNP in the gene that encodes one of the so-called P-450 enzymes, which is important for metabolizing nicotine, is more frequent among nonsmokers than heavy smokers. Slower metabolism of nicotine results in higher blood and brain levels, thereby—it is postulated—enhancing the initial unpleasant effects of nicotine, so that adolescents carrying this SNP may be deterred from taking up the habit. Moreover, adult smokers with the altered gene actually smoke fewer cigarettes, presumably for the same reason.

In the above and similar cases there is always the need to apply probability theory to make sure that the observed genetic differences between phenotypically characterized groups is not merely a chance association without real significance for addiction. And in each instance, if the SNPs in question are truly related to the addictive phenotype, what is the connection between the altered gene product and the actual neural and molecular mechanisms of the predisposition to addiction?

Summary

The practical significance of modern genetic research on addictive behavior is threefold:

(1) We have learned enough already to suggest that children of alcoholics should be advised never to touch alcohol; certainly they should be taught the special hazards that heavy drinking holds for them—hazards not shared by their peers. The same cautionary advice will be appropriate each time a hereditary component of a drug

addiction is established. Avoiding a drug at the outset is a sure way to avoid becoming addicted!

(2) When genetic techniques have been perfected for determining, person by person, who is especially at risk of addiction to a given drug, prevention efforts can be made more efficient by targeting the most vulnerable individuals.

(3) Every time a defective gene is discovered that contributes to a drug addiction, we are brought closer to understanding the biochemical basis of that addiction. The reason is that identifying a gene leads directly to the protein that is encoded by that gene. This, in turn, opens the way to understanding the role played by that protein in the addiction. As a result, we can come closer to developing novel strategies for rational prevention and treatment.

Part Two

The Drugs and the Addicts

8

Nicotine

As I was driving along the highway, a remarkable billboard advertisement caught my eye. Nearly filling the field was the weather-beaten face of a man in a cowboy hat. Nothing else was on the advertisement. And the only part of the product name that was not blocked by the man's face were two letters—"MC." What a remarkable exploitation of psychologic conditioning! Everyone seeing those two letters and that face could recognize instantly the symbol of MARLBORO COUNTRY.

The same evening, as I read the *Sunday New York Times* magazine section, my eye was caught by a very attractive, well-dressed, sophisticated woman, holding a cigarette delicately between the fingers of her left hand. "Portraits of Pleasure" was the title above the woman's face. Also displayed prominently was the legend "KENT: MORE FLAVOR IN LIGHTS" and the required Surgeon General's warning: "Smoking Causes Lung Cancer, Heart Disease, Emphysema, And May Complicate Pregnancy." How remarkable that this seductive advertisement, directed toward a highly intelligent readership, promotes a lethal product, one that in the United States alone kills over 400,000 people every year.

Although tobacco has been an article of commerce for hundreds of years, it became an addictive substance of major importance only in the last century. From the fifteenth-century importation of tobacco to Europe from America, and until the beginning of the twentieth century, pipes, cigars, snuff, and chewing tobacco were the principal vehicles for nicotine self-administration. Then, several technological advances opened the way to mass popularization of the cigarette. First, a new way of curing tobacco made the smoke less irritating to the air passages, so that deep inhalation became tolerable. Second, mechanization of cigarette production increased productive capacity, supporting a greatly expanded market. Third, the safety match, invented in the middle of the nineteenth century, and first mass-produced in the 1890s, was a necessary prerequisite to the successful spread of the cigarette. Fourth, new techniques of advertising and mass marketing were being perfected, and these were soon applied to this new commodity. Smoking had not been socially acceptable for women, but the women's suffrage movement and the rapidly changing status of women in society doubled the potential market, and females were recruited to cigarettes in vast numbers. With the rapid increase in cigarette smoking in the United States, followed by development of the export market, nicotine addiction became a health problem of worldwide scope.

To understand this historic development and to appreciate its relevance to policies concerning the regulation of other addictive drugs, we need first to understand the nature of nicotine addiction. This chapter discusses what we know about how this drug acts on the brain. It points out how the technique of deep inhalation, which is characteristic of cigarette smoking, changed the character of the addiction, and dramatically altered its health consequences. And finally, I summarize some methods of treating nicotine addiction.

The Fast Track from Lungs to Brain

About one percent of the weight of the tobacco leaf is nicotine. If all the nicotine in a single cigarette were absorbed quickly into the body, it would be very toxic or even lethal. Cigar and pipe smokers typically do not inhale, and nicotine is absorbed through the mucous membranes of their mouths. Cigarette smokers, on the other hand, usually inhale deeply and hold the smoke in their lungs before exhaling.

For any drug to reach the brain by the inhalation route, several key requirements have to be met. The drug must be a gas; or if it is to be smoked, it must be converted to a gas or carried on the smoke particles without being destroyed at high temperature. After inhalation, it must cross the thin partitions that separate the air sacs in the lung from the blood that passes by, so that it can be carried in the blood to the brain. And finally, it must be able to cross out of the capillary network in the brain, and penetrate into brain tissue, in order to reach the neurons that bear the nicotinic acetylcholine receptors.

A familiar medical example of this route of drug delivery is the use of inhalation anesthetics like ether or halothane to put patients to sleep on the operating table. Drugs taken by inhalation act fast because every breath fills the air sacs with a fresh supply, which passes into the blood before that breath is exhaled. A meshwork of fine capillaries surrounds each little air sac. All the blood in the body passes through the lungs—about five quarts every minute. From the lungs, all that blood goes directly to the left side of the heart, and from there, as it is pumped out, a certain portion goes to the brain. Consequently, blood that leaves the lungs arrives in the brain a few seconds later, carrying drug at full strength. The brain is swamped by a new drug spike immediately after each inhalation. After an intravenous injection, in contrast, the blood carrying the drug is first mixed in the right side of the heart with the large amount of drug-free blood returning from the rest of the body, and thus the drug is diluted before it reaches the brain. And after oral administration, absorption is slow, so the drug concentration in the brain builds up slowly.

If a drug is smoked, and its effect on the brain is pleasurable, each puff will produce a spike of immediate satisfaction in an unmistakable cause-and-effect manner (Figure 8.1), reinforcing the smoking behavior according to the classic rules of operant conditioning. In this respect, a smoker drawing on a cigarette is analogous to a rat pressing a lever in the standard self-administration experiments described in chapter 4. To observe this reinforcement in action, you have only to watch a nicotine addict draw smoke deeply into the lungs and hold it there; the instant gratification, as the nicotine spike hits the brain, is obvious in his or her facial expression.

An important feature of the inhalation route is its controllability. Because the drug reaches the brain in small spikes, the smoker can use the hedonic effect itself to regulate the rate of drug intake. For

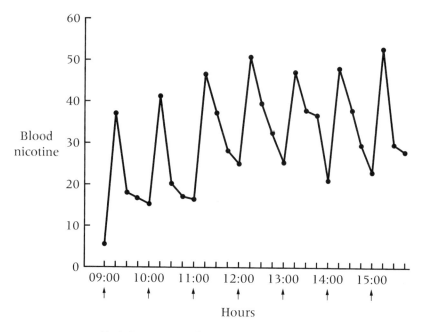

Fig. 8.1: Nicotine in blood after cigarette smoking. Subject smoked one cigarette every hour (arrows), and blood samples were taken every 15 minutes. Nicotine levels are in billionths of a gram per milliliter. (From M. A. H. Russell and C. Feyerabend, *Drug Metabolism Reviews* 8: 29,1978)

more effect, the user takes deeper or more frequent puffs. If a toxic concentration in the brain is being approached, the user (feeling dizzy or nauseated) simply stops smoking or slows down. This contrasts to other routes of administration, where a certain total amount of drug is put irretrievably into a vein, under the skin, or into the stomach. Thus, one great advantage of drug self-administration by inhalation is that dangerous overdoses can be avoided; this route is an especially important safeguard with illicit drugs, of unknown and variable strength, like marijuana, cocaine, or heroin.

Nicotine is metabolized fairly rapidly, disappearing from the body in a few hours. Therefore the addict starts each morning with a very low residual level in blood and brain—in other words, in a state of withdrawal. The first cigarette of the morning has a powerful effect because it brings relief of that withdrawal discomfort. Thereafter, each cigarette produces a sharp spike in the brain nicotine concentration. These spikes are superimposed on a gradual buildup of blood and brain nicotine, as each cigarette adds nicotine to what still remains in the blood and brain from the previous cigarette. By the end of the day, the residual nicotine concentration between cigarettes is quite high, associated with tolerance and dependence. It is interesting—and it raises some questions about nicotine patches (see below)—that the high nicotine level itself does not satisfy the smoker, who continues to enjoy each spike above that level. Then, during the night, the nicotine level drops gradually, and by morning the addict is in withdrawal and in urgent need of a cigarette.

A Low-key "High"

Nicotine passes from the blood into all parts of the brain, but it only acts where it finds high-affinity nicotinic acetylcholine receptors. It will be recalled, from chapter 3, that acetylcholine receptors are ion channels composed of five separate elements surrounding a central pore. Different receptor subtypes are composed of various combinations of these elements, designated by Greek letters and encoded in different genes. We now know which subtype has the highest affinity for nicotine—alpha-4, beta-2. These specific receptors have been located in animal brains by the radioreceptor binding technique, using radioactive nicotine. They are concentrated heavily in just a few brain regions, and PET scans (see chapter 3) show that nicotine stimulates neurons in just the areas of dense nicotine binding to the receptors. Moreover, selective nicotine receptor antagonists block the stimulation of sugar uptake by nicotine, showing that it is, indeed, the binding of nicotine to its receptors on certain neurons that stimulates those neurons. Most interesting, the same results are obtained in imaging experiments with humans. But the devil is in the details; still missing is a complete understanding of just how nicotine causes its hedonic effect. It is clear, however, that—like other addictive drugs—it acts in the mesolimbic reward pathway, causing dopamine release, especially at the nucleus accumbens.

For many years, it proved extraordinarily difficult to induce animals to self-administer nicotine, and this tended to reinforce the incorrect idea that nicotine was not addictive. Actually, the first exposure to nicotine tends to be so aversive that a rat will not readily repeat the lever-press that delivers that first dose. This initial unpleasant quality is well known to smokers, who can recollect vividly how their first cigarette made them ill—the nausea, heart palpitation, weakness, even fainting. Young people, just beginning to smoke, learn to become tolerant to these toxic actions by smoking only a little at first, then increasing their dosage very gradually; and the same method works for getting animals to self-administer nicotine. After a rat has been addicted successfully in that gradual way, the self-administration behavior becomes very persistent. Even after a period of forced abstinence, the animal self-administers eagerly when given the opportunity again, and readily becomes addicted again.

The behavioral effects of nicotine in humans are subtle; indeed, nicotine (and caffeine) cause the least behavioral impairment of all the addictive drugs. As one expert put it: "Nicotine and caffeine are the only addictive drugs about which I can say that it doesn't worry me if my airplane pilot uses them." Without any gross disturbances to measure, animal experiments have not been very helpful in determining the behavioral impact of nicotine. We have to depend on human experimentation, using subjective checklists for an account of what nicotine does to people. But here we encounter a problem. We would like to know about the direct effects of nicotine in smokers; but often, all we can measure are the effects of a small spike added to the nicotine level already in a smoker's blood. If we made volunteer subjects desist from smoking until their nicotine level fell off, and then tested the effect of a cigarette, we would be dealing with dependent addicts in withdrawal. Of course, nicotine will relieve the withdrawal distress, but that will tell us nothing about the initial direct effects of the drug.

Experiments with former smokers who are long past the discomfort of the withdrawal syndrome have confirmed what smokers themselves say about why they smoke. Double-blind comparisons of nicotine-free (or low-nicotine) with high-nicotine cigarettes implicate the psychoactive drug itself as the primary reason people smoke, rather than the oral or visual stimulation of smoking. Nicotine alleviates stress and anxiety, reduces frustration, anger, and aggressive feelings, and promotes a pleasurable state of relaxation. Many smokers suffer from depression, a comorbid condition that they may be trying to self-medicate with nicotine. How these effects relate to the pleasurable effects of other addictive drugs that stimulate dopaminergic reward systems is still unclear. Improvements in attention and in the ability to concentrate are also measurable, but these may well be secondary consequences of stress reduction. Small doses of nicotine produce no adverse effects on mental processes or psychomotor functions, so from the behavioral standpoint alone, the addiction does not pose any danger to the individual or to society, and in some respects may even be beneficial.

Smoking and Health

Although rapidity of action and controllability make smoking a preferred method of self-administering addictive drugs, a major drawback is that if the drug is contained in a natural product, something other than the drug has to be burned. Tobacco, marijuana, or coca leaves, like any combustible organic matter, produce a host of irritant and carcinogenic products with dangerous effects on the lungs. Thus, lung cancer and emphysema, caused by smoking, are not due to nicotine in tobacco, but to "tar" (i.e., combustion products of the leaves).

Before World War I, lung cancer was so rare that medical students flocked excitedly to the autopsy room whenever a patient died of it. Inexplicably to physicians at the time, however, the disease became increasingly common in the years from about 1920 to 1950. The study of epidemics is fascinating, and epidemiologists enjoy the mix of clinical medicine, medical research, and detective work that is involved in tracking down causes. As the epidemic of lung cancer cases seemed to be keeping pace with growth of the big cities, air pollution was blamed at first. When two things are correlated, one is often blamed on the other; this is a classic statistical trap, for the truth may be that either or both are related to some other, unknown, factor. A somewhat facetious example: There was an excellent correlation, over a period of many years, between the sale of bananas in England and the death rate from cancer; yet bananas do not cause cancer. Association is not the same as causality.

Finally, in 1950, medical researchers in England and the United States noted that cigarette smoking among men—but, significantly, not among women—had begun increasing rapidly some years prior to the onset of the lung cancer epidemic. And lung cancer was overwhelmingly a male disease. By studying a large number of hospitalized men with lung cancer, and comparing them with patients of the same age who suffered from other diseases, they found a far greater number of cigarette smokers in the lung cancer group. Most impressive was the relationship between lung cancer deaths and the amount smoked. Those findings, too, only demonstrated an association; they were not proof of causality. However, unlike the banana correlation, this one was corroborated by additional information that pointed to a causal connection—substances generated in burning tobacco were shown to be chemical carcinogens, which produced cancer when painted on the skin of mice.

Finally, convincing evidence came from a study of British physicians. That occupational group had smoked as heavily as any, but their professional training enabled them to accept very quickly the growing indications that cigarettes might be dangerous to their health. So while other groups in British society maintained and even increased their cigarette consumption, the physicians reduced theirs. The result was dramatic. While the lung cancer rate continued to climb in the population at large, it began to fall among physicians. Moreover, the chance of death from lung cancer fell steadily the longer a person had stopped smoking. The evidence from this research was not just correlational but truly showed that cigarette smoking was causing lung cancer. It also demonstrated that the damage caused by smoking is reversible—that it pays to stop, no matter how long the addiction has lasted. As women lagged about 20 years behind men in the extent of their cigarette smoking, it was predicted that the lung cancer rate in women would climb after a similar lag; and that is exactly what happened. Today the number of new cases of lung cancer in women is approximately equal to that in men, and lung cancer now kills more women every year than does breast cancer.

Lung cancer is a vicious killer, which ends the lives of more than 200,000 people every year in the United States. This cancer can spread throughout the body before the lung tumor itself is big enough to cause irritation and coughing. And since smokers usually have a chronic cough anyway, there is a dangerous delay before the victim seeks medical attention. By then it may still be possible to eradicate the cancer by removing a lung, but often it is too late.

Bronchitis and emphysema are the two noncancerous lung diseases caused by smoking. Inhaling deeply moves fresh air (and smoke) into finer and finer branches of the bronchial tree, until it finally reaches the delicate spongy meshwork of tiny air sacs, where oxygen passes into the blood and carbon dioxide passes out of the blood to be exhaled. The bronchial tubes are lined with millions of microscopic hairs called cilia, and are coated with a thin layer of mucus. The cilia are in constant movement, beating rhythmically and propelling the mucus layer upward toward the throat, where it is eventually swallowed or expectorated. In this way, dust and other foreign particles are prevented from clogging the system. At the same time, foreign substances are removed by scavenger cells of the immune system, which wander about engulfing particles (especially bacteria) that might otherwise cause infection. Unfortunately, irritants in tobacco smoke paralyze the cilia, the mucus flow stagnates, and the scavenger cells are damaged. More and more foreign matter accumulates, and the stage is set for bronchial infection.

The defective ability of smokers to clear foreign matter out of their lungs was demonstrated in an ingenious experiment. Nonsmokers and heavy smokers inhaled a harmless tiny amount of very fine magnetized particles; then periodically, a sensitive magnetic detector placed against the chest could measure how much of the original material remained in the lungs. The result was striking. After 11 months, only 10 percent of the magnetic dust remained in the lungs of the nonsmokers, but fully 50 percent remained in the smokers' lungs. This experiment demonstrated the impaired ability of smokers to clear foreign substances like dust and air pollutants from their lungs—an additional health risk from smoking.

Chronic bronchitis becomes emphysema when the thin walls of the air sacs actually break down. This becomes a life-threatening condition when the lungs are so damaged that the necessary transfer of oxygen into the blood can no longer occur. It is a dreadful disabling disease. The victim feels suffocated, and breathing becomes a terrible effort. In the long run, fatal complications ensue.

Although lung cancer is the most dramatic harmful effect of smoking, the actual numbers of smokers who die of cardiovascular disease caused by smoking is far greater. Smokers have more heart attacks, more narrowing and hardening of the arteries (arteriosclerosis), more strokes, more aneurysms (ruptures of damaged blood vessels), and more severe high blood pressure than nonsmokers. The risk of dying of lung cancer (an otherwise rare disease) is many times greater in heavy smokers than in nonsmokers, but the actual number of deaths is relatively small compared with all deaths from all causes. Cardiovascular disease, on the other hand, is very common with advancing age—in nonsmokers as well as smokers—so the difference caused by smoking appears less striking. In fact, however, the estimated actual number of excess cardiovascular deaths due to smoking—estimated at more than 200,000—is approximately the same as the total number of lung cancer deaths.

The serious, long-term effects of cigarette smoking on the heart and blood vessels may be caused by nicotine itself rather than other components of the smoke. This is still controversial; some think carbon monoxide (see below) is more important. One consequence of stimulating nicotinic acetylcholine receptors is certainly to cause spasm (narrowing) of small blood vessels, depriving the tissues of oxygen. Instruments that measure blood flow to the fingers and toes and to the skin elsewhere on the body demonstrate this effect after even a single cigarette. Some think that premature wrinkling of the skin in smokers may result from such reductions in the local blood supply.

Carbon monoxide is a product of incomplete combustion, and its concentration is high in the inhaled smoke. The blood of smokers always contains more carbon monoxide than does the blood of nonsmokers, except for those exposed occupationally to automobile exhaust. Carbon monoxide poisons the hemoglobin in the red blood cells, so oxygen can not be delivered to the tissues. This results in diminished capacity for exercise or physical work, shortness of breath, dizziness, impairment of mental capacities, and defective night vision. It also means that at the very time nicotine is reducing the blood supply to the heart muscle and other tissues, carbon monoxide is further reducing the oxygen supply. Thus, carbon monoxide poisoning, in conjunction with nicotine, is thought to play an important part in damaging the heart and blood vessels of smokers.

All the adverse health effects of smoking a pack (20 cigarettes) daily result in a probability of death from any cause in a given year about twice that of nonsmokers. Death from bronchitis, emphysema, or lung cancer is 10 times more likely in those who smoke a pack a day, and 20 times more likely in those who smoke two packs a day, than in nonsmokers. And as would be expected, the relative risk for the other health hazards is directly related to the amount smoked.

In pregnant women, nicotine affects the blood vessels in the placenta, and thus it interferes with oxygen supply to the fetus. Moreover, it passes readily from the mother's blood across the placenta, compromising the fetal blood circulation too. Women who smoke during pregnancy have a higher rate of premature delivery, as well as lower birth weight infants carried to term. There are more birth abnormalities, more sickness and death during infancy, significant damage to the infant's blood vessels, and possibly even retarded mental development. But can we be sure that nicotine is responsible for the adverse effects seen in human pregnancy? Can we even be certain that smoking is the culprit?

Proof that fetal damage is caused by a certain drug is hard to come by, not only for smoking but for any drug used during pregnancy. The problem is that women who are addicted to a particular drug differ in many ways from women who are not. Women who smoke, for example, exhibit higher anxiety levels and more hard-driving ("type A") behavior. Smokers are obviously less attentive to their health than nonsmokers (otherwise they would not smoke), and this leads to less concern about their bodies during pregnancy, less prenatal care, poorer diet, more use of alcohol and other drugs. Thus, it is difficult, when comparing the offspring of smokers with those of nonsmokers, to be sure that observed differences are due to smoking during pregnancy rather than to associated factors or to some innate characteristics of the mother. It is even possible that female smokers tend to choose different kinds of mates than do nonsmokers, so the paternal contribution to the genetic makeup of the offspring may also be different from that of infants born to nonsmoking mothers.

Administering nicotine to pregnant rodents does cause stillbirths, decreased birth weight, and numerous neurological and behavioral deficits in the offspring. But these effects occur at dosages that, if corrected for body weight, would correspond in humans to nearly 20 packs of cigarettes daily! Regrettably, as with animal toxicity studies in general, there is no sure way to extrapolate animal dosages to humans. Sometimes, however, when we lack scientific proof, we have to fall back on common sense and the best guesses we can make. Knowing what we do about how easily prenatal development of the human fetus can be disturbed, and knowing the adverse effects of drugs on fetal development in animals, common sense tells us not to expose a fetus to any drug—and certainly not to one like nicotine, which has known adverse effects on the blood vessels of the placenta and the fetus.

Finally, it has been established that inhaling secondhand smoke is not entirely harmless. Of course, the amount of smoke that actually reaches the lungs of nonsmokers is very much less than what smokers take in directly, so the adverse effects are very small compared with those in smokers. Nevertheless, data show that these effects are not negligible. Those exposed to secondhand smoke have detectable nicotine metabolites in their blood, demonstrating that the exposure to nicotine is real. Children of parents who smoke have a distinctly higher incidence of breathing disorders (including asthma) and respiratory infections—several hundred thousand each year in the United States—than do children in homes where neither parent smokes. It is estimated that if there were a linear relationship of toxicity to drug concentration at very low drug levels—a big "if"— secondhand smoke would cause some 3,000 lung cancer deaths each year in the United States. It must be noted, however, that many scientists are skeptical of this approach and its conclusions.

Treating Nicotine Addiction

If you know any nicotine addicts (maybe you are one yourself), ask them why they don't quit. At one time that would have been re- garded as an impolite, intrusive question, and the answer might well have been: "None of your business!" Or more humorously, they might have quoted Mark Twain: "Quitting is easy, I've done it many times." Attitudes have changed, and today's addicts are on the de- fensive. Now you will hear: "I am going to quit, tomorrow," or "I'm working on it." Right!

I hear these same pathetic replies from heroin addicts, too; "to- morrow" is a standard joke about quitting. Nevertheless, there is a certain sincerity about addicts' wish to be abstinent. They really do picture themselves free of the addiction some day, and they like what they imagine. But getting there is something else again. It is espe- cially hard to break an addiction to a substance that is not only readily available—usually only a few minutes away—and relatively cheap, but also (although to a decreasing extent) socially acceptable. Furthermore, by relieving stress and anxiety, nicotine may even im- prove performance. And except for the annoyance and very slight health risk of secondhand smoke to nonsmokers, and the occasional fire, the nicotine addict presents no threat to others. I advise heroin addicts to break all social connections, to get out of the heroin-using peer group, to move to a different neighborhood; all those steps are helpful in maintaining abstinence. But none of that is practical for nicotine addicts; they have to become abstinent in an environment that offers every opportunity to fail.

A typical nicotine addict smokes between 10 and 50 cigarettes every day. Each one is linked to a particular time, place, and activity in a way that is reminiscent of the place conditioning experiments described in chapter 4. For example, sitting down to the first morning cup of coffee is a conditioned cue to take out a cigarette and light it. Every meal ends with a cigarette. Sitting down at a desk to work evokes craving for a cigarette. Stepping into the lobby during intermission means light-up time. Just being near other smokers produces an automatic reaching for a cigarette. I call these situations conditioned association triggers because—in a pattern that is unique for each person—they trigger the self-administration of nicotine. Thus, the addict smokes on a regular schedule, repeating the pleasurable nicotine spiking pattern in the brain, and the conditioned association triggers make it difficult to break that pattern.

Millions—more than half of those who ever smoked—have become ex-smokers. Forty-five years ago, 57 percent of all U.S. males were smokers; today the figure is down to 29 percent. The number of female smokers then was 32 percent, and instead of continuing to rise, as it did for years, it has dropped to 26 percent despite the increasing social acceptance of smoking among females over that same time span. So quitting is certainly possible. On the other hand, the road to quitting is highly variable. Some can do it neatly and permanently; but others become abstinent only briefly, then relapse. Abstinence followed by relapse is a common pattern until at long last (and unpredictably) long-term abstinence—at least for some— is achieved. What usually causes relapse is some combination of unusual stress and one of the conditioned association triggers.

Ex-smokers (like other ex-addicts) who relapse are often so ashamed of themselves that they will not admit what happened. For this reason—as with all addictive drugs—a chemical test is absolutely essential to bring the problem quickly into the open for optimal treatment. If a problem is being denied, it cannot possibly be treated. There are three methods of testing: for carbon monoxide in the expired air; for thiocyanate (to which cyanide gas in smoke is converted in the body) in saliva; and for cotinine (a metabolic product of nicotine) in saliva, blood, or urine.

The "hard-core" addicts—those who have relapsed repeatedly— present a real challenge. People who have never smoked tend to belittle the difficulties, and worst of all are those who have become ex-smokers themselves; "I did it, why can't you?" is their unhelpful attitude. Hard-core addicts need sympathetic understanding, not preaching. For such people, who have tried to quit and have relapsed repeatedly, I advocate slow and deliberate reduction of intake as a realistic initial goal, putting off the ultimate quitting decision for later. This is known as a "harm reduction" strategy, which may be applicable, at least to some extent, to other drug addictions, too (see chapter 16). The rationale is simple. If a person who is smoking 30 cigarettes daily reduces that to 29, and maintains the new level, that smoker has actually accomplished a 3 percent reduction in all the health hazards of the addiction. If even one cigarette is removed permanently from the repertoire each week, in four months the health hazards will be reduced by half. Such a program requires discipline and motivation. It requires self-conscious analysis and modification of one's own behavior. One conditioned association trigger at a time has to be eliminated, by repeatedly skipping the cigarette associated with that trigger—the classic method of extinguishing a conditioned behavior.

In some quarters, "harm reduction" is used to justify continuing an addiction rather than attempting to cure it. Some people reject this strategy on the grounds that addiction is wrong, addictive drugs are bad, and one should not compromise with what is wrong and bad. Others reject it on the grounds that addicts, by their very nature, are unable to sustain moderate intake of an addictive drug, and quickly lose control if they try. This is the view held strongly with respect to alcohol addiction by powerful groups like Alcoholics Anonymous (AA), who are committed to total abstinence. In the face of this strong ideology, medical scientists have been afraid even to examine the question objectively; a few brave ones did and were pilloried for it. So although experience and common sense warn us that ex-addicts are at exceptionally high risk for relapse, we don't really have scientific evidence as to whether controlled drug use for a prolonged period could be a realistic option for some people in some circumstances, either as an end in itself or as a temporary expedient on the way to total abstinence. We know that the severity of drug dependence, and therefore the intensity of a withdrawal syndrome, are greater the higher the chronic drug dosage. Therefore, pharmacology tells us that slow and continuous dosage reduction ought to make eventual quitting easier.

Several kinds of pharmacological treatments are proving to have some value in aiding some hard-core nicotine addicts to become abstinent; but these drugs are useful only as adjuncts to behavioral therapy, and even then, none has an impressive long-term success rate.

Nicotine chewing gum was introduced some years ago as an aid to giving up cigarettes, and now it is available without prescription at the local supermarket. Furnishing nicotine in pure form was seen as a way to assist the addict in breaking the smoking habit completely, while avoiding withdrawal discomfort and sustaining the nicotine dependence. Then eventually, in this two-phase approach, the nicotine gum would be stopped. It turned out, however, that absorption of nicotine from the mouth was too irregular and unpredictable, a variable amount of nicotine was swallowed, and some failed to be absorbed at all. No doubt there are some smokers who broke their habit while chewing nicotine gum, but the long-term abstinence rate is very low.

Nicotine skin patches are more effective than nicotine gum, as are novel devices that deliver nicotine under the skin continuously. Patches are available now without prescription, and they smoothly establish nicotine blood levels comparable to what the smoker is used to. In principle, this approach makes some sense, but in practice it is only partly successful. If success is measured as numbers of patients who are still smoking a full year after removal of the nicotine delivery device, the record is unimpressive. Nicotine is clearly superior to placebo, but after the patch is removed, the one-year abstinence rate is only about 15–20 percent. On the other hand, there are no reliable data yet on the abstinence rate if the patch is not removed.

Some experts advocate a different philosophy. By analogy to the use of surrogate opiates like methadone in the long-term maintenance of heroin addicts, nicotine maintenance is being proposed for the hard-core group of smokers who seem unable to break their addiction. Unlike long-term methadone treatment, however, which has no known adverse effects, nicotine administration may cause cardiovascular problems, as noted earlier. If it really works, however, and if it is the only way to get someone to quit cigarettes, those addicts will at least be spared the bronchitis, emphysema, and lung cancer that are caused by smoking. That is the crux of an effective harm-reduction strategy.

Finally, as the smoker gets satisfaction from the spikes of brain nicotine concentration after every puff, a promising approach under development is a nicotine inhaler, a surrogate cigarette that delivers nicotine without any combustion products, thus avoiding the health damage caused by tobacco smoke.

Nicotinic receptor antagonists like mecamylamine can, in theory, prevent relapse from the abstinent state by blocking the rewarding effects of nicotine. The chief problem with antagonist therapy for any addictive drug is securing patient compliance in taking the medication regularly. This reluctance might reflect a dysphoria caused by blocking some normal actions of acetylcholine on the brain's nicotinic receptors.

If a smoker does discontinue abruptly, the withdrawal discomfort is worse the higher the chronic nicotine dosage (i.e., the more cigarettes smoked daily). There are numerous medications that reduce withdrawal discomfort sufficiently to allow complete cessation of smoking, but then the real problem is preventing relapse. Despite our armamentarium of pharmacological and behavioral tools, real success still cannot be counted on reliably.

More successful than most—but still falling far short of a perfect medication—are certain antidepressants. The trials with this class of drugs rest on the finding that more heavily addicted smokers than nonsmokers have suffered from episodes of serious depression in their lives. It may be, therefore (as noted earlier), that hard-core nicotine addicts are attempting to self-medicate their depression. If that is true, antidepressant drugs might relieve them of the need to smoke. One such drug, now used widely, is bupropion, an effective antidepressant that is marketed under the name Zyban as an aid to smoking cessation. Early results of controlled clinical trials with bupropion have yielded abstinence rates of 30 percent at one year, compared with 16 percent with nicotine or placebo patches.

Finally, the best way to rid society of nicotine addiction is obviously to prevent smoking in the first place. Progress in prevention research—not only for nicotine but for other addictive drugs—is discussed at length in chapter 15.

Summary

Nicotine addiction epitomizes many aspects of drug addiction in general. We know how and where the drug acts in the brain—on nicotinic acetylcholine receptors in the same dopaminergic reward pathway that is the target of other addictive drugs. The withdrawal syndrome is uncomfortable enough to maintain the addiction morning after morning, initiating the sequence of spiking brain levels that continues throughout the day as the background nicotine level builds up. It is a mystery given that nicotine seems to drive dopamine release in the same way as other addictive drugs, why it cannot substitute for heroin, cocaine, alcohol, or others.

Because nicotine, in cigarettes, is legal (except for children), readily available, and relatively cheap, all the societal elements for sustaining addictive behavior are present.

The inhalation route has ideal properties for maintaining an addiction—it is fast, and it offers drug delivery under the user's control. The most devastating health hazards are from the smoke rather than the nicotine; thus, a harm reduction approach might advocate a smokeless device for nicotine inhalation as a substantial improvement over cigarettes.

The treatment of nicotine addiction is a classic example of the complexities facing the therapist in the field of addiction. There is general agreement in the treatment community that whatever pharmacological means are used to assist in withdrawal, to suppress craving, or to prevent relapse, these have to be supplemented by expert face-to-face counseling. Finding conclusively, in controlled clinical trials, what combination of pharmacological and behavioral therapy works best—for whom, and at what cost—is the challenge for research on the treatment of nicotine addiction.

9

Alcohol and
Related Drugs

It is a typical foggy day in Manchester, England. Imagine that you are standing in an open field in the park, watching a pair of orange plastic road markers a few hundred yards away. A red double-decker bus comes barreling across the field, heading for the gap between the markers. You think: He'll never get through, it's too narrow for the bus. You are right. The bus knocks over one of the markers.

In this famous experiment, each experienced bus driver was first asked if he thought he could safely drive the bus through. If he said yes, he was asked to try it. If he said no, the markers were moved apart to a separation he thought adequate, and then he was asked to try it. On different days and with different drivers the experiment was done "cold sober" and—as in the run we were watching—after drinking a measured dose of whiskey. Under the influence of alcohol, the drivers actually needed a wider gap to maneuver the bus through than when they were sober, but at the same time they judged that a narrower gap was sufficient. This result demonstrates a characteristic double danger of alcohol—it spoils judgment at the same time that it ruins performance.

How does this simple molecule cause such profound disturbances in behavior? Why are alcohol and its pharmacological relatives (benzodiazepines, barbiturates, and volatile solvents) so widely used? What is the impact on the drinker and on society? What are the health hazards of long-term heavy use? How and where do these drugs act in the brain? What are the main features of alcohol addiction, and what is known about treating it?

Fermentation, Distillation, Intoxication

Alcohol is an ancient drug; fermentation has been recognized since the earliest agricultural civilizations. Throughout history, societies have accorded alcohol a position of special respect, hedging its use with restrictions as to time, place, and circumstance. In Judaism and Christianity, the sacramental use of wine illustrates this method of controlling a dangerous drug. Drunkenness is decried universally, whether in the biblical passage describing Noah's intoxication, or in Islamic law forbidding alcohol entirely. Even in a nonreligious context, the custom of drinking a toast on special occasions ("to health," curiously, in all languages) is a relic of the special status enjoyed by this drug in former times.

Fermentation is the process whereby yeast cells convert sugar to ethyl alcohol. It is self-limiting, because the yeast cells and yeast enzymes are destroyed when the alcohol concentration reaches about 12 percent. Therefore, wine cannot be stronger than that unless it is "fortified" by adding alcohol, as with port and sherry (about 20 percent alcohol). To achieve still higher alcohol concentrations requires distillation—boiling the alcohol out of the fermentation mixture (it boils at a lower temperature than water) and then condensing the alcohol vapor back to liquid in a still. An efficient still, which may yield nearly pure ethyl alcohol, can be put together from the simplest materials by anyone who wishes to produce bootleg liquor. Distilled liquors (e.g., vodka, gin, whiskey) are usually marketed at 80 to 100 proof (40–50 percent alcohol), and they are much more dangerous than wines (12–20 percent) and beer (usually 3–6 percent).

The history of drinking habits in England provides an interesting example of the relative dangers. As a beer manufacturing and beer drinking country, it did not experience alcoholism as a major public health problem until the introduction of cheap gin from Holland early in the eighteenth century. Then urban drunkenness, especially among the poor, became England's blight, as depicted so dramatically in Hogarth's famous engraving, "Gin Lane." There is a general principle here: The weaker (less concentrated) forms of all addictive drugs, in their natural state, are safer than the purified psychoactive chemicals themselves.

The easy availability of distilled liquors, and the erosion of the cultural protections surrounding alcohol use, have had devastating effects. Alcohol is the only addictive drug that alters behavior dangerously, yet at the same time is freely and legally available without a prescription. As it is so widely consumed, it causes users and society the most serious problems of all the addictive drugs.

Being Drunk

Intoxication by alcohol is a distinctive behavioral condition, dose-related and easily measurable. In both people and laboratory animals, the blood concentration of ethyl alcohol is a good indicator of the concentration bathing the brain. And alcohol vapor in the breath reflects, quite accurately, the concentration in the blood flowing through the lungs. This is the basis of the Breathalyzer technique for measuring blood alcohol; and the close blood-brain relationship is the basis for setting a presumptive blood-level standard for "driving while intoxicated." A level of 0.08 percent (becoming accepted universally) is justified by results obtained in driving simulators; and 0.05 percent is being advocated as safer. People differ, of course, not only in how many drinks it takes to reach the legal limit—for some people, one drink suffices. People differ also in their behavioral sensitivity to alcohol, i.e., their behavioral impairment at the same blood alcohol level. Testing by breath or blood sample provides useful and accurate information about whether—for the average person—psychomotor behavior is likely to be disrupted by alcohol at the time the sample is taken. In contrast, urine tests for any drug provide a historical record, proving that a drug entered the body at some prior time.

In alcohol research the single drink is used as a unit of measure because typical single drinks of all kinds are roughly equivalent in alcohol content. For example, a typical small jigger (an ounce and a half) of 80-proof (40 percent) distilled spirits contains 18 milliliters of alcohol. The same amount of alcohol is contained in a 12-ounce can of strong (5 percent) beer—but most commercial beer is 3–4 percent—or a 5-ounce glass of wine (12 percent). This is the dose that people usually take at the outset in social drinking, because it represents the smallest amount of alcohol that has a psychoactive effect. Of course, individual differences (especially of body weight) modify this initially effective dose, and women, in general, require lower doses than men.

The popular belief is that alcohol produces harmless relaxation at low doses and significant behavioral toxicity only at higher doses. That is not true. The very first drink disrupts complex mental abilities and psychomotor coordination; tests requiring calculations, quick memory recall, vigilance, and the like, all show decrements in performance. Harder to measure are the subjective effects, the very ones that people seek from social drinking: loss of inhibitions, a relaxed mood, loquaciousness, and easy sociability. Unfortunately, these sought-after hedonic effects are accompanied by poor judgment and greater risk-taking behavior, as the Manchester bus drivers demonstrated.

After a few drinks, the fine control mechanisms that maintain our sense of balance are disturbed. This is the basis for tests like "walking the line" and eyes-closed sway. The disturbance of equilibrium is thought to be due—at least in part—to an action of alcohol in the cerebellum; in this part of the brain, incoming signals bringing position information from the muscles, and balance information from the inner ear, are coordinated with outgoing signals to the numerous muscles involved in the control of posture. Animal tests for this action of alcohol are popular because they are so easy to carry out in the laboratory. One such test uses a horizontal rod driven by a motor that makes it rotate slowly. A normal mouse or rat placed on the rod has no difficulty maintaining its balance; it walks continuously as the rod turns under its feet. A slightly intoxicated animal falls off the rod. This behavioral deficit can be scored quantitatively—number of falls, time to falling, critical speed of rotation—and those scores relate directly to the blood and brain concentration of alcohol.

In humans, as the alcohol dose is increased, speech becomes slurred and incoherent; balance is severely impaired; and inappropriate, foolish behavior develops. Loss of inhibition leads to boastfulness ("Sure, I can drive!") and enhanced aggression ("I can fight him with one hand tied behind my back!")—a particularly dangerous combination. It is estimated that alcohol plays a role in more than half of all homicides, in most domestic violence, and it is the cause of half the motor vehicle deaths. Still higher doses cause profound sedation, deep sleep, respiratory depression, eventually coma and death. Alcohol-induced "sleep" (not a normal sleep, but rather an immobility like that seen with anesthetics) is easy to measure in animals; the duration of immobility and loss of the righting reflex are related to the alcohol dose.

Where and how in the brain does alcohol cause its psychoactive effects, which make it so attractive to so many people? Gamma-amino butyrate (GABA) is an abundant inhibitory neurotransmitter. Its receptors are ion channels (see chapter 3), composed of several protein subunits arranged to permit the passage of negatively charged chloride ions. When GABA is released from a nearby nerve ending, it binds to this receptor complex, opening the channel. The sudden inrush of chloride ions increases the negative electric charge inside the neuron, making it more refractory to neurotransmitters that ordinarily would stimulate it. Alcohol enhances these actions of GABA. At the same time, it inhibits the function of excitatory brain receptors such as the nicotinic acetylcholine receptor and the NMDA subtype of glutamate receptor, which are also ion channels. Some of the effects on receptor function (for example, on the nicotinic acetylcholine receptors) occur at very low concentrations, corresponding to mildly intoxicating levels in laboratory animals or humans. Alcohol also acts directly within neurons, bypassing the receptors and the cell membranes, and stimulating or inhibiting enzymes that regulate the neuron's activity, such as those that attach or detach regulatory phosphate groups to receptors. Whatever effects of alcohol one considers, if they occur only at high concentrations that would be toxic in the whole organism, they cannot be relevant to the hedonic or addictive properties of alcohol.

As the several receptors affected by alcohol are found in so many parts of the brain, we should not be surprised that alcohol has very complicated effects in different brain regions. Acting on GABA receptors in the cerebellum, for example, it could disturb equilibrium and posture. In the hippocampus, it could disturb memory formation and retrieval. The depression of breathing and of blood pressure in alcohol coma is due to the drug's action on the lower parts of the brain that regulate these vital activities. Finally, and not surprisingly, alcohol stimulates the same dopaminergic reward pathway that mediates the pleasurable effects (positive reinforcement) of other addictive drugs. This action seems to be enhanced by the endogenous opioids that act on the mu opioid receptor.

Other Drugs in the Alcohol Family

Barbiturates and benzodiazepines (e.g., Valium)—although their effects are not identical—both cause a behavioral intoxication very much like that due to alcohol, so it is significant that these drugs, too, enhance the effects of GABA on its receptors. Barbiturates were widely prescribed as sleeping pills before the 1960s. Their easy availability made them favorite drugs of abuse; accidental deaths from overdose were not uncommon, as well as intentional suicide. Addiction was a problem, too. Even today, barbiturates remain useful for euthanasia and assisted suicide in terminally ill patients. As for the treatment of insomnia, barbiturates were never really effective. Regular use causes dependence, and then attempts to sleep without the medication are frustrated by withdrawal disturbances—which include, ironically enough, insomnia. A colleague who is an expert on sleep disturbances puts it this way: "Sleeping pills cause insomnia."

Benzodiazepines have their own specific binding site on the GABA receptor complex, different from the barbiturate binding site. The end result is like that caused by alcohol—to enhance the effect of GABA in opening the ion channel in the receptor, thus allowing chloride ions to rush in. Indeed, in contrast to the complex multiple actions of alcohol on various receptors, virtually all the effects of benzodiazepines seem to be mediated by GABA receptors. In the late 1960s, with the abandonment of barbiturates for treating insomnia, and their diminished use for treating anxiety, the first benzodiazepines came onto the market and quickly replaced them, becoming the most widely prescribed drugs in the United States. Advantages of the benzodiazepines over the barbiturates are their safety (overdose deaths are virtually unknown), lesser tendency to dosage escalation and dependence, and less dangerous withdrawal syndrome. In the view of some experts, however, they were greatly overprescribed, both for insomnia and for anxiety; without doubt, many people became addicted to them. Population surveys 20 years ago showed that about one adult in ten was using a benzodiazepine occasionally (usually Valium); and one in seven of those (especially the elderly) was using daily for at least a whole year and became dependent. In an overreaction to these findings, prescribing was drastically reduced, so that now—according to a report from the American Psychiatric Association—benzodiazepines are not prescribed nearly often enough, even for legitimate needs.

Certain benzodiazepines—especially flunitrazepam (Rohypnol, "roofies")—have become popular among young people as party drugs, especially at college campuses. What makes them attractive is that, like alcohol, they relax social inhibitions but without the taste, odor, or local irritant action of alcohol. These properties have led to the designation "date rape drug"—a woman can be attacked sexually after this potent benzodiazepine, slipped into her drink, has incapacitated her. Recent statistics also show this drug present (rather than or in addition to alcohol) in 10 percent or more of "driving while intoxicated" cases. A similar "party drug," which also acts on GABA receptors, is gamma-hydroxybutyrate (GHB).

The third member of the alcohol family comprises the inhaled nitrites (amyl nitrite and related compounds), gaseous anesthetics, and volatile solvents. The nitrites relax smooth muscle, causing a sudden increase of blood flow to the extremities, the sexual organs, and the brain. Relaxation of the anal muscles makes them especially popular for homosexual intercourse. The nineteenth century saw ether, chloroform, and nitrous oxide ("laughing gas") become fads for obtaining a quick "high," and these compounds are still abused by medical professionals. They have a long history as mood-altering agents, and their psychoactive effects are quite similar to those of alcohol, barbiturates, and the benzodiazepines. The volatile solvents are used chiefly by children, who have easy access to glue, correction fluid, paints, fuels, and the like. These inhalants seem to act on brain receptors in much the same way as alcohol does; but basic research on their mechanism of action has been remarkably scanty. The "high" they produce is much like alcohol intoxication, but their immediate and long-term effects are far more dangerous. Sudden death may occur from heart stoppage; and chronic use is toxic to the liver, kidneys, and other organs. Repeated exposure can also cause permanent brain damage, manifested initially by loss of balance, tremors, and visual disturbances in the absence of any intoxicating agent.

Are There Alcohol Receptors?

How, in the brain, do the many and diverse effects of alcohol, especially the psychoactive ones, come about? Ethyl alcohol is a very small—one might say nondescript—molecule, containing only two linked carbon atoms, one oxygen atom, and six hydrogen atoms. No alcohol receptor has yet been identified conclusively, and some scientists doubt that a receptor could bind such a simple ligand in a specific manner. Controversy has raged for years concerning alcohol's molecular mechanism of action in the brain.

One point of view stresses the ability of alcohol, at intoxicating concentrations, to disorder (fluidize) nerve cell membranes. These membranes, in which receptors, ion channels, enzymes, transporters, and other functional molecules are embedded, are composed of two layers of lipid (oily fat), with long chains of carbon atoms called fatty acids arrayed in a densely packed parallel manner that gives the membrane a highly ordered structure. The various receptors and other functional proteins in the cell membrane are very much affected by the state of this oily environment in which they float. The researcher can insert labeled fatty acid (called a reporter group) into the membranes. Then an appropriate instrument will detect vibratory motion in the vicinity of the label. Such motion measures the rigidity or fluidity of the membrane, expressed quantitatively as an order parameter.

Five key findings support the idea that membrane fluidization, directly or indirectly, may be responsible for the psychoactive effects of alcohol.

(1) The biological potency in a series of alcohols is strictly correlated with solubility in lipids, as though it is the amount of alcohol in the lipid cell membranes that determines the biological effect.

(2) Not only in the family of alcohols do many compounds—isopropyl alcohol (rubbing alcohol) is an example—share many psychoactive effects of ethyl alcohol. Volatile solvents and anesthetic gases also share these effects, and some of them have even fewer atoms than ethyl alcohol—nitrous oxide ("laughing gas" is an example). The extreme case is the rare gas xenon, which is but a single atom, yet nevertheless produces many psychoactive effects that are indistinguishable from those of ethyl alcohol. All these substances

dissolve in neuronal cell membranes, and the striking lack of specificity is quite at variance with what we expect from ligands that bind to receptors.

(3) In attributing a drug effect to a particular molecular interaction, pharmacologists look closely at drug concentrations. We know what concentration of alcohol in the fluid bathing the brain (about 0.1 percent) is required to cause the characteristic hedonic effect and mild intoxication. At very much higher concentrations, even above the lethal range, alcohol disturbs numerous biochemical processes, but such actions cannot be relevant to the addictive or intoxicating effects. The alcohol concentration required to produce even the mildest of its actions is millions of times higher than the effective concentrations of typical receptor ligands. So, if there is an alcohol receptor, it must have remarkably low affinity for alcohol. We accept as possibly important the actions of alcohol on membrane fluidity because the alcohol concentrations needed for that effect are in the pharmacologically relevant range.

(4) Strains of mice bred for high natural resistance to alcohol ("short-sleep" mice, see chapter 7) have neuronal membranes that are resistant to the disordering effect.

(5) Brain membranes from mice that have been made tolerant to alcohol by long-term exposure are less readily disordered by alcohol than they were at the outset.

The measured disorder is quite small; one wonders if it could be sufficient to account for the psychoactive effects of alcohol. Especially hard to explain is the fact that a small increase in body temperature causes membrane disorder of comparable degree yet does not cause intoxication. It may be, therefore, that the observed small fluidizing effect, which represents an average disorder across the whole membrane, is an important indicator, but obscures a much greater disordering action at certain critical sites. Indeed, such sites could be the lipids that closely surround important receptors, or even lipid (hydrophobic) regions of those receptors themselves. In this way, the disordering effect could be reconciled to the effects of alcohol on receptors.

Research during the past decade supports the concept that certain brain receptors may be direct targets of alcohol. There is, after all, an enzyme in liver—alcohol dehydrogenase—which accommodates alcohol in a binding site. Therefore, we cannot summarily dismiss the idea that a brain receptor might have a binding site for alcohol, albeit of low affinity. Experiments support this idea. In a series of alcohols with longer and longer chains of carbon atoms, potency increases with chain length, as noted above. However, a length is reached at which the potency drops off abruptly. This "cut-off" effect suggests that a pocket of limited size accommodates the alcohols presumably a cavity in a receptor rather than the entire lipid environment of the nerve cell membrane. The idea of size-limited cavities on certain receptors is further supported by the fact that the cutoff is different for different receptors; for example, at a chain length of 10 carbon atoms for glycine receptors, but seven for GABA receptors.

Yet another hypothesis regards alcohol as a pro-drug that gives rise to a more reactive and more potent compound, which is the actual functional drug. Over the years, much effort has been devoted to confirming this idea. As alcohol is converted directly to acetaldehyde, this highly reactive product itself has been a promising candidate. Moreover, acetaldehyde reacts with dopamine and other neurotransmitter amines to yield complex chemical products (alkaloids), any of which might be a high-affinity ligand for some key receptor in the brain. Experiments in progress at this writing reveal that rats will inject acetaldehyde into their own VTA at the origin of the dopaminergic reward pathway—in other words, that acetaldehyde is reinforcing. Moreover, although alcohol is also self-injected, the concentration required is more than 200 times that of acetaldehyde. This makes it plausible to believe that a tiny amount of acetaldehyde formed from alcohol within the VTA (or an alkaloid derived from acetaldehyde) accounts for the rewarding effect of alcohol there.

Alcohol Dependence and Withdrawal

Chapter 6 outlined the history of alcohol dependence research, and chapter 7 presented some of the evidence for a role of genetics in the predisposition to alcohol addiction. To become addicted requires a pattern of repeated heavy drinking, and this typically develops over a number of years. Most people who enjoy social drinking in moderation, to obtain a mild degree of behavioral disinhibition, do not enjoy—indeed, may even be disgusted by—

being drunk, and they dislike losing control. Alcoholics, in contrast, evidently like being drunk, and they drink to get drunk.

Chronic exposure to alcohol produces physical dependence in animals and in people. When someone has been drinking heavily for a long time and then abruptly discontinues, the withdrawal syndrome can be severe to the point of death. Bursts of electrical activity in the brain occur, accompanied by convulsions and sometimes by psychotic phenomena like hallucinations (delirium tremens). With respect to the withdrawal syndrome, alcohol and related substances are the most hazardous of the addictive drugs. The withdrawal disturbances are instantly relieved by alcohol, by benzodiazepines, or by barbiturates. In like manner, the withdrawal syndrome caused by chronic exposure to either benzodiazepines or barbiturates is relieved by alcohol. This cross-dependence is entirely consistent with a common site of action of these drugs—for example, on the GABA receptor complex.

Probably because of its unpleasant taste and the way it irritates the mouth, esophagus, and stomach, mice and rats will not readily drink enough alcohol, in a free-choice arrangement, to become dependent. In order to produce alcohol dependence in experiments like those described for opiates (see chapter 6), mice have to be exposed continuously for at least several days. This can be accomplished by housing them in an inhalation chamber, an airtight plastic cage, through which alcohol can be furnished in a continuous flow as a vapor in the airstream. The concentration in the vapor can be held steady at whatever level is desired. The blood level of alcohol is measured from time to time in a drop of blood taken from the tail. At various times after removing mice from the chamber, the withdrawal syndrome can be elicited by lifting a mouse by the tail, provoking a convulsion—a response never seen in normal animals. Such studies show a direct relationship between the alcohol concentration in blood during development of dependence and the intensity of the subsequent withdrawal disturbance, analogous to the findings on opiate dependence in animals and humans. Tolerance develops simultaneously with dependence, and both phenomena are reversible over a period of about 24 hours after stopping alcohol administration. Thus, the time course of alcohol tolerance and dependence in mice is much like that seen with opiates.

Health Hazards of Alcohol Use

A consequence of long-term heavy use of alcohol is liver cirrhosis, a condition in which damage to the cells leads to their replacement by scar tissue, until eventually the liver fails entirely, and the addict dies. A complication on the way to that final outcome is severe bleeding, which can be fatal. Blood circulating from the gut normally flows into the liver on its way back to the heart; but as the liver becomes more scarred and hardened, resistance to the blood flow increases, veins in the stomach and esophagus become distended, and hemorrhage results.

In addition to its psychoactive effects, alcohol—even at ordinary doses, but more significantly as dosage is increased—disturbs the regulation of several hormone systems in the body. Prominent among these effects is a suppression of sex hormone production. In women, menstrual irregularities are common. In men, sexual potency is reduced during intoxication; and long-term drinking causes degeneration of the testicles and diminished production of testosterone, enlarged breasts, and decreased sex drive.

Curiously, numerous studies have demonstrated an association between moderate drinking and a lowered risk of coronary heart disease. Association, however, is very different from causality; there is as yet no conclusive proof that drinking is the protective factor. People who abstain, or who drink heavily, differ in many ways from moderate drinkers—in physical activity, diet, use of other drugs, various lifestyle behaviors, and possibly also genetic vulnerability to heart disease. Unless further research dictates otherwise, the prudent advice of the National Institute on Alcohol Abuse and Alcoholism (NIAAA) should be followed: People should not be encouraged to drink for health reasons; and if they do drink, should not exceed one or two drinks daily. Furthermore, as explained below, pregnant women (or women likely to become pregnant) should not drink at all.

A special toxic effect of alcohol addiction is the fetal alcohol syndrome, recognized only since 1973. If a woman drinks heavily during very early pregnancy, she is likely to miscarry. But if the fetus escapes that fate, the newborn infant will have low birth weight and the various medical problems that accompany low birth weight. Growth of the infant is abnormally slow, and in later years there are various degrees of mental retardation, hyperactivity, attention deficits, and learning disorders. The characteristic marker of fetal alcohol syndrome is a special kind of malformation—a flat face, a thin upper lip, and a peculiar appearance of the eyes and nose.

Recent studies with rats reveal a clear and disturbing analogue of fetal alcohol syndrome. Alcohol, by overstimulating GABA receptors and blocking NMDA receptors, triggers a widespread degeneration of neurons in the forebrain. Even transient exposure to alcohol during the period—both before birth and during postnatal development—when synapses are being formed, kills millions of nerve cells. Consistent with the rat findings, when infants with fetal alcohol syndrome were followed into adolescence and adulthood, with periodic testing of intelligence and mental functioning, the facial abnormalities were found to be accompanied by permanent brain damage, as evidenced by poor test performance. In one study—a prospective one—pregnant women were queried, before they gave birth, about their alcohol use early in pregnancy and also in the month before they knew they were pregnant. Then their infants were examined on the first day of life and again periodically until seven years of age. This research showed that even moderate drinking in the earliest weeks of pregnancy had small but measurable and lasting effects on behavior of the newborn, even when the facial abnormalities of the severe fetal alcohol syndrome were not present. Behavioral deficits, learning difficulties, short attention span, impulsivity, and numerous other inappropriate behavior patterns symptomatic of brain damage were correlated with the extent of maternal drinking. Most important, these problems persisted throughout childhood.

The conclusion of this research—that pregnant women should not drink at all during pregnancy—is generally accepted, but still controversial. An unavoidable weakness of all such studies is that they depend on self-reporting of drinking during pregnancy, and self-reports are likely be on the low side of the truth. Therefore, bad outcomes may be mistakenly attributed to very low alcohol consumption when, in truth, much more was imbibed. Furthermore, some investigators have failed to demonstrate any adverse effects on the newborn when maternal alcohol consumption during pregnancy was less than three drinks daily on average. Until these uncertainties are resolved, the safest course is obviously for women to avoid alcohol throughout pregnancy.

There is a general problem here, which applies to all drugs that affect fetal development. In a regular 28-day menstrual cycle (Figure

9.1), ovulation occurs about 14 days from the start of the previous menses, and then the ovum can only be fertilized within the next couple of days. The time of greatest sensitivity of the developing fetus to serious damage by any drug is during the formation of the body organs, which begins early—only 20 days after fertilization. Since ovulation and fertilization occur in the middle of the menstrual cycle, this critical time would begin barely a week after the expected start of the first missed period. That is also the earliest time a pregnancy test is likely to turn positive. What this means is that even with perfectly regular periods—and the situation is much worse if periods are irregular—a woman who is using any drug cannot be sure she is pregnant early enough to prevent serious damage to her fetus. Clearly, then, it is not safe for her to continue addictive drug use, planning to stop if she discovers she is pregnant. Furthermore, if the pregnancy is unplanned, and the woman drinks heavily, she will not even be alert to the urgency of trying to stop in time. This state of affairs really points to a stark truth—that all female addicts of child-bearing potential are at risk of producing abnormal offspring if they use drugs. This issue will be revisited in connection with cocaine in chapter 11.

Treating Alcohol Addiction

Gaining solid information about how best to treat any addiction is beset with problems. In addition to the usual technical challenges in carrying out clinical trials, addicts are often poorly motivated and uncooperative, are not often amenable to long-term follow-up, and tend not to be truthful in self-reporting about abstinence. Thus, clinical trials on the treatment of addiction to alcohol (and other drugs) are difficult and controversial. One cannot simply assign patients randomly to different treatment modalities, as one would like to do in order to obtain valid comparisons. The reason is that most addicts have strong preconceptions about what treatment is best. Moreover, it would be ethically impermissible to deprive anyone of treatments thought to be beneficial merely in order to establish untreated controls against which to measure the effects of treatment. Adding to the difficulty, addicts tend to switch impulsively from one treatment to another, and from treatment to no treatment. And finally, complicating matters further, powerful political constituencies are committed single-mindedly to one approach—total absti-

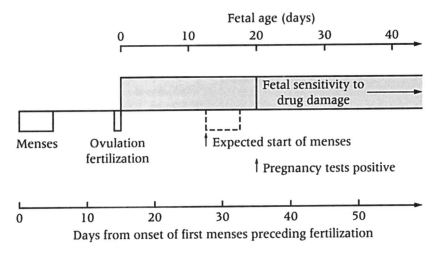

Fig. 9.1: Critical period for drug damage to the fetus, normal 28-day menstrual cycle. (From A. Goldstein, L. Aronow, S. M. Kalman: *Principles of Drug Action,* Harper & Row, New York, 1968, Fig. 12–3.)

nence through a 12-step program like that originated by Alcoholics Anonymous (AA). It is not surprising, given this situation, that there are no convincing experimental data to tell us which treatments are most effective.

Nevertheless, there is a shared impression among many professionals that 12-step programs are effective for many (if not most) alcohol addicts. The method rests on peer support, honest self-examination, self-accusation, confession, and acceptance of guidance by a "higher power." The only requirement for AA membership is a desire to stop drinking. These are the 12 steps, from the official AA manual:

1. We admitted we were powerless over alcohol—that our lives had become unmanageable.
2. Came to believe that a Power greater than ourselves could restore us to sanity.
3. Made a decision to turn our will and our lives over to the care of God as we understood Him.
4. Made a searching and fearless moral inventory of ourselves.
5. Admitted to God, to ourselves, and to another human being the exact nature of our wrongs.
6. Were entirely ready to have God remove all these defects of character.
7. Humbly asked Him to remove our shortcomings.

8. Made a list of all persons we had harmed, and became willing to make amends to them all.
9. Made direct amends to such people wherever possible, except when to do so would injure them or others.
10. Continued to take personal inventory and when we were wrong promptly admitted it.
11. Sought through prayer and meditation to improve our conscious contact with God as we understood Him, praying only for knowledge of His will for us and the power to carry that out.
12. Having had a spiritual awakening as the result of these steps, we tried to carry this message to alcoholics, and to practice these principles in all our affairs.

Step 12 may well be the most important one, for it makes every alcohol addict a member of a peer support group, reaching out to help others. Furthermore, central to the AA philosophy is the concept "once an addict always an addict," meaning that one can become a "recovering alcoholic" but never an "ex-alcoholic." Pithy slogans guide the progress of treatment. "One day at a time" addresses the addict's ambivalence about never being able to use alcohol again. "Easy does it" stresses that recovery from a drug addiction is a long process, requiring patience. "Keep it simple" puts the focus on not drinking, on attending meetings, and on reaching out to help other alcoholics. "First things first" is a reminder that staying sober has top priority. Usually rejected in the AA treatment plan is any pharmacotherapy at all, although it is by no means obvious why medications are incompatible with the AA approach. Indeed, some 12-step programs do advocate medications to aid in maintaining abstinence. Also rejected is the idea that controlled and moderate drinking may ever become possible. The tenets of 12-step programs are realistic and practical, and they are consistent with much of what we know about addiction. Moreover, motivation is strengthened by the evangelistic enthusiasm with which AA groups operate. Yet, as AA's approach to the treatment of alcohol addiction does not rest solidly on a scientific foundation, and does not subject itself to objective outcome testing, we cannot really assess its effectiveness.

Certain it is that many alcohol addicts have given up drinking through adherence to these programs. Certain it is, also, that many drop out, and that long-term abstinence rates are low; but relapses are accepted as part of the disease, and those who fall by the wayside are encouraged to become abstinent again. Despite the AA clarification that "God" is only a symbolic name for the "higher power," to which alcoholics may attach any meaning they wish, some cannot accept this religious aspect of the basic philosophy; and others find the regimentation and rituals unacceptable. The prime enemy of success, as in all drug addiction treatment, is ambivalence in the motivation to remain abstinent.

Disulfiram (Antabuse)

Disulfiram is a pharmacological agent that has been used widely and has had partial success in treating alcohol addiction. Its discovery, more than 50 years ago, illustrates how serendipity can lead to new pharmacotherapies. Disulfiram was an industrial chemical being tested as a possible medication to eradicate parasitic worms. In the course of trying it on themselves to assess its safety, two Danish pharmacologists noted that drinking alcoholic beverages made them ill. They recognized the possible value of this reaction for discouraging drinking, and they carried out extensive studies on the mechanism of action.

Alcohol is metabolized by two enzymes in the liver. The first, alcohol dehydrogenase, converts alcohol to acetaldehyde, which is extremely toxic. The second is acetaldehyde dehydrogenase, which converts the toxic acetaldehyde to harmless acetic acid. Ordinarily, acetaldehyde is changed to acetic acid almost as fast as it is formed, so very little accumulates even after heavy drinking. Disulfiram destroys the acetaldehyde dehydrogenase, so acetaldehyde does accumulate—but only if alcohol has been consumed. Thus, alcohol in the presence of disulfiram produces symptoms that mimic the "Oriental flush" (see chapter 7)—a reaction that is due to an inherited deficiency of the same enzyme.

If disulfiram is taken by mouth once daily, even a single drink will cause a dreadful aversive reaction. The face and other parts of the body become hot and flushed, and an intense throbbing headache develops, with nausea, vomiting, sweating, dizziness, and trouble breathing. In extreme cases, the blood supply to the heart is affected, the blood pressure collapses, and the patient goes into shock and may even die. The rationale for disulfiram use is that an addict who, in the sober state, is motivated to take it regularly will be unlikely to succumb to the craving for a drink, knowing (perhaps from one bad experience) what is bound to happen. Thus, we have the paradoxical criterion of therapeutic success—that the pharmacological effect of disulfiram should never be seen.

Experience has shown that alcohol addicts who take disulfiram regularly are able to maintain abstinence reasonably well. But compliance is a major problem. Those with poor motivation either discontinue entirely and relapse, or they skip disulfiram periodically, for several days at a time, in order to be able to drink with only minimal discomfort. It follows that intensive counseling, as well as methods of monitoring compliance objectively, is an absolute requirement in disulfiram treatment.

This is a drug with several limitations. It is not highly selective for acetaldehyde dehydrogenase; some drug-metabolizing enzymes are also destroyed, so that dosages of other medications become difficult to manage. Moreover, patients vary unpredictably (probably on a genetic basis) in their disulfiram dose requirement. A further significant limitation is that disulfiram is toxic to the liver—especially in the presence of liver disease, which many alcohol addicts have. Various other toxic effects probably reflect the poor selectivity for the acetaldehyde dehydrogenase. Finally, a constant danger is that an addict may impulsively indulge in a drinking binge, and suffer very serious consequences.

Studies of large numbers of alcohol addicts fail to show consistent efficacy in preventing relapses, primarily because of failure to take the medication regularly. The challenge for drug discovery is to develop a long-lasting, selective, nontoxic aldehyde dehydrogenase inhibitor or an effective delivery system for disulfiram itself. The challenge for the therapist is to find effective ways of encouraging compliance. In chapter 10, a similar compliance problem is discussed—how to get heroin addicts to take naltrexone as part of their treatment. In the stark choice between an addictive drug and a medication that effectively blocks the hedonic effects of that drug, the addict—by the very nature of the addiction—often makes the wrong choice.

Naltrexone

There is an interesting relationship between alcohol intake in free-choice experiments in mice or rats and the endogenous opioid systems. Low doses of opiates increase alcohol preference; strains of mice with naturally high endogenous opioid activity display high alcohol preference; and opioid antagonists tend to reduce alcohol consumption. Moreover, mice without mu opioid receptors ("knockouts," chapter 3) show a decreased preference for alcohol, as do animals treated with the specific opioid antagonists naloxone and naltrexone. The mechanism of these effects is not yet fully understood, but the findings indicate that the pleasurable and addictive effects of alcohol are somehow mediated by (or enhanced by) the mu opioid receptors. That the opioid system may play a central role in the workings of the dopamine reward pathway—whichever addictive drug stimulates it—is a major and unexpected finding of recent research. Thus, it was logical to test whether the opioid antagonist naltrexone might be useful in the treatment of alcohol addiction.

In double-blind placebo-controlled clinical trials, alcohol addicts, after becoming abstinent, were assigned randomly to receive daily naltrexone or placebo by mouth. In addition, both groups received supportive counseling that included behavioral training in methods of preventing a single lapse from leading to full-blown relapse. The trials were continued for three months with regular measures of alcohol consumption by Breathalyzer, by self-report, and by reports of family members. Craving was also measured, by self-report. As the subjects were given naltrexone (or placebo) pills to take at home, it was necessary to confirm that they actually took the pills. This was accomplished cleverly, in one study, by incorporating a fluorescent vitamin in the pill, so that a simple measurement of urine fluorescence would confirm that a subject had taken the medication.

The results of this first clinical trial were so encouraging that other researchers quickly replicated it, with the same favorable results. Naltrexone has no striking effect in preventing subjects from taking single drinks, but it is dramatically better than placebo in preventing single drinks from triggering binges. Most important, it reduces craving, it is safe, and it is acceptable to the subjects. However, naltrexone is not a miracle cure; it must be accompanied by intensive counseling. About one-quarter of the subjects on naltrexone did relapse during the first year, as compared with well over half of a placebo-treated group. Lack of compliance is the major stumbling block; a naltrexone implant to provide long-lasting protection has been developed recently.

Acamprosate

This is another anti-craving medication, like naltrexone in its effects on relapse in alcohol addicts. Animal studies showed its efficacy in reducing alcohol preference in laboratory animals. Extensive large-scale clinical trials of acamprosate in Europe have had very favorable outcomes, leading to widespread clinical use there. In one very large trial, a full year after a one-year course of treatment was completed, 39 percent of the subjects were still abstinent, compared with only 17 percent of those who received placebo.

Acamprosate is acetyl-homotaurine, a sulfur-containing amino acid somewhat related to GABA. Its mechanism of action is still virtually unknown; apparently it acts on excitatory NMDA type glutamate receptors. At the moment, it exemplifies an old practical principle of drug development—that if a drug works, it doesn't matter why it works. Indeed, before the modern era of molecular biology, most medications came into clinical use first, and their mechanisms of action were only clarified years later.

Summary

Alcohol is by far the most dangerous of the addictive drugs, both to users and to society. It interferes with judgment at the same time that it degrades performance. It causes a loss of normal restraint and inhibition, and it promotes aggressive behavior; thus, it is involved in most domestic violence, in fully half of all homicides, and in half of all traffic fatalities. Moreover, it is a legal commodity (except for children); and it is so available (to children, too!) that worldwide, more people use it, abuse it, and are addicted to it than to any other addictive drug (except possibly nicotine).

Probable targets of alcohol in the brain include the GABA, glycine, nicotinic acetylcholine, and NMDA receptors, but the molecular mechanisms of action remain controversial, and lively research continues. Of great interest is the recent unexpected finding of a close functional relationship in the dopamine reward pathway between alcohol and the endogenous opioid system.

Alcohol addicts suffer serious long-term—often fatal—damage to their body organs, as well as serious disruption of their social relationships and economic well-being. A special danger is the heavy use of alcohol during pregnancy, which can cause permanent brain damage to the unborn child (fetal alcohol syndrome).

Other drugs closely related to alcohol in their psychoactive effects and addiction liability include the benzodiazepines (such as Valium), barbiturates, and inhalants (volatile solvents). Of these, the most important from the standpoint of danger to health are the volatile solvents, used very widely and with dire consequences by children.

Even after moderate chronic use, withdrawal discomfort (as with other addictive drugs) drives the motivation to drink again. Sudden cessation of use after a long period of heavy drinking causes a very severe withdrawal syndrome, which may even be fatal unless treated properly.

Treatment of alcohol addiction—as of all addictions—is difficult, with relapse prevention the major challenge. Disulfiram (Antabuse) offers promise of relapse prevention, but it is potentially toxic, and compliance with the medication schedule is very unpredictable. Naltrexone and acamprosate are two new medications that seem to be useful in reducing craving and preventing relapses. Many alcohol addicts benefit from a drug-free environment and peer support, such as offered by 12-step programs; but here, too, compliance is a major problem.

10

Heroin, Morphine, and Other Opiates

A passage in *The Odyssey* faithfully captures the peculiar quality of the psychoactive effect of opiates. The scene is the palace of Menelaus, king of Sparta. Telemachus, depressed and miserable after his long and vain search for his father Odysseus, is being entertained at dinner. Then Helen, we are told,

> had a happy thought. Into the bowl in which their wine was mixed, she slipped a drug that had the power of robbing grief and anger of their sting and banishing all painful memories. No one who swallowed this dissolved in wine could shed a single tear that day, even for the death of his mother and father, or if they put his brother or his own son to the sword and he were there to see it done.

What Are Opiates?

This family of drugs includes morphine (the chief active component of crude opium from the opium poppy), heroin (a laboratory-produced derivative of morphine), and numerous potent synthetic morphinelike compounds used in medicine. These are powerful painkillers in the hands of physicians, and as the quotation above suggests, they dramatically relieve emotional as well as physical pain.

Heroin is a late nineteenth-century invention. Before the middle of the century, the addict ate or drank concoctions of raw opium. The introduction of the hypodermic needle and syringe into medical practice at the time of the Civil War allowed morphine to be injected under the skin or into a vein, flooding the bloodstream with the potent pure drug quickly and efficiently. During the last half of the century, many people—mostly middle-class housewives—were maintained on morphine by their physicians and became dependent. This practice probably represented an attempt to treat chronic anxiety, much in the way benzodiazepines like Valium are used today.

When morphine is injected under the skin or into a muscle, it reaches the brain slowly. Heroin floods the brain within seconds after injection into a vein; its chemical structure favors more rapid passage than morphine from blood into brain tissue. That heroin could produce a rapid spike of concentration in the brain made it attractive to a new class of addicts, who sought its euphoriant actions and self-administered it without medical supervision. Heroin quickly became the opiate of first choice for addicts everywhere, and nearly a million people in the United States are now addicted to it.

In recent years, with expansion of heroin production in many countries, and with competition forcing the price down, purer and purer heroin has become available on the street. Twenty-five years ago, street heroin was only about 3 percent pure, "cut" with sugar and other adulterants; today it can be nearly pure. This makes it possible to use heroin effectively by smoking or snorting. As a result, young people who would balk at intravenous use see these routes as less bizarre and more acceptable. Certainly, smoking is less risky than putting impure materials and possibly viruses or bacteria into a vein, but the addiction liability is the same.

How does a person typically progress from first use of an opiate to full-blown addiction? How can heroin addicts be treated most effectively? Is methadone a solution or is it part of the problem? This chapter addresses these questions, both by reviewing the research findings of others and by citing my own experiences treating heroin addicts with methadone.

Relief of Physical and Emotional Pain: "Keys of Paradise"

Even after thousands of years, morphine and its synthetic "look-alikes" are unexcelled for relief of severe physical pain. This characteristic makes them some of the most important drugs at the physician's disposal. Because of their remarkable calming effect on extreme stress and anxiety, they are also used routinely to prepare patients for the operating room. Millions of hospitalized patients have received opiates and have even become physically dependent on them while in the hospital, but after their discharge they almost never seek out opiates again. Thus, medically caused addiction is today truly a rarity, practically a myth. The reluctance of many physicians to use opiates at sufficient dosage and frequency to control pain is therefore unjustified. It is especially absurd for physicians to refuse opiates in sufficient dosage to patients suffering the pain of terminal cancer for fear of addicting them.

When self-administered intravenously, morphine (and even more effectively heroin) acts rapidly upon the brain to produce an intense feeling of sublime pleasure—a "rush," which is sometimes compared with orgasm. Then, as the initial drug spike declines, a second phase sets in—a peculiar dream state, an emotional disconnection from reality. If morphine or heroin is injected under the skin rather than intravenously, or if morphine is taken by mouth, the initial brain spike with its associated "rush" does not occur; instead, the predominant effect is the tranquil mood of the second phase.

In *The Man with the Golden Arm,* Nelson Algren describes the "rush":

> It hit all right. It hit the heart like a runaway locomotive, it hit like a falling wall. Frankie's whole body lifted with that smashing surge, the very heart seemed to lift up-up-up—then rolled over and he slipped into a long warm bath with one orgasmic sigh of relief. . . . All he had to do the rest of his life was to lie right here feeling better and better with every beat of his heart till he'd never felt so good in all his life.

Thomas De Quincey, in his classic *Confessions of an English Opium-Eater,* comments on the calming effect of smoking raw opium: "Thou has the keys of Paradise, oh just, subtle, and mighty opium!"

A carefully designed and meticulously executed experiment on intravenous self-administration of pure heroin by addict volunteers was carried out in a closed research ward. Standardized checklists were employed to follow mood changes. The result, in scientific prose, lacks the Romantic hyperbole of the literary descriptions, but makes the same point about the hedonic effects that follow the "rush." Subjects reported themselves significantly more carefree, relaxed, calm, elated, clear, and "stoned."

I have asked many addicts to recollect and describe for me their first experience with heroin, which usually occurred during adolescence. They tried to explain what the feeling was like—an overwhelming sensation of otherworldly bliss—but words seemed inadequate. All of them, at the time, had known perfectly well the dangers of addiction but succumbed to curiosity (often after urging by friends), rationalizing that although others might become addicted, they would not. But you cannot just try heroin, the way you might try a new breakfast cereal from the supermarket. Someone who is experienced has to teach you the ropes: how and where to buy it, how to dissolve it over a flame in a bent spoon, how to filter it through cotton, how to acquire the syringe and needle. You have to be taught how much to use, an uncertain business because of the unknown strength of the powder you have bought. You have to be shown how to use a tourniquet to make a vein stand out, how to slip the needle into the vein and draw back blood to make sure it is in the vein, how to release the tourniquet, how to inject, and how fast. In other words, heroin use necessarily starts out as a very social affair with its own special rituals and techniques.

The first injection of heroin usually provokes nausea and vomiting (as happens also with the first cigarette or the first drink), but your friend will assure you that this side effect disappears with subsequent injections. One might imagine that if something makes you sick, you would avoid it in the future. Not so with heroin. The drug's effect suppresses the emotional distaste of the nausea and vomiting. Many addicts have told me: "You don't mind puking behind heroin!"

The idea of "just trying it once" is readily set aside when the second opportunity arises, perhaps the next weekend. After using heroin weekly for a while, with the unpleasant consequences no longer occurring, you somehow find yourself taking a "fix" in the middle of the week. Gradually the intervals become shorter, leading to tolerance and dependence, as described in chapter 6, and soon you are using daily. One morning you awaken with what seems to be a cold—running nose, a slight feeling of chilliness. You mention it to a friend, who says: "That's no cold. Try some heroin and see how fast it goes away. You're hooked!"

Once you have learned what a mild case of opiate withdrawal is like, and how dramatically it is abolished by heroin, you begin to crave heroin intensely at the very mildest feeling of "being sick." Gradually, as the weeks go by, you find yourself needing more and more heroin to relieve the sickness and to achieve that marvelous feeling of satisfaction. Eventually you become fully addicted. Now you are using heroin three or four times a day, and the cost of each dose, which was originally a reasonable few dollars, has escalated to many times that amount. You have to spend more and more of your time between injections just finding a supply. As a result, you may have trouble holding down your job; but even if you manage that, heroin may be eating up more and more of your income. Unless you are extremely wealthy, you may very well be tempted by the kinds of illegal activity that will raise money quickly—prostitution, theft, robbery, embezzlement, and so on.

The process has to end. Either you are caught and begin a long relationship with the criminal-justice system, or you decide to quit your habit before you are caught. In either case, you have to be detoxified; your system has to rid itself of the opiate. This can be done "cold turkey," but that requires a kind of discipline and perseverance not often found among addicts. Withdrawal never kills, but it is extremely uncomfortable, something like a very severe case of the flu. And all the while you know that there is an instantaneous cure for the discomfort (heroin, of course!), so you are very likely to give up the attempt to detoxify. It is universally recognized that detoxification on an ambulatory, outpatient basis—even though the worst of the withdrawal discomfort can be relieved by medicinal means—nearly always ends in relapse to heroin use even before the planned 10-day or 21-day detoxification program is completed.

There is an alternative and more effective way to become drug-free—the "half-way house," a disciplined and closed residential therapeutic community in which drugs are not available. The addict who spends enough time (typically at least six months) in such a facility, can become drug-free while there, at the same time receiving the many rehabilitative services that are needed to reconstruct a normal life. Unfortunately, this method is not acceptable to most addicts (so the dropout rate is generally at least 75 percent of all admissions), it is quite expensive, and it remains unclear what proportion of those who are "cured" remain abstinent (and for how long) after they return to the larger community.

The Opioid Receptors

The three subtypes of opioid receptor—mu, delta, and kappa—are widely distributed, not only in brain but in almost every organ system of the body. In the nervous system, they are not confined to the brain and spinal cord, but are found even at the endings of sensory nerves—out in the fingertips, one might say. Pain relief by morphine was long thought to involve only brain sites but was later found to be mediated also at several levels of the spinal cord, and by opioid receptors in the sensory nerves. In surgery of the knee, for example, morphine injected directly into the knee joint is effective for pain control without reaching the brain at all.

The opioid receptors and their functions have been studied extensively (see chapter 3). We know how they inhibit the release of neurotransmitters from many kinds of nerve endings. We know how, in the dopaminergic reward pathway, they stimulate dopamine release by suppressing the ongoing inhibition of dopamine neurons. The pleasurable effects are due chiefly to the mu subtype in the brain. Animals that are born without mu receptors ("genetic knockouts") will not self-administer morphine, nor does morphine relieve them of experimentally produced pain.

Although at low doses morphine acts chiefly on the mu receptor, higher doses interact with the other subtypes. Activation of kappa opioid receptors produces generally opposite (aversive) effects. Delta receptors seem to be involved in regulation of breathing, blood pressure, and similar automatic processes. Thus, the effects of morphine and other opiates can be extremely complex.

Much useful information has been obtained recently about how an agonist ligand like morphine binds and "turns on" a receptor whereas an antagonist (like naltrexone, see below) binds but does not. As the opioid receptors have all been cloned, their fine structure can be modified by mutating single amino acids, in order to study in fine detail how opioid ligands interact—both endogenous peptides and compact molecules like morphine. Recent findings indicate that different opioid receptor subtypes may combine—mu and delta, for example—to yield a mixed dual receptor with somewhat different properties than either of its separate components.

Naltrexone: A Medication That Is Too Good?

In previous chapters, I described the opiate antagonists naloxone (Narcan) and naltrexone (Trexan). Both are extraordinarily effective and potent in blocking the opioid receptors, both are remarkably nontoxic, and both are useful in treatment, albeit for different purposes. Naloxone cannot be given by mouth because it would be carried in the bloodstream directly to the liver, where it is rapidly destroyed. Its main therapeutic value is for resuscitating victims of heroin overdose. In that application it is the most dramatic antidote known to medicine, instantaneously restoring life to people already at death's door.

In contrast to naloxone, naltrexone is effective by mouth. Pretreatment with it (chapter 4) can completely abolish the effect of a subsequent intravenous injection of heroin. Taken by mouth, naltrexone lasts a few days. This means that if a person drinks a naltrexone solution a few times a week, that person is very unlikely to use heroin; heroin would be pointless, a waste of money. Like many technologic advances, this one breaks down in the face of human behavior. An adequate dose of naltrexone is, indeed, 100 percent effective in blocking the hedonic effect of heroin. Therefore, it could be completely effective in preventing heroin use. Too effective, perhaps! Faced with the stark choice between naltrexone and heroin, most addicts give up the naltrexone and revert to heroin use. As with medications used to prevent relapse to drinking in alcohol addicts, compliance is the main problem. However, in addition to the desire for the heroin "high" there may be another reason: Studies have shown a subtle but measurable dysphoric effect of naltrexone, even in normal volunteers. This is presumably due to blockade of the endogenous opioids that mediate normal feelings of well-being. In people who are very strongly motivated to remain abstinent, naltrexone has nevertheless proved extremely effective; the typical example of such a favorable result is in an addicted physician, nurse, or pharmacist, whose continued licensure is contingent on complete abstinence from opiates.

Methadone Maintenance

For 40 years prior to the 1960s, addiction had been wholly the concern of law-enforcement officials. Physicians had been frightened away from treating addicts by sanctions dating back to the time when opiates were first brought under legal control by the Harrison Act of 1914. Of course, physicians were permitted to use morphine for pain control, but they were expressly forbidden from giving an opiate to an addict for the purpose of maintaining the addiction. Physicians who violated the regulation risked losing their medical license and facing criminal charges. Heroin addicts were regarded as nothing more than manipulative schemers, criminal sociopaths who had to be locked up to protect society from their predations. Just after World War I, clinics had been opened in some parts of the country to give addicts morphine, on the pragmatic grounds that if they would not give up their habits, they could at least avoid whatever criminal activities they were carrying out to obtain the drug. These clinics were all shut down by federal government authorities.

In the 1960s, in New York, Marie Nyswander (a psychiatrist) teamed up with Vincent Dole (a biochemist) to develop a novel approach to treating heroin addicts. They wondered at the addicts' compulsive, seemingly irrational, irrepressible drive to obtain and use heroin, even in the face of grave health risks and repeated incarcerations. Addicts behaved, they speculated, as though they had a real physical need for heroin. Was it possible that their bodies actually needed an opiate to function properly? This heretical hypothesis—that heroin addiction is a "metabolic disease"—suggested that addicts might improve if they were maintained and stabilized on a long-acting opiate taken by mouth. Such an opiate—methadone—had been studied at the U.S. Public Health Service narcotics hospital in Lexington, Kentucky. Methadone had been developed during World War II in Germany to replace morphine, the supply of opium from abroad having been cut off. Methadone was active by mouth, its pain-relieving action was like that of morphine, and a single oral dose lasted nearly 24 hours. Moreover, it was not toxic to any body organs, even on prolonged use, provided reasonable dosages were not exceeded.

What was discovered in those first trials in New York has been substantially borne out with hundreds of thousands of heroin addicts all over the world. Dole and Nyswander reported that after stabilization on a sufficient daily dose of methadone, the addicts stopped their frantic search for heroin, seemed to be normalized physically and psychologically, and began to accept rehabilitative services leading to honest employment and reintegration into family life and the community. Over the decades since then, the safety and efficacy of long-term methadone maintenance has been established. All indicators of general health improve, and abnormalities of body systems (for instance of the hormones) tend to normalize. Most important is the fact that methadone maintenance has no adverse effects on cognitive or psychomotor function, performance of skilled tasks, or memory. Indeed, if former addicts maintained on methadone are in the same room as nonaddicts, no observer or psychologic test can pick them out. Court judgments have established in law that methadone patients may not be barred, solely because of taking methadone, from any kind of employment, including—in one famous case—driving a New York subway train.

In 1969 I established the first major methadone maintenance program in California. This was based in San Jose, a city of half a million at the time, about 50 miles from San Francisco. My purpose was twofold. First, I wanted to confirm what was being claimed about methadone in New York, and to study certain aspects of the use of this drug under rigorously controlled conditions. Second, I saw an opportunity to offer needed help to addicts, who were being hounded and harassed in California as they had been in New York and elsewhere. My colleagues and I had no idea, at the outset, how many heroin addicts there actually were in San Jose and its vicinity. We soon discovered how to find out. By opening a methadone clinic under conditions the addicts would regard as safe, by offering them respect and anonymity, and by making it clear that our aim was to treat rather than harass, we quickly found that a great many, who previously had concealed their addiction, would make themselves known by registering for the program.

Planning and carrying out research in the community and on the streets is far more difficult than doing research in the laboratory. Before we could open the first clinic, my colleagues and I had to enlist the cooperation of the police—the very police whose previous experience with addicts was in a never-ending cops-and-robbers game. Unless the police stayed away from the clinic, we realized, the addicts would not risk attending. Before we could deal with the police, we had to establish a solid citizen support group, an effort that required extensive educational efforts, inasmuch as methadone maintenance was still a novel idea. We also had to get the support of the county mental health center as the official agency that would operate the clinic. And that, in turn, meant convincing the county commissioners and the city council of the expected benefits, especially the likelihood that property crime could be reduced, as the New York experience suggested.

Rigorous clinical research has to be conducted within an ethical framework. Informed consent of the subjects is always required. If a treatment is known to be efficacious (as experience in Chicago by then, as well as in New York, indicated), it may not be denied. It would have been impermissible, for example, to have an untreated control group while another group was being given methadone. On the other hand, as optimal dosage was at that time unknown, blind comparisons of different dosages were appropriate.

A special requirement for conducting rigorous research on addicts in a therapeutic setting is to train the treatment staff to comply with research protocols. In the laboratory this problem does not arise because the students, research fellows, and technicians who carry out the work have an educational background in the natural sciences and expect to apply their skills to the research at hand. In contrast, the staff in treatment programs are nurses and counselors, who usually have little or no training in scientific methodology and no prior research experience. Moreover, their primary commitment, quite appropriately, is to the welfare of their patients. Therefore, unless they understand the ethical justification for the research and its ultimate benefit to addicts, they are unlikely to insist on the prescribed research procedures, especially if patients object. Moreover, addicts tend to identify those in charge of the research with officialdom, whose edicts and demands they are expert at evading. The only solution to this problem—though I have never seen it work perfectly—is to create an atmosphere in the clinic that commands the respect and confidence of the patients. Insisting on following protocol, and enforcing that even to the point of discharging a recalcitrant patient or staff member, is effective in commanding the respect of the patient group as a whole. In short, clinic personnel must avoid being manipulated—and this rule applies to all addiction treatment, whether or not it includes a research component.

We implemented strict protocols for random urine testing. The primary purpose of methadone maintenance is to reduce, and if possible eliminate, the use of heroin. Therefore, the only objective measure of success is the presence or absence of morphine (to which the body converts heroin) in the urine. Some methadone programs expel or otherwise penalize patients with "dirty" (i.e., morphine-positive) urine—a curious way to react to a treatment failure. However, even in programs that operate on a more helpful philosophy, patients devise the most amazing ways to cheat on a urine test. The incentive to cheat is always present if a condition of parole or probation is never to use heroin. And even in a research program without penalties, cheating may occur simply because it has become a way of life. A simple way to cheat is to drink so much water or beer before coming to the clinic, that the morphine in urine is too dilute to detect. Another way to cheat is to carry someone else's urine. The only way to avoid being fooled, in the early days, was for a counselor to observe, carefully and directly, the act of urination. But that is an invasion of privacy of a most demeaning kind; and even so, the clever patient who wishes to cheat can easily embarrass the staff monitor into turning away.

The whole situation troubled me, so I devised a better system of urine collection. We established a pass-through window with a sliding shutter between the lavatory and the dispensing station, where a nurse was always on duty. Freshly voided urine is at body temperature. Body temperatures do vary somewhat among people, so we first measured hundreds of samples to establish the range of temperatures of freshly voided urine. We also noted the rate of cooling in standard containers. We were then in a good position to assess whether a urine specimen had come directly from a subject's bladder. Someone else's urine strapped to the thigh (for example) was never warm enough. Heating a cold sample with a cigarette lighter usually made it too hot. Of course, the system was not unbeatable, but it gave us reasonable assurance of the validity of the urine tests while preserving the dignity of our patients.

Knowing that a urine specimen was genuine, we next needed an immediate method of determining whether morphine was present. Denial is typical; and a patient cannot be helped if he or she is not facing reality, right there, on the spot. Unfortunately, the existing method of testing, called thin-layer chromatography, had to be carried out in a chemical laboratory, and it usually took about a week to get a result back. Thus, although urine tests were still useful in documenting the efficacy of the program, the loss of immediacy compromised their therapeutic value. A way was needed to get a test result instantaneously, right at the clinic, in order to confront patients then and there about their use of heroin. I devised a way to do this, based on the principle of immunoassay (chapter 3). However, as immunoassay was then practiced, it required measuring a radioactive ligand bound to an antibody. That, in turn, required separating the bound ligand from the free (unbound) ligand, usually by means of a centrifuge. For obtaining an instantaneous result, such manipulations would be unacceptably slow.

A free radical is a molecule that has an extra electron, which can be detected in a device known as an electron spin resonance (ESR) spectrometer. The method I invented for instantaneous detection of morphine in urine works like this: When morphine labeled with a free radical is bound to an antibody, the ESR spectrometer shows very little. If unlabeled morphine is added, as in a "dirty" urine specimen, the labeled morphine is displaced from the antibody on the principle of competition. That labeled morphine, no longer bound to the bulky antibody molecule, is now able to spin freely and rapidly in the solution, giving an immediate signal in the instrument. The new method was all one could hope for. A drop of urine added to a tiny tube containing free-radical morphine, bound to the antibody, gave the answer—reliably, in a few seconds. This was one of the first homogeneous immunoassays—assays that do not require physical separation of free ligand from bound.

Unfortunately, an ESR spectrometer is a very large and costly machine—out of the question for low-budget methadone clinics. Luckily, the method was superseded by a cheap and efficient homogeneous immunoassay based on color development by an enzyme; that new method (called EMIT) came into widespread use in clinics everywhere. But there is an interesting twist to the story of the free-radical test. Heroin use had become a major problem for our troops in Vietnam. To avoid returning actively addicted soldiers to the United States, the Army wanted to detoxify them first; but that required a quick and reliable method of identifying heroin users. Within a few days of the authorities hearing about my instantaneous detection method, ESR spectrometers were on their way to Vietnam. For the Department of Defense, needless to add, the cost was of no concern!

To find out what dosage of methadone was appropriate for treating heroin addicts, we undertook double-blind experimental comparisons of different dosages. Patients could report whether the methadone "held them" for the full 24-hour period, or whether they felt the early symptoms of withdrawal when they came for their morning dose. These studies and several like them elsewhere established that the proper dosage of methadone for most patients is at least 60 to 80 milligrams daily. Occasionally, more or less is needed. But addicts tend to view themselves as great experts on drugs; so to avoid being misled by their often inaccurate beliefs, double-blind design is critically important in studies of this kind. Fortunately, there is no great danger in exceeding a dosage of 80 milligrams, as tolerance will develop anyway; and it has been shown that some people metabolize methadone unusually rapidly, so they actually do need more. On the other hand, too low a dosage—as with any medication—is always disastrous. State or federal regulatory authorities have sometimes interfered inappropriately with the practice of medicine by decreeing a maximum dosage—sometimes as low as 40 milligrams. Then the patient may be at the very edge of withdrawal, methadone fails to suppress the craving for heroin, and the program is doomed to failure. It is noteworthy that outcome studies conducted under government auspices have consistently shown that the programs with the poorest results are those that mandate the lowest doses.

Later in the 1970s we tested an improved long-acting methadone, called LAAM. Taken by mouth, like methadone, this opiate lasts for up to 72 hours. We found that patients who had previous experience with methadone uniformly preferred LAAM because—they said—it made them feel more stabilized. As LAAM was not yet approved for general use, but only as an experimental drug, we conducted extensive toxicity studies on over 100 subjects and found no untoward effects. Our conclusion, at the end of these studies in 1979, was that LAAM was safe and efficacious and ought to replace methadone for routine use, while methadone should be kept available as an alternative for any patients who might react adversely to LAAM. We tested LAAM in a couple of hundred patients; and altogether, throughout the country, LAAM was given to over 4,000 patients in carefully monitored trials, and the same conclusion was reached. However, LAAM had no patent protection, and no pharmaceutical company saw sufficient profit motive to bring it through the elaborate minefield of FDA requirements to final approval. The National Institute on Drug Abuse took up the project but, as happens so often with government agencies, ran into bureaucratic obstacles again and again. Finally, after years of effort, LAAM was approved and brought to market for the maintenance treatment of heroin addiction.

An important advantage of LAAM over methadone is that because it need be taken only three times weekly, pressure for "take-home" doses can be resisted fairly easily. With methadone, the need to come to a clinic every day to drink a solution of the drug made it impractical for many addicts to lead normal lives and hold down regular jobs. Consequently, the practice of "take-home" medication began. Most patients handled this responsibly, but some did not. An ordinary dose, to which the patient has developed tolerance during the induction phase of treatment, is lethal for a nontolerant person. There were even instances of children being killed by a "take-home" dose. Furthermore, there has always been, and continues to be, insufficient funding to offer treatment to all addicts who want it. Consequently, "take-home" methadone was sometimes divided, and part of it sold on the street as a means of preventing withdrawal during an untreated addict's frenetic hunt for heroin. In summary, LAAM offers benefits to society as well as to the addict being treated.

This is a good place to clear up the chief misunderstanding about methadone or LAAM—that they are "just addictive opiates, just heroin substitutes." This is pharmacological nonsense; methadone and LAAM are not heroin substitutes at all, because they do not provide the main hedonic effect of heroin that is sought by the addict. Let me explain. Yes, it is true that methadone occupies the same mu opioid receptors as do morphine and 6-acetylmorphine, the two active products of heroin in the brain. But the essence of heroin's action, as described above, is the spiking "high," the "rush." And this simply does not occur when the same receptors are occupied in a continuous and stable manner. It is this stabilizing effect of methadone (and even more so of LAAM) on brain chemistry that makes them therapeutic for addicts, that prevents the destructive cycle of "high" and "sick" that drives the addict's compulsive use of heroin. To watch this change take place in a new patient, day after day, as the methadone or LAAM dosage is raised into an effective range is a rewarding experience for physicians, nurses, and counselors.

A newly approved medication for maintenance treatment of heroin addicts is buprenorphine, closely related to morphine in its chemical structure. This is an unusual opiate, which combines agonist and antagonist properties in an interesting way, and is very potent. It blocks heroin effectively, while at the same time it offers the kind of stable satisfaction produced by methadone or LAAM. Its potency makes it possible to administer the small required dose in a sublingual tablet once every day or two. One tablet formulation cleverly takes advantage of a difference in absorption between buprenorphine and naloxone. The combination with naloxone in the same tablet, prevents its unauthorized intravenous use; naloxone is ineffective by mouth but precipitates a withdrawal syndrome if used by vein in a person dependent on heroin. Another unusual feature of this medication is that it reduces cocaine use as well as heroin use in patients with dual dependence on both drugs. It is too soon to predict what niche it will occupy in the armamentarium of treatments for heroin addiction.

Long-term Results of Methadone Maintenance

In the remainder of this chapter, I shall not mention LAAM specifically; everything I say about methadone applies equally to LAAM. People often ask if methadone "works." To answer that question we need a more precise definition of efficacy; what should we measure to find out if it works? The simple definition given earlier was that during methadone maintenance, the use of heroin is discontinued or at least greatly reduced. That favorable outcome can be expected only if the dosage is adequate and the clinic environment offers additional support. That means practical counseling about job training and employment, about relating appropriately to the criminal-justice system, about family problems, and about other aspects of daily living.

A different criterion of success has also been proposed—that addicts be able to get off methadone and lead drug-free lives without it. I find this criterion destructive because it promotes premature attempts at abstinence. It is noteworthy that the need for lifelong treatment with a drug is not questioned for diseases like diabetes or schizophrenia. So in principle, from the medical standpoint, nothing would be wrong with lifelong methadone maintenance, if it is necessary for a patient's well-being. According to the "metabolic disease" hypothesis, addicts might actually have some kind of physiological need for an opiate in order to function normally. And in earlier chapters I discussed recent advances in neurochemistry that suggest a possible basis for such a view. It is certainly conceivable that addicts—either on a genetic basis or as a consequence of chronic insult to their brains by heroin—actually have a deficiency in their endogenous opioid (endorphin) systems. If this is ever proved to be true, the arguments against lifelong methadone maintenance ought to subside. In the meantime, we have to adopt an agnostic position on this issue while we resist pressure to terminate methadone maintenance prematurely.

Patients themselves, though ill-advised, try to reduce their dosage and repeatedly discontinue treatment, thus defeating the whole purpose of stabilization, which is the key to the beneficial effect of methadone maintenance. A common pattern is for a patient to manage for a while without methadone but then to relapse to heroin use and return to methadone treatment. I recall one such case that was truly dramatic. A San Jose man—let's call him Joe Campbell—had a history of years of heroin addiction and difficulties with the law. On methadone maintenance, he was able to discontinue heroin completely. To remove himself from the influence of old associates who were still active addicts, he moved to Detroit, where he knew no one. Finding a good job in the automobile industry, he led a stereotypic middle-class life. He fell in love, married, bought a little house and a new car, started a family. Life seemed perfect—for all of four years. Then one day, on his way home from work, he met an old friend from San Jose. "I've got some good stuff in my room," the man volunteered, "come and have a taste." Campbell refused, but the "friend" pressed him, arguing that "one fix for old times' sake" could do no harm. Of course, that one injection soon led to another, and another. Within a few months, Campbell had lost job, home, car, and wife. A broken man, he returned to methadone maintenance.

The story of Joe Campbell is typical of what can and often does happen. His behavior seems so irrational, it defies our understanding. It shows the extreme vulnerability of former addicts to relapse; and this is true regardless of which drug is the culprit. It also tells us that some ex-addicts can indeed function well for varying periods after quitting methadone maintenance, but that we must always be ready to reinstate them in a methadone program—quickly, without question, and without red tape—if they relapse.

Anecdotes are not data. What about systematic studies to find out what eventually happens to heroin addicts who enter a methadone program? How many continue to do poorly and end up dead or in prison? How many change their lifestyles and give up heroin, whether or not they remain in methadone treatment? How long do favorable results last? How frequent is relapse? Follow-up studies on heroin addicts are extraordinarily difficult and expensive to carry out, but several have been done. In general, researchers find some kind of treatment is always better than no treatment; but a skeptical interpretation would be that this is because people who are better motivated, who are more likely to succeed anyway, are just the ones who choose to enter treatment. Results are quite similar regardless of the treatment modality—methadone or a drug-free residential program; but this may only mean that different people require different approaches, and they all choose what suits them best. A global summary of all outcome studies, including our own five-year follow-up in San Jose, might go something like this: About one-third do very poorly, continue illegal activities, often drink heavily, and end up either dead or in prison. Another one-third do well periodically, then relapse, and spend many years—perhaps their whole lifetimes—on and off methadone maintenance. The final one-third become truly rehabilitated, put heroin and other drugs behind them (although many continue taking methadone), and become upright citizens in their community. There is no known way to predict at the outset which group a person will fall into.

At the Foot of Sandia

Sandia at sunset is one of the most beautiful sights in the world. The red glow turns the mountain into a huge open watermelon—its name means "watermelon" in Spanish. Here in the New Mexico desert, everything is so incredibly vast, it is hard to get one's bearings. The blue sky seems endless, with scattered puffy white clouds, and you can see for hundreds of miles. Then, as you adjust your vision to put things into a human scale of dimensions, your gaze shifts down from Sandia's crest to the sprawling city at its foot. Albuquerque, once a mere stop on the railroad, is now a city spreading over the desert floor, across the Rio Grande, and onto the western side of the river.

Shortly after starting the methadone maintenance program in San Jose, I was asked by colleagues in Albuquerque to come and advise them on starting a methadone program there. Just as the availability of methadone treatment brought a thousand heroin addicts out of the woodwork (so to speak) in San Jose, the same thing happened in New Mexico. Within three years, more than a thousand addicts had registered for methadone in this city, which at that time had a population of 300,000. What eventually became of them? A long-term follow-up would be impractical nowadays in most places; the extreme mobility of American urban society would make it very difficult to find people. But Albuquerque is different. It is isolated in the vastness of the New Mexico desert. It has a large Hispanic population with a strong network of extended families. Its people tend to stay; and if they do leave, they tend to return. It seemed possible to track those first thousand methadone patients, to find out how many were still (or again) on methadone, how many were dead (and why), how many were in prison (and why), how many were still (or again) actively using heroin, and how many had been integrated into normal society and were no longer drug addicts at all.

Some of the methodological pitfalls are worth describing. My aim was to track down the first thousand addicts who entered treatment in 1969, 1970, and 1971. The first task, of course, was to find out who they were. The original treatment records had long since been lost or placed in archival storage; just finding them took a year and a half. I felt like a sleuth rather than a medical researcher as my helpers and I rummaged through the University of New Mexico archives. Let me give a few small examples of the kinds of special difficulty one runs into in tracking heroin addicts. The straightforward method of tracking by names is unreliable because aliases are so common among a group in constant trouble with the law. Date of birth, a customary means of identification, also proved unreliable rather often: a person would give dates that differed by a day or a month or a year on different occasions. Fortunately, those who registered for treatment 22 years before were assigned sequential numbers from 1 to 1,000, so we at least knew when a number was missing from our list. Eventually, we attached a name to all but six of the sequential numbers, and the real tracking could begin.

Of the original thousand, we were able to account for 77 percent. Fifty-six percent of these were alive, of whom we interviewed more than half. Six percent were in prison. Forty-four percent of those found (one-third of the original number) were dead; and the most frequent causes of death (according to death certificates) were violence, drug overdose, and alcoholic liver disease. Considering that the average age of this group 22 years earlier was only 26, this is an amazingly high death rate. It illustrates strikingly the life-threatening quality of heroin addiction and of the associated circumstances of life (including alcoholism) for so many heroin addicts.

Nearly one-half of the original thousand appeared on the records of the probation and parole office—and half of those had committed significant crimes of violence or property crimes more than five years after their initial entry into treatment. Many continued to be regular clients of the criminal-justice system, on and off supervision, in and out of prison.

An honest assessment of this record tells us how difficult a disease this is to treat. A substantial fraction—at least one-quarter—continued on methadone maintenance at one time or another during the final five years of the study, more than 17 years after their initial entry into treatment. There is no doubt, therefore, that opiate dependence, whether on heroin or on methadone, is a lifelong condition for a considerable fraction of the addict population. The good news—and the most important finding—was that most people we were able to locate and interview did best, from any point of view, during periods on methadone maintenance. One can easily think of other chronic diseases (rheumatoid arthritis is an example) in which no cure is known, and treatment success has to be measured by small improvements. Often it is those who comply conscientiously with treatment requirements who enjoy the best long-term success.

What about the 23 percent of the original Albuquerque group, whom we were unable to locate? Have they done well or poorly? Here we encounter a general methodological problem in addiction treatment follow-up: The people with the poorest outcomes are naturally easiest to find, as indicated in the three categories just listed. The ones with the best outcomes are hardest to find; the ethics of confidentiality prevent one from tracing such people by the most effective methods, such as inquiries of their families, friends, and associates. Ex-addicts who have been off methadone and drug-free for years, who are well integrated into the community, who have become respected citizens, do not wish to be tracked and found. They wisely want nothing to do with the drug scene. Their present acquaintances—even close members of their families—may not have any inkling of their heroin-addict history.

Thus, the outcome of such a follow-up is necessarily biased in an unfavorable direction. Despite our best efforts, we cannot put a reliable number on the probability that a heroin addict in Albuquerque in 1970 would be an abstinent ex-addict 22 years later. However, we do know, for certain, that there are former addicts who, whether or not still on methadone, have put illicit use of addictive drugs behind them. The experience of one of them—let's call him Michael Romero—makes a hopeful ending to this chapter.

At the age of 32, a typical unemployed street addict, Romero registered for methadone maintenance in 1970. At first, his sights were set on becoming drug-free without methadone, but it never worked. Whenever he was getting methadone, he stopped using heroin completely. Whenever he quit methadone, he found himself using heroin again. After two years of this, he took stock and made a decision that determined his future and probably saved his life. As he explained: "My life didn't seem to be going anywhere without methadone. Why couldn't I just look at methadone as my own insulin, and stop trying to live without it?" Twenty-two years later, Romero owns his own business, a machine shop, in a small town about 75 miles from Albuquerque. His annual personal income is about $50,000. He is a prominent citizen in his community. He has a wife and three children, the eldest of whom is attending university. Once every two weeks he drives 75 miles to Albuquerque to pick up 13 daily doses of methadone, drink one dose, and leave a urine sample. At the time of our interview, he had not touched heroin for nearly 20 years. Few of his friends or associates know that he was ever a heroin addict or that he now takes a dose of methadone every day.

Summary

This chapter describes the main features of heroin addiction—how it begins, how it progresses, and how it can be treated. It documents that this addiction is a chronic and often lethal brain disease. It is exceedingly difficult to treat, and success is unpredictable and often only partial.

The most effective treatment is long-term maintenance on methadone or LAAM (and possibly buprenorphine). The criterion of treatment success is cessation of heroin use, making physical and social rehabilitation possible. Some addicts do achieve eventual long-term abstinence without continuous pharmacotherapy and without relapse, but that should certainly not be a primary goal of treatment.

Methadone and LAAM are not heroin substitutes; they are medications that occupy mu opioid receptors in a nearly continuous fashion, thus stabilizing the chaotic fluctuations in neurochemistry that are induced by heroin. It does not produce the "rush" or other hedonic effects that addicts seek in heroin.

Naltrexone is an effective antagonist, and it blocks the pleasurable effects of heroin, but it is not acceptable to most addicts. Buprenorphine is the newest addition to the armamentarium of treatments for heroin addiction.

11

Cocaine and

Amphetamines

"They give all that they possess, in order to indulge their mad craving," wrote the German physician and medical researcher Louis Lewin in 1887 about cocaine addicts. That comment is just as apt for cocaine users today as it was a century ago, and is true of amphetamine addicts as well. Chapter 4 described how monkeys, given free access to cocaine, self-administer it to the exclusion of all other activities until they reach a state of sleepless exhaustion and die in a couple of weeks. One sees the same frantic, compulsive behavior in cocaine addicts on a binge, the chief difference being that their supply of cocaine is usually (but not always) exhausted before they can kill themselves.

The Most Powerful Stimulants

Amphetamines were the stimulants of choice from the 1930s, when they were first synthesized and introduced into medical use. This is a class of drugs containing many synthetic compounds that are chemically similar and share the same mechanism of action. Included are amphetamine itself (formerly allowed in inhalers and other over-the-counter cold medications), methamphetamine ("speed," "crank," "crystal"), methylphenidate (Ritalin), and a pure form of methamphetamine ("ice") that can be smoked. Epidemics of intravenous amphetamine use raged in Japan after World War II, and in Sweden and America during the sixties and seventies. The pharmacological actions of the amphetamines are very similar to those of cocaine, though not identical in all respects. Amphetamines, like cocaine, act on the reward pathways to increase dopamine in the synapses (see chapter 4); whereas cocaine does this primarily by blocking its reuptake into the neurons, amphetamines also stimulate dopamine release at nerve endings. Drug discrimination experiments show that experienced human subjects cannot distinguish amphetamines from cocaine, as found also with animals.

Cocaine is a natural substance found in coca leaves. In the nineteenth century, the active principle, cocaine, was purified and its chemical structure identified. It is a compact molecule of complex structure, well suited to be the ligand of a specific receptor. The coca leaf has for centuries been chewed by natives in the Andes highlands. It was believed to prevent fatigue and to increase energy for laborious physical labor. No doubt its stimulant effects produced a subjective impression of enhanced work capacity, but careful experiments have failed to confirm such an effect objectively in the absence of fatigue. Like caffeine (chapter 13), cocaine does reverse impairments of performance caused by fatigue.

Chewing coca leaves produces effects that are quite different from the "rush" and "high" obtained from cocaine by snorting, smoking, or intravenous use. The contrast between chewing tobacco and cigarettes is analogous. It had been thought that absorption of cocaine from the mouth was poor, but this is not the case. As with other addictive drugs, it is a question of slow and steady brain levels as compared with repetitive spiking ones. Some of the same people, moving to Lima after years of coca chewing in the mountains, start using pure cocaine, intravenously or by snorting, and lose control very quickly as they become typical urban cocaine addicts.

Cocaine was early found to be a powerful local anesthetic, especially for numbing the mucous membranes of the nose, throat, and eyes. Thus it found a legitimate use in medicine, but its mood-altering effects did not escape attention. A leading exponent of the recreational use of cocaine was Sigmund Freud, who denied it was addictive. Lewin's years of research, documenting the powerful grip of cocaine on users, helped to counter Freud's misconceptions. Nevertheless, in Europe, and later in North America, the use of cocaine as a "tonic" spread widely. As late as 1900 it was still a component of Coca-Cola and similar products. The stimulant actions were well recognized by the public, and Coca-Cola was even referred to in the vernacular as "dope."

Amphetamine was invented by laboratory chemists in the pharmaceutical industry, but a fascinating discovery of the 1970s revealed that nature makes its own amphetamine. An East African shrub called khat contains a substance (cathinone) in its leaves that is almost identical to amphetamine, differing only by a single atom. The natives of Ethiopia and Somalia have chewed khat leaves since ancient times, much as the Peruvian highlanders chew coca leaves. Cathinone is quite unstable, so the leaves have to be fresh and young; and cathinone is destroyed rapidly in the body. Although all the psychoactive, cardiovascular, and toxic effects of cathinone are identical to those of amphetamine, it is metabolized so rapidly that it is difficult for the khat user to establish high brain levels. Khat is certainly addictive, but it is much safer than intravenous or smoked amphetamines, much as chewing coca leaves is safer than using pure cocaine.

Cocaine—together with other popular psychoactive drugs, especially opiates—was placed under legal restrictions in the Harrison Act of 1914. Its legitimate use in medicine as a local anesthetic for mucous membranes was retained; but synthetic analogues like procaine (Novocaine) and lidocaine, which deaden the nerves locally if injected under the skin, have largely displaced it. Their primary advantage over cocaine is that they do not readily enter the brain, so they are not psychoactive. Cocaine continued in use as an illicit stimulant; but until the 1980s it was considered a luxury drug because of its expense, and amphetamines were the illicit stimulants of choice for all but the wealthiest. Then increased supply made the price of cocaine fall, and a cocaine epidemic in the United States began to spread; it peaked in 1979, when 9 percent of young adults were using the drug at least once a month. Then the numbers fell steadily, for reasons that no one really understands, to less than 2 percent by 1998.

There are two chemical forms of cocaine, the hydrochloride salt and the free base. Cocaine itself is the biologically active material in both, but the two forms have different physical properties and are absorbed differently into the body. Cocaine hydrochloride dissolves in water; it is used by the nasal route ("snorted") or intravenously. "Crack" (a form of free base cocaine) cannot be dissolved, but it can be smoked; and this fact, which makes it easy and efficient to use, greatly expanded the illicit market. Typically, a simple glass pipe is used; a water pipe, which filters the smoke, is also effective because free base cocaine does not dissolve when the smoke passes through water. Like nicotine in cigarette smoke, crack cocaine reaches the brain within a few seconds (even faster than intravenous cocaine hydrochloride). Dosage is controllable by varying the puff frequency and depth of inhalation, and the "rush" is immediate. An important advantage—especially in view of the AIDS epidemic—is that smoking eliminates the danger of transmitting blood-borne diseases by needles and syringes.

Crack became enormously popular, from 1985 on, for two main reasons. First, it was manufactured as convenient little "rocks" that could easily be smoked and were individually fairly cheap. Second, inexperienced people—especially young people—who would not even consider putting a needle into their veins, were willing to try a new drug by a long-established and socially accepted route of administration.

The immediate effect of a small dose of cocaine or amphetamine is an extremely intense pleasurable sensation (the "high" or "rush"), a magnification of normal pleasures (especially of sexual feelings), a release of social inhibitions, talkativeness, and an unrealistic feeling of cleverness, great competence, and power. Enhancement of sexual activity and of the intensity of orgasm evidently plays a major role in the attractiveness of these stimulants. Extravagant sexual fantasies are common, and are often acted upon, so that all sorts of uninhibited and aberrant sexual behaviors may be indulged in, which the user would not ordinarily condone.

Nationwide studies on many thousands of cocaine addicts have revealed characteristic patterns of behavior, which foster the spread of AIDS. These include enhanced sexual activity, with modes of sexual contact that favor transmission of HIV; frequent exchange of sex for money or drugs; and sex with intravenous drug users.

By whatever method cocaine is administered, it is rapidly destroyed in the bloodstream—so rapidly that the effects of a single moderate dose last only ten minutes or so. Amphetamines, by contrast, are destroyed slowly, with the effect of a single dose lasting more than an hour. With both drugs, a special kind of rapid tolerance develops, within minutes: The pleasurable effects die away even before the drug concentration in the blood falls significantly. This phenomenon encourages dosage escalation and binges in some users, who attempt desperately to keep the "high" going. The blood levels attained during binges—especially in the presence of alcohol—can cause irregular heartbeats and even heart stoppage, and sometimes a stroke because of spasm of blood vessels in the brain. The widely publicized sudden deaths of a few famous young athletes in the prime of physical condition are attributable to one or another of these causes. Binge use can also lead to frankly psychotic behavior, such as extreme paranoia, visual and auditory hallucinations, a belief that bugs are crawling under the skin, and other sensory distortions. This kind of bizarre reaction, in an individual whom the drug has made to feel extraordinarily powerful but whose judgment is seriously affected, can produce dangerously aggressive, even homicidal, behavior.

Although continuous administration of cocaine leads to tolerance (as expected by analogy to other addictive drugs), intermittent administration produces sensitization. Here a given dose has an exaggerated effect on both motor activity and (most important) on reinforcement. Sensitization has been studied principally in rats, but it probably also occurs in people during the process that leads to a typical binge. The opposing effects of sensitization and tolerance complicate our attempts to understand fully the way full-blown cocaine addiction develops.

A cocaine binge may last 24 sleepless hours or more (even longer with amphetamines), with several "hits" per hour, followed by a "crash" when the drug supply is exhausted. Intense craving follows, and finding a fresh supply of drug becomes an obsession. Then another binge is initiated. Only a fraction of users go on to this extraordinary, self-destructive, compulsive pattern of use; but as with other addictive drugs, we cannot predict who will go out of control in this way. One experienced clinician in this field, writes: "Human cocaine addicts report that virtually all thoughts are focused on cocaine during binges; nourishment, sleep, money, loved ones, responsibility, and survival lose all significance."

Not Addictive?

The myth that cocaine was not addictive enjoyed wide currency throughout the medical profession and in society at large for many years. Some accepted this notion as late as the 1980s, despite the knowledge that regular users experience intense and irresistible craving. The confusion arose because in contrast to withdrawal from opiates and alcohol, the cocaine withdrawal syndrome is not dramatic, obvious, and physical, but primarily behavioral. The immediate "crash" upon exhausting the drug supply is followed by depression, anxiety, agitation, and suspiciousness (sometimes actual paranoia). As abstinence continues, there is extreme boredom, lack of motivation, and depression. Recalling what the "high" was like provokes intense craving, as do numerous conditioned cues (people, objects, and situations associated with cocaine or amphetamine use). Often these conditioned association triggers (as I call them) provoke a new binge, and vulnerability to relapse may persist for a lifetime.

A Drug To Drive You Crazy

A remarkable experiment at Vanderbilt University in 1971 taught us something important about amphetamine. In animal testing, amphetamine had seemed to be a reasonably safe drug; and regular administration for a long time had not produced any remarkable toxicity—no liver damage, no kidney failure, no heart stoppage, no cancer. As the drug was popular as an illicit stimulant, and at that time was still available in over-the-counter dieting aids and cold remedies, it was important to find out if regular use caused any significant adverse mental effects. Heavy users were known to become psychotic on occasion; but arguments raged over whether that was a direct effect of the drug, whether it was due to other drugs used at the same time, or whether amphetamines only caused psychotic behavior in those already prone to serious mental illness.

In order to meet the ethical requirement of not introducing anyone to an addictive drug for the first time, only subjects who had used amphetamine before were recruited. Then only the most stable of these were selected, with no history of mental illness, and healthy in all other respects. In order to ensure complete control of drug intake, and for safety, the subjects were housed in a closed hospital ward. Nine young men, volunteers, were maintained under close observation for six weeks to make sure that all drugs were eliminated from their bodies, and that no drugs of any kind were taken. Careful baseline measurements were made of physical and psychological status. Then amphetamine was administered and continued for up to five days. Dosage was high from the start, but not out of the range used by many street addicts.

All subjects showed increases of blood pressure and heart rate and a low-grade fever. No big surprises there! But amazingly, a full-blown psychosis developed before the fifth day in eight of the nine subjects. They became hostile and paranoid. They believed that the investigators were engaged in a conspiracy against them. They thought they were being poisoned. One complained of a giant oscillator in the ceiling, placed there to control his thoughts and behavior. Another insisted on guarding the window and door against an imaginary hired assassin. Two subjects believed they were being discussed on television, and one that he was being photographed through a mirror. In similar experiments carried out elsewhere, the same kinds of reaction occurred, which are much like those seen in classic paranoid schizophrenia. The more suspicious of the subjects had powerful delusions of persecution, were terrified of what might be done to them, and even expressed homicidal or suicidal thoughts. Meticulous inspection of the surroundings—as though looking for dangerous concealed items—was a common expression of the paranoia. The subjects also felt they were gaining sudden insight into "deep meanings" of common objects that were not apparent before. For example, one of them used a magnifying glass to examine every period and comma in a newspaper article to discover secret codes.

Of course, in these experiments the amphetamine was stopped immediately when a psychotic reaction occurred. Then, as the drug was eliminated from the body, over a period of 24 hours, the mental states of all the subjects returned to normal. At the end of the experiment the investigators carried out exhaustive psychological testing but found no evidence of persistent abnormality. And the subjects, looking back on their experience, recognized it for the abnormal reaction it was. However, after amphetamines or cocaine are used for a long time and then stopped, it is not unusual to find persistent depression, lack of energy, anhedonia (inability to experience pleasure), and episodes of intense craving. As with the long-term aftermath of addiction to other drugs, we cannot yet say whether this clinical depression reflects long-term neurochemical brain damage caused by the drug, or whether a preexisting deficit in the dopamine reward pathways contributed to the excessive use of stimulant drugs in the first place.

The important lesson of the experiment described above is that continuous intake of an amphetamine at high-dosage can eventually produce psychotic behavior in everyone; no special predisposition is required, nor any prior mental instability. Similar experiments have not been conducted with cocaine, but in view of the close pharmacological similarity to amphetamine, it is likely that everyone who uses cocaine at high dosage is at risk for psychosis.

Firing Up the Reward Systems

Cocaine and amphetamines do not combine directly with any of the receptors for brain neurotransmitters (see chapters 2–4). Instead, their specific receptors are the transporters that remove neurotransmitters from the synapses and return them to their respective neurons. Blockade of their specific transporters causes dopamine, serotonin, and norepinephrine to accumulate in the synapses. Consequently, the receptors for those neurotransmitters are overstimulated. The hedonic effects were at first attributed to overstimulation of dopamine receptors alone, but this is evidently an oversimplification. Knockout mice that lack dopamine transporters have greatly elevated dopamine levels in their synapses, as expected, and the animals are extremely hyperactive. If the reinforcing effect of cocaine were due entirely to its blockade of dopamine transporters, cocaine should be ineffective in the knockout mice. Contrary to expectation, however, these animals did self-administer cocaine, and they responded positively to cocaine in the conditioned place preference procedure. Thus, dopamine transporter blockade cannot alone be responsible for the psychoactive effects. Suspicion now attaches also to blockade of the serotonin transporter.

As a consequence of receptor overstimulation—especially of the dopamine receptors in nucleus accumbens—there is long-term decrease in receptor number, as well as numerous other adaptive changes. Some specialized proteins act as regulators of gene transcription, and some of these—especially one called CREB—are "turned on" by the short-term effects of cocaine or amphetamines. Altered activity of genes is, of course, what underlies long-term changes in brain chemistry, which long outlast the presence of cocaine. Thus, they offer a possible explanation for the long-lasting depression of mood that follows withdrawal. It is even possible that some such changes are irreversible and could play a role in relapse after long periods of abstinence.

The possibility that the psychostimulants may have persistent or even irreversible effects in the brain raised a concern about their use in treating attention deficit hyperactivity disorder (ADHD) in children, because the drug commonly used for treatment (methylphenidate, Ritalin) falls into this class. Well controlled prospective studies indicate that children diagnosed with this disorder—whether or not they are medicated—are much more likely than age-matched controls to become drug users (nicotine, cocaine) and to engage in some antisocial activities in adolescence and adulthood. However, children treated with methylphenidate are not more likely than untreated children with the same diagnosis to become cocaine addicts later in life; indeed, the therapeutic effect of this drug in ADHD substantially reduces the comorbid risk of substance abuse disorders.

Treating Cocaine and Amphetamine Addiction

In the United States, immediate toxic reactions to cocaine and amphetamine account for nearly half of all drug-related episodes (excluding alcohol) seen in hospital emergency rooms, and for half of all medical examiner cases (unexplained sudden deaths) in which a drug is involved. Immediate treatment for cocaine users suffering a serious immediate toxic effect—especially on the heart—consists of life-saving measures by medical response teams and at the hospital emergency room. Antibodies to cocaine and amphetamines are becoming available, which can quickly reduce the circulating drug levels. Most treatment, however, is directed toward alleviating withdrawal symptoms in addicts who are trying to discontinue the drug. As withdrawal is characterized by profound depression, standard antidepressant medications are used. However, as these do not take effect for two or three weeks, the initial period after stopping cocaine or amphetamine self-administration is the most difficult to manage. Later in the post-withdrawal phase, antidepressants can reduce craving and increase the abstinence rate.

As with most addictive drugs, detoxification can be carried out fairly easily; but preventing relapse is the heart of the problem. Recent research has focused attention on conditioned association triggers, which were described in connection with nicotine addiction in chapter 8. Brain imaging studies on craving have produced remarkable results. Abstinent cocaine addicts were exposed to audio tapes, video tapes, and play acting, depicting situations that had been associated with securing and using cocaine. For example, a video presentation might show an addict preparing cocaine hydrochloride powder for injection. Actors might pretend to be purchasing crack or smoking it. These cocaine-associated cues—but not neutral cues—provoked craving, and also selectively increased blood flow in certain regions of the brain (such as the amygdala) that are known to function in the storage and retrieval of memories with high emotional content. This finding supports the common-sense view that craving leading to relapse must be based on activating memories of the pleasurable effects of the drug.

One approach to relapse prevention, then, is to decondition, to bring about extinction of the behavior. In this procedure, the conditioned stimulus is presented, but not reinforced; thus, craving is provoked but no cocaine is available. Abstinent cocaine addicts were hospitalized for two weeks in a closed ward while cocaine cues were systematically presented in daily "extinction sessions." Subjects were then exposed to such sessions on an outpatient basis for another eight weeks. Classic psychologic theory based on studies of animal behavior predicts that by doing this repeatedly in a situation where the reinforcer (i.e., the drug) is not available, the conditioned association triggers should lose their power to evoke craving.

The experimenters measured the drop in skin temperature (reflecting emotional arousal) that is typically evoked by cues associated with cocaine administration. Neutral stimuli had little effect, but cocaine-related stimuli caused significant skin temperature change. Craving, as measured by subjects' reports on a numerical scale, was virtually abolished by the extinction sessions, and the ability of cocaine cues to cause a drop in skin temperature was also reduced. Then, for seven months after completion of the 28-day treatment, the researchers conducted follow-up assessments of abstinence, confirming self-reports by urine tests. Subjects who had participated in the extinction sessions had a higher proportion of cocaine-free urine samples at follow-up than did control subjects who had also been in treatment for 28 days but without the specific deconditioning program.

Is full hospitalization required during the initial stage of treatment, or could a less expensive alternative work? Arguing from common sense (but without regard for treatment cost), many professionals have advocated round-the-clock hospitalization as the best way to provide a drug-free environment in which to establish abstinence. But common sense must always give way to actual experimental proof. Experiments showed that coming to the hospital for several hours a day but being free to return home in the evenings was at least as effective as full hospitalization. Half of the subjects reported no cocaine use at the 7-month follow-up, and abstinence was confirmed by urine test—an unusually good outcome.

Another question that often arises is whether treatment must be conducted by fully trained professional psychologists and psychiatrists or whether standard drug counseling by paraprofessional staff suffices. Here again we are dealing with an issue of great practical importance because of the relative costs. Some studies have suggested that standard drug counseling—especially behavior modification techniques directed toward relapse prevention—work as well as more sophisticated individual psychotherapy.

Animal experiments have revealed that long-term cocaine administration causes an irreversible destruction of dopamine neurons. This has suggested that depression and craving even after years of abstinence might be due to a persistent dopamine deficiency. Accordingly, numerous attempts have been made to prevent relapse by long-term treatment with standard antidepressant medications, which modify the dopamine or serotonin systems, and some groups have reported favorable outcomes. There is also an ongoing search for some kind of long-acting cocainelike surrogate agonist that would be analogous to methadone in heroin addiction.

Recent animal studies suggested that naltrexone or other opiate antagonists (especially the agonist-antagonist buprenorphine, chapter 10) may have therapeutic value in cocaine addiction. Although the mechanism is not understood, these drugs do cause animals to reduce their cocaine intake in self-administration experiments. They also make cocaine less effective in conditioned place preference.

One therapeutic approach is to destroy the cocaine or amphetamine in the blood stream or prevent it from passing into the brain. The dream is to develop some kind of effective vaccination. But typical antibodies raised by vaccines have only to neutralize tiny amounts of an infectious agent, whereas cocaine is used at dosages millions of times higher. One way around this obstacle may be the technology of catalytic antibodies. These are antibodies deliberately fashioned to combine specifically with a certain molecule (in this case cocaine) and at the same time destroy it much faster than it is destroyed by enzymes already present in the blood and liver. Although the mechanism would be entirely different, the principle of these approaches is really a variation on the naltrexone theme (chapter 10)—based on the idea that depriving a drug of its rewarding effect will cause the addict to give it up.

There seems to be general agreement that, pending some breakthrough in pharmacotherapy, rehabilitation counseling and 12-step programs such as those used for alcohol addiction (chapter 9) will remain the mainstays of treatment. A "magic bullet" to prevent or cure cocaine addiction does not seem to be on the horizon.

"Crack Babies"

It is early dawn in New York City. A faint light gives the bridges across the East River a mystical hushed beauty. Not far from the river, at Bellevue Hospital, a woman in the seventh month of pregnancy appears, alone, in the emergency room. She is writhing in pain, obviously about to go into premature labor. Her last crack binge ended barely an hour ago and she is still "high" on the drug. She reaches the delivery room only just in time to give birth. Her baby is not only premature, its weight is low even by standards of prematurity. Its head is small, it has trouble breathing, it seems to have some kind of congenital heart malformation, and its chance of survival is uncertain even with all of modern medical technology thrown into the battle to rescue it. The physician in charge, when satisfied that the baby's condition has been stabilized, goes to the ward to report to the mother. The sun has just risen. The woman is gone.

Scenes like this are enacted every day in every large city. The intensity of the "mad craving" can be judged by the astounding, totally unbiological behavior of a mother abandoning her newborn infant to go out in search of cocaine. The media have reported extensively on "crack babies" and their future; in a few instances, mothers who used cocaine during pregnancy have even been prosecuted for harming their unborn offspring. But are there really "crack babies," babies permanently harmed by a mother's cocaine use?

We do know that cocaine causes spasm of blood vessels, and very large doses given to pregnant rats provoke premature delivery. And there is no doubt that cocaine use by a pregnant woman can cause complications due to spasm of her own blood vessels, including those of the placenta, where such a spasm can result in miscarriage. Moreover, the disturbances of placental circulation could well cause damage to the fetus, for its health and normal development is dependent on a normally functioning placenta. We do know that babies exposed to cocaine in utero are often premature and abnormally small and have unusually small heads.

But to what extent is cocaine responsible? As can well be imagined, many women addicted to cocaine do not maintain adequate nutrition, do not get prenatal care, use other drugs that harm the fetus, and neither breast-feed nor establish normal maternal bonding with their newborn. Then, when developmental deficits occur in the growing child, it is very difficult to say with certainty what role was played by these associated factors rather than by cocaine itself. Problems of methodology extend even to evaluating the published information, for researchers tend not to report and publish negative results (i.e., results that show no adverse effects), so that the medical literature is bound to give an exaggerated picture of fetal harm. On the other hand, real drug-induced abnormalities may be missed for a long time; for instance, the very existence of the fetal alcohol syndrome—now an undisputed reality—went unrecognized until nearly 30 years ago.

Contrary to the impression one gains from the media, several well designed prospective studies show no difference at all between children who were exposed to cocaine prenatally and those were not— provided other influences were matched properly. For example, each cocaine-exposed child was compared with a child of a mother who did not use cocaine but lived in the same inner-city neighborhood, had the same socioeconomic and educational status, was of the same ethnicity, and so on. The result of intelligence testing and standard measures of childhood behavior was clear—at least during the first couple of years of life, the group exposed to cocaine did not differ from the matched control group. Strikingly, however, the entire distribution of IQ and other scores—for both groups—was shifted significantly to the left as compared with general population norms. Thus, inner-city poverty might endanger the next generation, but we do not know enough yet to support all that has been claimed about "crack babies." But research into this controversial issue continues, and there are some indications now that subtle negative effects of exposure to prenatal cocaine or amphetamines can, indeed, be seen as the children grow older.

I must end this section with a caveat. Knowing the truth is essential for making sensible decisions and for not overreacting to perceived drug problems. But nothing said here should be misinterpreted as indifference to the many dangers of using cocaine or amphetamines (or other addictive drugs) during pregnancy. Indeed, the best, safest, and most obvious advice for pregnant women is not to use any drug whatsoever.

Summary

Cocaine and amphetamines are powerfully addictive drugs with seriously disruptive immediate effects on behavior (including a dangerous paranoid psychosis at high doses) and with potential for unpredictable lethal toxicity. Relapse, even after prolonged abstinence, is common, driven by conditioned association triggers.

These same drugs are relatively harmless when taken into the body by chewing the leaves (coca, khat) but have very different pharmacological effects and consequences when spiking brain levels are produced by intravenous injection, smoking, or snorting.

The hedonic effects are mediated by increased levels of neurotransmitters (especially dopamine) in synapses of the reward system, the consequence of blocking the transporters that normally return dopamine, serotonin, and norepinephrine to the neurons from which they were released.

These psychostimulants initiate a cascade of neurochemical changes, including effects on gene expression, which persist long after the drugs are withdrawn, and which may possibly contribute to craving and relapse.

No specific treatment has yet been developed. The opiate antagonist naltrexone and the agonist-antagonist buprenorphine are useful for some patients. The continuing search for effective pharmacotherapy—perhaps for a maintenance agonist analogous to methadone—continues. Meanwhile, the mainstays of treatment remain counseling, 12-step programs, and other methods of strengthening motivation to remain abstinent. As with other addictions, any treatment is better than no treatment, but no single treatment modality stands out as better than another. The greatest present need is for a pharmaceutical agent that would reliably suppress relapse.

"Crack babies" are to some extent a creation of the media. Some controlled studies have failed to demonstrate any major adverse effect specifically resulting from prenatal exposure to cocaine. Other studies do find indications of subtle but real cognitive disturbances as the children exposed in utero grow older. It is clear that other characteristics (socioeconomic, educational, environmental, etc.) of women who use cocaine during pregnancy are associated with defects of intellectual and behavioral function in their children. Other drugs commonly used by pregnant women who use cocaine (especially alcohol and nicotine) are known to harm the fetus. The best advice for pregnant women is to abstain from all drugs.

12

Cannabis (Marijuana)

A professional airplane pilot sits in a simulator, the kind used to check the abilities of the men and women who fly for the military and the airlines. The task is to bring an aircraft safely down onto a runway through clouds or fog without being able to see anything outside. As the aircraft descends, the pilot has to watch for the smallest deviations of instruments on the panel, and correct for them quickly with more or less power or with slight movements of the control yoke. A continuous scan of instruments is required to make sure that all aircraft systems are operating correctly. The pilot must consult an approach chart continuously without interrupting the other tasks to which he or she is attending. And while all this is going on, the pilot has to communicate by radio with a controller on the ground and must be prepared to carry out unexpected instructions. Furthermore, if in the pilot's judgment anything at all seems wrong, an immediate climb must be initiated, rather than gamble on reaching the runway safely.

Before the test begins, the pilot reports that he feels up to par, that he would feel comfortable flying a real airplane right now, and that he has no doubt about his ability to carry out the standard instrument landing procedure. But he is wrong. His performance is so poor that if he were flying an actual airplane there might be real danger. Yet the only thing different today is that—as part of an experiment—he had smoked a single marijuana cigarette, and that single exposure to cannabis had occurred 24 hours before. While cannabis—marijuana and hashish—is not as dangerous as some other addictive drugs, it clearly impairs judgment, and long-term heavy use may have adverse consequences

Marijuana and the Brain

The leaves of the hemp (cannabis) plant contain many chemicals, of which tetrahydrocannibol (THC) is the principal psychoactive one. Typically, THC is self-administered by smoking cigarettes packed with finely ground cannabis leaf. The concentrated hemp resin called hashish can also be smoked, usually in a pipe; and because THC does not dissolve in water, a water pipe is often used to filter the smoke. Finally, marijuana is sometimes taken in edible form, as in baked goods. The THC content of cannabis leaves varies greatly; most wild hemp is derived from plants originally grown for fiber, which contain less than one percent THC. Strains cultivated for their psychoactive effect may contain five percent or even more, while hashish and "hash oil" are even richer in THC. Whatever the THC content, as with nicotine (chapter 8), smokers can adjust their intake to obtain the desired effect by inhaling more or less frequently and deeply. THC is very potent; a few milligrams taken into the lungs with smoke, and entering the brain readily, suffices to activate the cannabinoid receptors. Pure THC is used primarily in research because one wants a standard dosage, and because it is almost impossible to make laboratory animals inhale smoke. The evidence to date suggests that THC produces the same biological effects as smoking the whole leaf. Nevertheless, like other addictive plants that are smoked (e.g., tobacco leaf, coca leaf), a very large number of different chemicals is present; so it remains a question whether smoked marijuana may have some biological actions that differ from or modify those produced by THC.

THC acts on a seven-helix receptor (chapter 3) called CB1, which has been identified in those parts of the brain that mediate the changes of mood and perception caused by marijuana. A closely related receptor called CB2 is found chiefly in organs and tissues outside the brain; its functions remain unclear. The story of CB1 is reminiscent of the opioid receptors and their endogenous ligands. A natural brain chemical called anandamide is the natural ligand of the CB1 receptors in the brain; another, very similar chemical (2-arachidonyl glycerol) may also play a role. Unlike the opioid peptides, anandamide is a compact molecule structurally similar to the hormones called prostaglandins. It will be recalled (chapter 2) that the plant product morphine, which binds to the opioid receptors, has a chemical structure quite different from the endorphin peptides in brain, which are the natural ligands. In an analogous manner, the plant product THC, the active constituent of cannabis, binds to the anandamide receptor CB1, even though its chemical structure is quite different. Of course, chemicals of different families, which may look very different on paper, can nevertheless have the necessary common shapes and reactive groups to fit a pocket in a specific receptor.

A potent CB1 antagonist, called SR141716A, has shed light on a hitherto unsuspected role of CB1 receptors. In rats, analgesia can be produced by electrical stimulation of the area of the brainstem called the periaqueductal gray. In chapter 2, I described the key experiment in which an opiate antagonist prevented this stimulation-produced analgesia, thus demonstrating pain regulation by a natural opioid system. Now a similar experiment, using the CB1 antagonist, has revealed the presence of a natural cannabinoid system of pain control, parallel to the opioid (endorphin) system but also interacting with it in interesting ways that are not yet fully understood. For example, the opioid antagonist naloxone blocks some rewarding actions of THC. Moreover, THC reduces the intensity of the opioid withdrawal syndrome. As with morphine and other addictive drugs, withdrawal from THC after a period of daily administration results in reduced activity of the midbrain dopaminergic neurons. THC withdrawal, precipitated by the CB1 antagonist, elevates the levels of corticotropin releasing hormone in the brain, a typical stress response.

With respect to the pleasurable and addictive properties of marijuana, activation of the CB1 receptors by THC or endogenous anandamide increases the dopamine level at the nucleus accumbens in the forebrain, apparently by blocking the dopamine transporter, much as cocaine does. Consistent with this action, THC is rewarding in animals—for example, in the conditioned place preference test. Knockout animals lacking CB1 receptors not only become indifferent to all the rewarding actions of THC, they also show reduced responses to morphine and other opiates. Finally the well-known stimulation of appetite by marijuana in humans has its counterpart in experimental animals, apparently by increasing the rewarding value of foods.

Behavioral Effects

That a single exposure to cannabis the previous day can disrupt a pilot's performance on the complex flight-simulator task may sound like the kind of scare story used to frighten children about the dangers of marijuana. But it is not. The same result was confirmed with many other pilots. Marijuana users know that performance on complex tasks suffers after smoking a "joint"; when simulator tests were carried out immediately after smoking, the pilots themselves realized they were impaired. However, the marijuana "high" is largely gone a few hours after a single joint, as the blood levels of THC fall to a point supposedly below what is needed to cause mental effects. But experiments like the one with pilots showed not only that subtle disturbances of judgment and coordination persist for a very long time—but of even greater concern, that such persistent effects may not be recognized by the individual. This finding contradicts a common belief among cannabis smokers. "When you're drunk," they say, "you think you can do anything perfectly, including driving a car or flying an airplane. But when you're high on grass, you know better than to try." No doubt that statement is true during the period of obvious intoxication, but the simulator experiments point to a dangerous false optimism that persists after the obvious "high" has disappeared.

Why do people use cannabis? They seek a sense of well-being (euphoria)—a relaxed, calm, drowsy, dreamlike state, with a feeling of disconnection from the ordinary world. Thoughts ramble out of control. Things seem funny to the smoker that are not especially humorous to an observer. The most obvious behavioral abnormality displayed by a subject under the influence of cannabis is difficulty in carrying on an intelligible conversation, perhaps because of an inability to remember what was just said. The disorder has been described as "impaired ability to think in a connected fashion to a goal."

A characteristic feature of being "stoned" is a distortion in the sense of time, associated with profound deficits in short-term memory and learning. In experiments to define these effects more precisely, it was found that new information is learned very poorly or not at all while under the influence of the drug. This is obviously relevant to the education of students who smoke marijuana.

A consequence of the memory and time-sense disruptions is loss of the alertness, coordination, and judgment that are required for complicated tasks. Thus, operating a car, train, airplane, or any other complex equipment is seriously impaired; and numerous studies have found, among drivers involved in highway accidents, a disproportionate number with detectable THC in the blood. Data are underestimates here because unlike on-the-spot alcohol detection by Breathalyzer, there is no comparable method of measuring THC levels on the highway.

The marijuana smoker typically has a sense of enhanced physical and emotional sensitivity, including a feeling of greater interpersonal closeness. Increased sensitivity to all kinds of sensory stimuli can be demonstrated, and this may be related to reports of enhanced sexual pleasure. Increased sex drive is also claimed, but this is controversial; it is unclear which reported effects of cannabis, as perceived by the user, are objectively real, and which are merely part of the altered mental state.

Especially confusing in assessing the immediate effects of smoking marijuana is a very strong influence of expectation. A study compared a group of subjects who had never tried marijuana with a group of experienced chronic smokers. At the very same dosage, the experienced smokers showed greater effects than the first-time smokers. This curious phenomenon had been observed frequently and had been attributed to some sort of pharmacological sensitization by the drug. However, when placebo "joints" were included, a very different light was shed on matters. The first-time smokers reported very little effect from the placebo cigarettes, but the experienced smokers described many typical cannabis effects. Thus, social setting, previous experience, and expectation contribute heavily to how chronic users react.

Ordinary dosages cause increased heart rate and dilation of blood vessels in the eyes; but redness of the eyes may be caused in so many different ways that this effect is not useful in the diagnosis of marijuana use. High levels of cannabis intake can cause psychotic reactions, with hallucinations, paranoia, depersonalization (the feeling of being outside one's own body), and panic attacks.

THC remains in the body for a very long time, and some of the behavioral disturbances linger surprisingly long, as in the experiment with pilots. The long persistence is due, in part, to storage of THC in fatty tissues, with traces leaking out into the blood (and excreted in the urine) for many days, even for weeks, after stopping intake. For this reason, although urine tests tell positively that a person did smoke cannabis, they tell little about when that was. Also, differences among people in their sensitivity to THC make it hard to set sharp legal standards for likely impairment. This contrasts with alcohol testing, where breath or blood analysis tells the concentration of alcohol to which the brain is exposed at the moment the test is conducted, and the relationship of the measured levels to known deficits in psychomotor performance have been well established.

Long-term Use

Does regular use of cannabis for a long time have serious long-term adverse consequences? Why is there so much controversy surrounding this question? In trying to decide if an addictive drug has long-lasting behavioral toxicity, the fundamental difficulty is that we never know what users were like before they first tried marijuana. How could we? With current users we can never distinguish cause from effect; whatever behavioral abnormalities we see might not be due to the drug at all, but might have been present before drug use began—indeed, might have been factors predisposing to the addiction in the first place. And to conduct a proper prospective study, we would have to start with a large number of children, before they begin using drugs, deliberately expose a randomly chosen group of them to a drug for many years, and then test the outcome. Moreover, the young subjects in such an experiment would have to be isolated in a closed environment—just as experiments with volunteer adult subjects have to be done in a closed ward—to guarantee that the drug and control (no-drug) conditions were maintained. I mention such a fantasy experiment with children only to highlight the problem; any study of that kind would, of course, be unethical as well as impractical.

Let's look at one famous example of a controversial study. Nearly

2,000 Egyptian prisoners were studied—those who had been long-term cannabis users and those who had not. The ones who had used prior to their incarcerations did more poorly than the others on tests of psychomotor performance and visual coordination. The conclusion was drawn that chronic use of cannabis by these Egyptian prisoners had affected their brains adversely. Studies like this, with any addictive drug, have political impact—and that makes it doubly important that the science be good, that the results be valid. People who believe passionately that cannabis is dangerous and should be tightly controlled cite studies like this one in support of their position. People who believe cannabis is harmless and should be legalized find plenty to criticize. In this case, as the two populations were not necessarily comparable to start with, how can cannabis be blamed for the difference? Could one not argue just as well that the less capable people were just the ones who had turned to cannabis in the first place?

Cannabis smoke contains more carcinogens than tobacco smoke, so lung damage and cancer are real risks for heavy users. Disturbances of hormone balance have been well documented, especially of the sex hormones; these effects result from actions of THC in the hypothalamus, the part of the brain that controls the secretion of pituitary hormones. Repeated administration of THC under controlled conditions to normal volunteers caused a reduction of sperm count, a depressed testosterone level, decreased libido in males, and menstrual cycles in females were disturbed. All these effects were reversed when the drug was discontinued.

In one experiment, when monkeys were forced to inhale the smoke of a single marijuana cigarette every day, five days a week for six months, structural damage was evident in their brain cells. In a similar experiment, the monkeys were found to have a significant reduction in the number and size of brain cells, with the result that the ventricles (the central cavities) of the brain became dilated—an indication of tissue loss. Comparable findings were reported in rats after administration of THC by mouth for 90 days, at a dose that established blood levels comparable to those found in smokers of several marijuana cigarettes daily. The microscopic changes observed in the brain were evident principally in the hippocampus, where the nerve cells were shrunken and the number of synapses reduced. This finding was consistent with long-term effects on rat behavior, which were similar to what happens if parts of the hip-

pocampus are destroyed. Furthermore, it is of interest that cannabinoid receptors are especially dense in the hippocampus and cerebral cortex, areas of the brain specialized for memory and
cognitive skills. The other brain area rich in CB1 receptors is the
cerebellum, a region thought until recently to be concerned mainly
with balance and fine control of muscle movement. We know now
that the cerebellum also participates in memory processing and decision making. On the other hand, cannabinoid receptors are virtually absent from parts of the brain that control the heart rate, the
constriction or dilation of blood vessels, and the rate and depth of
breathing; this may well account for the lack of immediate serious
toxic effects on these vital systems—no overdose deaths due to marijuana have been reported.

Even though brain damage has not been shown convincingly in
humans, the findings in rats and monkeys are disturbing. They indicate that although occasional use of this drug has relatively mild
effects, frequent high-dose use for a long time could have serious
permanent consequences. One claimed long-term effect, about
which there has been much controversy, is the "amotivational syndrome." The existence of such a syndrome is not supported by scientific evidence; and, unfortunately, relevant scientific evidence is
impossible, in principle, to obtain. No doubt chronic heavy marijuana users often reject the goal-directed lifestyle and ethos of our
modern urban civilization. It is impossible to say if that is a consequence of cannabis use, or a cause of cannabis use in the first place.
Whichever it is, therapists do know that some fraction of users—
evidently a larger fraction than thought in the past—become compulsive users; and as with other addictive drugs, they seek treatment
when they become so heavily involved that cannabis seems to dom-
inate their lives to the exclusion of other activities.

On discontinuance of chronic THC administration in animals,
there is a profound reduction in activity of the dopaminergic reward
pathway. In humans, after chronic heavy use of cannabis, the withdrawal syndrome consists of irritability, restlessness, loss of appetite,
sleeplessness, tremor, perspiration, and sometimes nausea, vomiting, and diarrhea. Most of the withdrawal symptoms are behavioral
rather than physical, much as with nicotine or cocaine; and
therefore, in the past, the very existence of a withdrawal syndrome
was controversial.

The special problem of possible fetal damage requires consideration with any drug, and marijuana is no exception. Animal experiments indicate that—at least at high dosages—the course of pregnancy can be affected adversely; and some neurochemical changes in the dopamine reward pathway of the fetus may last well into adult life. These results, in rodents, raise serious concerns about marijuana use by pregnant women. THC crosses the placenta readily, and prematurity and low birth weight are associated with maternal marijuana use. However, as other drugs (especially alcohol, caffeine, and nicotine) are usually also being used, the specific role of marijuana is nearly impossible to establish with certainty. This is the same issue discussed at greater length in connection with cocaine (see chapter 11).

Medical Marijuana: What Is the Evidence?

Cannabis is like the opiates in being an addictive substance with potential (though limited) therapeutic uses. Controlled clinical trials with THC—not smoked marijuana—have shown a beneficial effect in relieving nausea and vomiting during cancer chemotherapy. How much of the anti-nausea effect is selective and how much is secondary to feeling "high" remains uncertain. If no effective alternative medications existed, one might argue that if it works, it works, and never mind if it disturbs mental processes. However, other medications have been developed, which have proved exceedingly effective in suppressing nausea and vomiting without psychoactive side effects.

Marijuana is also effective as an appetite stimulant in wasting diseases like AIDS. Here weight gain is an objective measure of efficacy, and there is no doubt that these seriously ill—often terminally ill—patients feel better and enjoy food more. This condition may present the strongest case for medical marijuana. There may also be value in spastic muscle disorders, such as multiple sclerosis. Claims of therapeutic efficacy in glaucoma are not borne out by rigorous clinical trials.

A major contraindication to medical marijuana is that smoking the leaf is harmful in the long term—harmful to lungs and with at least the same risk of cancer as in smoking tobacco leaves. It seems reasonable to argue that in terminal conditions, these long-term risks are not relevant; and if marijuana gives dying patients pleasure, so much the better. A panel set up by the National Institutes of

Health examined the scientific evidence concerning medical marijuana, as did a committee of the Institute of Medicine of the National Academy of Sciences. Both reports stressed the unacceptability of delivering medication by smoking a plant leaf, and therefore the need for a THC inhaler, which would deliver the medication quickly and in pure form. Some would still say it is arguable whether pure THC really delivers all the same benefits as the mixture of chemicals in the cannabis leaf.

How Dangerous Is Cannabis to Society?

There is a curious discrepancy with regard to some addictive drugs between actual danger to the individual or to society and the perceived danger, as reflected in their legal status and the severity of penalties for violating the laws. This discrepancy, with respect to nicotine and alcohol, was noted in previous chapters; considering the seriousness of their harmful effects, the law treats them very leniently. Cannabis presents a discrepancy in the other direction; considering what we know about the harm it causes, the law seems excessively harsh. Even today, in some states, people are serving prison terms for uncomplicated possession of small amounts for personal use.

Governmental commissions are established from time to time to study the cannabis question, and they always arrive at the same conclusions and recommendations. As long ago as 1894 the Indian Hemp Commission, appointed by the British parliament, published an exhaustive report of 3,281 pages, which concluded that moderate use of cannabis was not injurious to the majority of users. The La Guardia Commission in New York City in 1944 found no evidence that cannabis was the terrible menace it was claimed to be at the time.

In 1962 a White House Panel on Narcotic and Drug Abuse reported:

> It is the opinion of the Panel that the hazards of marihuana per se have been exaggerated and that long criminal sentences imposed on an occasional user or possessor of the drug are in poor social perspective.

Similar findings emerged from official committees of inquiry in the subsequent two decades in Britain and in Canada. The periodic reports of such expert groups do not oppose legal restrictions on cannabis; they certainly do not suggest that it is a safe drug for general use. But they do address—and forcefully—the discrepancy between true danger and perceived danger, as reflected in the law. In this connection chapter 18 describes an interesting alternative to the U.S. system of cannabis regulation.

Summary

Marijuana (cannabis) and the cannabis resin, hashish, contain an active principle, tetrahydrocannabinol (THC), which stimulates the brain reward system to release dopamine at the nucleus accumbens in the forebrain. This action—similar to that responsible for the "high" produced by other addictive drugs—accounts for the hedonic effects of THC.

There is a natural cannabinoid system in the brain, consisting of CB1 receptors and two endogenous ligands, anandamide and 2-arachidonyl glycerol. This brain cannabinoid system plays a role in pain control and in numerous other brain functions still under active investigation. The cannabinoid system influences and is influenced by the endogenous opioid system.

People self-administer marijuana or hashish, usually by smoking, otherwise by mouth. The "high" (being "stoned") is a peculiar relaxed and disinhibited state. The user is at risk in operating any kind of complex machinery (e.g., driving) because judgment, time sense, learning, and memory are seriously impaired. Subtle disturbances of mental function persist for 24 hours or more.

High dosages continued for a long time may lead to serious brain damage, with psychotic symptoms. Serious addiction, requiring medical intervention, does occur, though infrequently. There is no valid evidence of an "amotivational syndrome" caused by marijuana, although many users do reject conventional standards of study and work.

Despite all expert medical opinion supported by research data, and regardless of the conclusions of government commissions, the dangers of this drug have been greatly exaggerated. Criminal sanctions are out of all proportion to the actual harm done to individuals and society.

Cannabinoids have a very limited medical use in suppressing the nausea and vomiting that accompany chemotherapy, in stimulating appetite in wasting conditions such as the terminal phases of AIDS, and in improving function in multiple sclerosis and similar spastic diseases. For long-term use, a THC inhaler will need to be developed to avoid the risks of smoking.

13

Caffeine

It is 7 P.M. Twenty Stanford medical student volunteers are sitting around a conference table, pencil and paper at the ready, intent on a large movie screen on the wall. The film rolls. The screen is blank. Suddenly, in the upper left corner, the number 15662 flashes for a fraction of a second, and the screen goes blank again. The students try to write down all five digits of the number. Unpredictably, a few seconds later, the number 70597 flashes—this time at the center bottom of the screen. After 50 random numbers have been flashed in this way, at random intervals and random positions on the screen, the room lights go up. The subjects have abstained from coffee since breakfast. Now everyone drinks a coded sample of instant coffee, which may or may not contain caffeine. Later, the group gathers around the table again for another test with 50 new numbers. The same subjects go through this procedure on nine nights, each subject receiving sometimes caffeine and sometimes placebo.

The above is a scene from one of many experiments I conducted to see if caffeine enhances performance. In other experiments I studied sleep disturbance, hedonic effects, and how dependence and withdrawal are manifested.

Effects on Performance

Caffeine is the most popular and least harmful of all the addictive drugs. Others are either illicit (cocaine, heroin, marijuana, hallucinogens) or have a social stigma attached to heavy use (alcohol, nicotine), and this complicates research. Because caffeine is legal and so widely used (by 90 percent of the population), it is relatively easy to find subjects for experiments. Also, the oral route of administration makes it possible to give subjects coded samples to take at home, as for experiments on sleep. Most important, research on caffeine addiction is not confounded by the sorts of social factors that complicate research on illicit drugs. Consider the key question of why some people become addicted heavy users of a drug, whereas others do not. With illicit drugs, not everyone has equal access to them in the first place; and even among those who do, the willingness to break a legal taboo may vary in ways unrelated to any biological predisposition to use and become addicted. With caffeine, on the other hand, virtually everyone (except in families with religious scruples) has socially acceptable access during childhood or adolescence, following which, by self-selection, only a few become chronic heavy users, and a very few become addicts.

My own first studies on addiction, over 30 years ago, like the one described above, were experiments with caffeine on volunteers. To prepare for double-blind experiments, my colleagues and I had first to develop coded caffeine and placebo samples that were truly indistinguishable by appearance or taste. Starting with a decaffeinated instant coffee base, we added caffeine in the usual amount to one set of samples, a bitter white powder (to match the color and taste) to the other set. We set up a coffee bar in our medical school lounge, and we offered everyone free coffee on the condition that they examine and taste two coded samples and tell us immediately which they thought was real coffee and which decaffeinated. Day after day, we made adjustments to the mixture until the students were guessing right only half the time, by chance, and expressing no consistent taste preference. Then we were ready to start the experiments.

People presumably take caffeine to obtain a rewarding effect, usually described as feeling more alert and competent. But are they really more alert and competent, or do they only feel that way? The procedure using flashing numbers, as described above, is a form of vigilance test. To see and read a number flashed so briefly ($\frac{1}{32}$ second) requires extraordinary vigilance because a subject does not know when or where it will appear, and a momentary lapse of attention will result in missing the number entirely. To inspire maximum effort, I offered a monetary prize for the best performance at each of the nine sessions.

Another test required good eye-hand coordination and fine control. Subjects had to draw a continuous line through a zigzag maze on paper as fast as possible. Scoring was based on speed of completion, with penalties for touching the edges of the maze. Finally, a questionnaire surveyed mood. The two performance tests and the mood survey were administered once before and then again 90 minutes after drinking the coded coffee sample.

Caffeine did not enhance performance on either of the tests. Nonetheless, subjects reported feeling more alert, more active, and better coordinated after caffeine than after placebo. The chief effect was a favorable mood state, unaccompanied by any improvement in performance. As a well-known effect of the drug is to enhance the state of wakefulness, improvements in performance are seen best in subjects who are fatigued and sleepy, whose performance is already degraded.

Numerous other experiments carried out since my initial studies have confirmed the description of caffeine as a mild stimulant that, by overcoming fatigue and boredom, can improve vigilance and the performance of some mental and physical tasks. Likewise, athletic performance is generally unaffected when maximum exertion is required for a very short time, as in a 100-yard dash, but is improved if continuous prolonged effort is called for, as in a marathon.

Caffeine enjoys a reputation as a pain reliever. However, animal and human experiments show no beneficial effect of caffeine in pain after surgery, or in other kinds of severe pain. The drug does relieve headache pain, and there is clearly an adjuvant effect when administered in conjunction with aspirin and related mild analgesics. Thus, the way it is marketed in over-the-counter combinations is supported by the data. The mechanism of action in the brain is uncertain; it may be due to an indirect stimulation of cholinergic neurons.

Sleep Disturbance

Ask any group of people if caffeine affects their nighttime sleep. You will hear a confusing multiplicity of answers, ranging from "If I drink any coffee after noon, I toss and turn all that night," to "I can drink coffee all evening and sleep like a baby." According to their own accounts, people differ greatly in their sensitivity to the drug. My aim was to find out whether sleep disturbance by caffeine was real, and if so, whether people actually differed as much in their sensitivity as their accounts suggested. I gave out coded coffee samples to medical students, asking them to drink one before bedtime, and then the next morning to fill out a questionnaire about how well they had slept.

Caffeinated coffee (containing the usual amount of caffeine) did cause wakefulness, as compared with placebo, in most of the subjects. But there were large and consistent differences in sensitivity; "consistent" means here that if a subject was kept awake (or not kept awake) by caffeine, the same result was obtained on several nights. Were the intrinsic differences among people due to differences in brain sensitivity to caffeine, or did they reflect differences in absorbing and metabolizing the drug? To answer that question I measured caffeine in the subjects' blood after the standard dose, and found only minor differences. Therefore, since the blood bathing the brain contained about the same amount of drug in all subjects, I could conclude that the brain itself is responsible for a person's sensitivity to caffeine.

Another double-blind study was carried out with 239 young women, mostly wives of students. They drank coded coffee samples shortly before bedtime, and they filled out questionnaires each morning. The habitual coffee drinkers described coffee as an enjoyable, pleasant-tasting beverage that helps one to wake up and get going, that gives one a feeling of well-being and a certain lift, and that also induces relaxation and reduces irritability. Those who habitually drank the most coffee were the least disturbed in their sleep. One's first reaction to this finding might be that it demonstrates tolerance. Not necessarily. A quite different interpretation would be that these people are intrinsically less sensitive to caffeine, and were that way even before they began using the drug. That would explain why they have to drink so much coffee to get the desired stimulant effect in the daytime, and why coffee is less disturbing to their sleep at night.

Here, again, we confront the familiar "chicken-and-egg" problem in the study of addictive drugs. Which came first, relative insensitivity to caffeine, or heavy caffeine use leading to tolerance? One way to distinguish the two possibilities would be to test children before their first contact with caffeine, make a record of their sensitivity, then follow them to adulthood and see how their drug-using habit develops. This would be nice, but as previously noted, such experiments would be difficult to conduct, very expensive, perhaps entirely impractical. Another way would be to recruit addicts who are willing to abstain from caffeine for long enough to allow the withdrawal syndrome as well as any drug-induced tolerance to dissipate, and then to carry out the controlled trials. But getting addicts to give up their addiction for the sake of science is a dubious proposition, and it would also require regular testing of urine to confirm abstinence. Furthermore, even with so mild an addictive drug as caffeine, some would think it unethical to readminister it for experimental purposes to ex-addicts who might wish to remain abstinent.

Important advances in sleep research have been made in recent years, and careful quantitative measures have added greatly to the precision of sleep experiments. My own sleep studies described above, however, despite their crudity, were conclusive; they illustrate an interesting point about scientific method. Good science does not necessarily require expensive sophisticated equipment and highly precise measurements. Four things are needed: (1) a testable hypothesis, (2) a sound experimental design, (3) a clear decision in advance about what are to be the outcome measures, and (4) valid statistical analysis of the results. A useful result can never come from a poorly designed experiment, no matter how precise the measurements. A well-designed experiment, which (as with the double-blind technique) has eliminated all sources of subjective bias, can yield decisive results even when the measurement technique is crude—as here, just asking subjects how well they slept the night before.

Taking advantage of technological developments in sleep research, other investigators have measured sleep latency—the time required to fall asleep, where sleep was defined by changes in the brain wave pattern. Time to bed and time to wake in the morning were strictly standardized, and a device that could record movements was attached to the wrist in order to measure periods of activity and inactivity. At 9 A.M. each day, subjects were given caffeine or placebo. Then at several times during the day they were placed on beds in a quiet darkened room and instructed to relax and fall asleep. If they did, the time it took was recorded, and they were awakened immediately; otherwise, after 20 minutes, the attempt was terminated. Interspersed with these opportunities to fall asleep were two vigilance tests. One was a 15-minute visual presentation on a computer monitor, much like our flashing-number procedure. The other was a 40-minute auditory vigilance test, in which the subject had to detect long tones presented randomly during a continuous series of short tones. Caffeine consistently increased the sleep latency as compared with placebo; in other words, caffeine made it harder to fall asleep. The drug also improved performance on the auditory vigilance test.

Rewarding Effects

Although extracts of coffee beans were probably consumed for at least a thousand years in East Africa and Yemen, the custom of drinking coffee first flourished in the urban centers of the Middle East in the late fifteenth century. One of the earliest descriptions notes that "it drove away fatigue and lethargy, and brought to the body a certain sprightliness and vigor." Coffee reached England in the middle of the seventeenth century, and coffeehouses were established on the Middle Eastern model. The founder of London's first coffeehouse advertised that coffee "quickens the spirits, and makes the heart lightsome."

When a novel psychoactive drug enters a society, it often arouses opposition. Despite the mildness of caffeine's stimulant actions, coffeehouses were the objects of suspicion from the beginning. In 1511 they were actually prohibited for a short time by the religious authorities in Mecca. And in England in 1675 they were shut down by Charles II in response to a strong temperance movement, coffee being regarded as a kind of intoxicant, one that made people too lively and loquacious, and which promoted dangerous literary and political discussions.

Recently, preference for caffeine over placebo was tested in the following experiment. Pure caffeine at various doses (or a placebo) was packaged in distinctively colored capsules. The experimental design was a three-day sequence. A subject might be given a blue capsule on day 1 containing (for example) a low dose of caffeine, on day 2 a red placebo capsule. Then on day 3 both colors were presented. Of course, neither the subjects nor the experimenters knew the color code, and it was different for each subject. The question was whether, on the basis of subjective effects experienced on the first two days, a subject would choose caffeine or placebo.

There were 12 subjects, 10 independent trials at each dose level, and four doses were tested—truly a major undertaking. Questionnaires about subjective effects were filled out a few hours after taking a capsule, and again later the same day. Saliva tests were done to determine caffeine levels in the blood. If caffeine had neither rewarding nor aversive effects, a subject would be expected to choose caffeine over placebo about half of the time.

At the low dose (100 mg, the amount in a cup of weak coffee), caffeine was clearly reinforcing, as compared with placebo, for four of the 12 subjects, and was aversive to none. Reported subjective effects were "stimulated, energetic, talkative, vigorous." As the dose was increased, the preference for caffeine over placebo decreased in most (but not all) subjects, as aversive effects became predominant ("jittery, nervous, shaky"). This phenomenon is described as a bell-shaped (inverted U) dose-response curve, and it was characteristic of caffeine in all subjects; but the most pleasurable dose (the peak of the curve) varied from person to person. This elegant experiment demonstrated the following: (1) The mild stimulant effects of caffeine are reinforcing for some people, chiefly those who are of a calm and relaxed temperament. (2) Caffeine becomes aversive to most people as the dose is increased to the amount contained in about six cups of coffee, and very likely it would be aversive to everyone at some higher dose. The principal negative effects of high doses are anxiety and jitteriness. (3) People differ widely in their sensitivity to caffeine. It has been shown independently that these individual differences chiefly reflect intrinsic sensitivities of the brain to a given blood concentration of the drug, rather than differences in blood concentrations at a given dose.

Caffeine on the Brain

Caffeine binds as an antagonist to receptors for the neurotransmitter adenosine. Of the four adenosine receptor subtypes, the A2A subtype has highest affinity for caffeine. These receptors are on GABA neurons (see chapter 3). Adenosine stimulates GABA release, which in turn inhibits the release of dopamine in the reward pathway. So the caffeine effect is another example (as with opiates) where inhibiting inhibition causes stimulation. By blocking the effect of adenosine, caffeine reduces GABA release, thus disinhibiting (stimulating) dopamine action in the reward pathway. If this sounds remarkably complicated—yes, brain chemistry works in complicated ways!

For a drug that is as widely used as caffeine, it may seem foolish for scientists to devise complicated experiments to show that it is a reinforcer. After all, it is freely chosen by millions of humans, and free choice is the criterion used to demonstrate that a drug is a primary reinforcer in animal experiments. Animals will self-administer it, and it is reinforcing in the conditioned place preference test. But the drug is certainly not a powerful reinforcer.

Caffeine resembles cocaine in some respects. Like cocaine, it is a psychostimulant, but a mild one. It also sensitizes animals to the effects of cocaine, and rats actually confuse it with cocaine in drug discrimination tests. Yet in contrast to the binge pattern characteristic of cocaine self-administration, dosage escalation does not occur—perhaps because of the aversive effects of higher doses. In humans there is a very high correlation of caffeine use to alcohol and nicotine use, but the reasons for this correlation are unclear. Twin studies have revealed that preference for caffeinated beverages is to a considerable extent genetically determined.

This is probably a good place to note an aspect of the dopamine hypothesis that puzzles some neuroscientists, including me. All the addictive drugs discussed so far in this book—nicotine, alcohol, opiates, cocaine, cannabis, and now caffeine—appear to provoke an increase of dopamine at the nucleus accumbens in the mesolimbic reward pathway. But these drugs differ from one another in so many ways! One has to believe that dopamine is responsible for the one thing they have in common—namely, their reinforcing and addictive properties. One has to suppose that the striking differences in their behavioral effects are due to other interactions in the brain. But if this were correct, all the addictive drugs should be interchangeable—nicotine should satisfy heroin addicts, alcohol addicts should gladly switch to caffeine, and so on. That does not happen, so dopamine must be only one piece of the addiction puzzle, with much more still to be learned.

Toxicity and Dependence

In my studies, people who habitually drank the most coffee complained of headache, drowsiness, fatigue, and a negative mood state on awakening in the morning. These withdrawal symptoms were quickly relieved by morning caffeine, but they became worse after morning placebo. The existence of a caffeine withdrawal syndrome has been confirmed again and again, with its characteristic triad of headache, drowsiness, and fatigue. Most interesting, mild withdrawal symptoms of the same kind have been documented even in some subjects who take (in coffee, tea, or caffeinated soft drinks) less than the equivalent of a single cup of coffee a day. Since 90 percent of the population, including young children, take caffeine daily, one has to conclude that a large fraction of the entire population is to some degree dependent on this addictive drug. In a survey of 162 randomly selected caffeine users, more than half met an explicit psychiatric criterion of drug dependence—that they strongly desired to stop using, or had actually attempted unsuccessfully to stop.

The addition of caffeine to soft drinks has resulted in regular caffeine intake by young children. Most, on a body weight basis, consume the daily equivalent (for an adult) of less than a cup of coffee daily. For a few, however, the amount is equivalent to six or more cups. Several studies have revealed that discontinuing caffeine intake in children—especially those who consume the most caffeine—produces typical withdrawal symptoms. In the United States, the food labeling regulations mandate that the presence of added caffeine be stated, but not the amount. Medical scientists are requesting the Food and Drug Administration to change the labeling rules so that parents can know how much caffeine their children are consuming.

How concerned should one be about this nearly universal dependence on caffeine? Much effort has been expended in large-scale epidemiological studies throughout the world to see if caffeine is a "risk factor" for coronary heart disease, high blood pressure, or cancer. To say that coffee drinking is a risk factor for coronary heart disease, for example, would mean that a greater proportion of coffee drinkers than of abstainers develop this serious medical problem. It would not mean that coffee drinking causes the disease: The term "risk factor" merely denotes an association, nothing more. Sophisticated statistical procedures try to tease out what other factors may also be associated, and to remove them from the analysis. For example, coffee drinkers often smoke, and smoking is certainly associated with heart disease. Then the question is: After accounting for the effects of smoking, do coffee drinkers still have a higher likelihood of developing heart disease? No matter how many other factors can be recognized and accounted for, one may still be left with unknown associated factors. After all, coffee drinkers are different, in many aspects of lifestyle and personality, from people who do not drink coffee. For example, coffee drinking is associated, for unknown reasons, with a diet high in animal fat—itself a risk factor for heart disease.

These large-scale studies show that no toxic effects of any kind have been attributed unequivocally to modest use of caffeine. Only at extremely high dosages may the drug cause irregularities of the heartbeat, anxiety states, and occasionally mental confusion. Moreover, caffeine—like nicotine but unlike alcohol, cocaine, marijuana, or hallucinogens—causes no socially dangerous disruption of behavior. And finally, when caffeine is used on a long-term basis—unlike alcohol or tobacco—it causes no evident damage to brain or other organs.

The possible risk of caffeine use during pregnancy, however, requires special consideration. Many drugs that are harmless to adults at moderate dosages can be dangerous to the fetus, especially during the very early period of organ development, which takes place even before a woman can know she is pregnant. Caffeine consumption at a very high level—for example, more than 10 cups of coffee daily—can cause miscarriage and premature labor, as well as chromosome abnormalities, congenital malformations, respiratory difficulties, and problems with the heart and circulation of the newborn. At moderate dosages, however, the finding of fetal damage is subject to all the uncertainties arising from factors associated with the use of a drug (as discussed already in earlier chapters), such as differences in lifestyle, prenatal care, nutrition, and use of other drugs.

Animal studies help to resolve some of the ambiguities, but extrapolation to humans is problematic because of the many differences between species in responses to any drug. With that caveat in mind, we can summarize the animal experiments as follows: When monkeys were given caffeine in their drinking water at a dosage corresponding (on a weight basis) to about five cups of coffee daily in humans, early fetal death and stillbirths occurred more often than with controls. Numerous experiments in rats have shown deleterious effects of maternal caffeine intake, but only at dosages corresponding to about 10 cups of coffee daily in humans. These effects included reduced body weight of the newborn and delayed development of the pups, as well as depressed motor activity and sleep disturbance, but no significant changes in learning or memory. The pups did have an increased number of adenosine receptors in their brains, a condition associated with increased sensitivity to adenosine; this would be expected from long-term exposure to an adenosine receptor antagonist like caffeine. In discrete brain areas a decrease in dopamine content was also observed. Taken together, the human and animal data are suggestive enough of fetal damage to indicate that—as with some other addictive drugs—the prudent course is to avoid caffeine entirely during pregnancy, and to begin that abstinence regimen (if possible) even before conception.

A key problem for study is the extent to which genetic predisposition accounts for the striking differences in habitual caffeine self-administration and in sensitivity to the alerting and wakefulness caused by the drug. This question is relevant to all the addictive drugs, as discussed in chapter 7, but it might be studied most easily with caffeine, for the reasons outlined at the beginning of this chapter.

Summary

Caffeine is a mild psychostimulant, which is pleasurable and reinforcing consequent to its activation of the dopaminergic reward pathway. It is an adenosine receptor antagonist, which indirectly causes dopamine release in the reward pathway. High doses are aversive, causing anxiety, jitteriness, and sleep disturbance; this probably accounts for the fact that dosage escalation is rare.

The most prominent psychoactive effect is a feeling of energy and efficiency, with enhanced ability to concentrate. Objectively, there is little or no evidence of improved performance, except when performance is already degraded because of fatigue, boredom, or sleepiness.

People differ greatly in their intrinsic sensitivity to caffeine, especially in the sleep disturbance caused by the drug.

Chronic intake leads to dependence and to a withdrawal syndrome on discontinuing. Prominent withdrawal symptoms are headache, fatigue, and sleepiness.

A very large fraction of the population consumes caffeine in coffee, tea, and caffeinated soft drinks. Among these are children—

even very young children—some of whom take large amounts daily and become dependent.

High dosages taken regularly during pregnancy cause fetal abnormalities, so abstaining entirely from caffeine is the prudent course for women who are pregnant or intend to become pregnant.

14

Hallucinogens

An anthropologist studying a native tribe in the jungles of South America observed the ceremonial use of an intoxicating drink called ayahuasca, made from a certain vine. "The natives," he wrote, "see big snakes curling upward on their house posts, and on the walls appear colored butterflies and creatures that are aggregates of snakes, jaguars, and birds. . . . A man saw a cat climbing a wall, then turning into a leopard, when in fact, not even the cat existed." To understand the custom better, he drank some himself. The world around him took on an extraordinarily vivid appearance. Colored geometric designs seemed to soar before his open eyes. With his eyes closed he saw quickly moving small figures, as in a cartoon— abundant imagery, with bright-colored red-green or blue-orange contrasts. There were long dreamlike sequences. Buzzing sounds occurred. Most remarkable was the superimposition of images on walls, or imaginary scenes and objective scenes appearing simultaneously.

The ritual use of hallucinogens is embedded in many cultures. Indigenous peoples in all parts of the world have discovered natural products that could alter the sense of time and place, and produce visual, auditory, and other sensory distortions. Some hallucinogens may not be addictive in the sense of producing an irresistible craving or leading to a frank withdrawal syndrome. Yet one, at least, is powerfully addictive; and some addictive drugs of the other families may cause hallucinations at high doses. At the end of this chapter I shall consider the arguments about their classification. But let us first examine the hallucinogens for the light they shed on how psychoactive drugs can disorder normal brain function.

Hallucinogens on the Brain

There are two groups of hallucinogens with effects like those just described, and the compounds in both groups are chemically akin to neurotransmitters. The first group contains chemical structures related to serotonin (also called 5-HT), the other to dopamine and the closely related amphetamine structure. Both groups seem to activate—directly or indirectly—one of the 14 or more subtypes of serotonin receptor, the one called 5-HT2A. These receptors belong to the 7-helix family (see chapter 3). For substances chemically related to serotonin, this mode of action is not surprising; but it is not understood why compounds with structures related to dopamine and amphetamine should behave in the same way. Compounds of both groups cause a massive discharge of serotonin from the endings of the serotonin neurons, followed by prolonged depletion of this neurotransmitter.

The receptors are concentrated in the higher brain centers such as the cerebral cortex and the nucleus accumbens, which process cognition, perception, and mood. Another area rich in these receptors is the locus coeruleus, a cluster of nerve cells containing the neurotransmitter noradrenaline; its neurons branch out widely to numerous areas of the brain. It is an ideal target for hallucinogens because it plays a central role in processing and filtering sensory inputs; and it does seem to be an important site of action of the hallucinogens. Directly or indirectly, as a consequence of serotonin release, excitatory neurotransmission by glutamate is enhanced in the cerebral cortex, an effect thought likely to explain the psychoactive effects. Still a mystery, however, is the fact that serotonin itself, acting on the same 5-HT2A receptors, does not cause effects like those of the hallucinogens. As it is almost impossible to study hallucinations in animals, research on the mechanisms of action has progressed very slowly, but the recent development of brain imaging techniques offers hope of better progress.

Some effects of the hallucinogens resemble some symptoms of schizophrenia, and therefore much research has been devoted to trying to understand this connection. Indeed, there is even some evidence that the use of hallucinogens can precipitate schizophrenia in vulnerable users who were not diagnosed previously with a psychosis.

Substances Related to the Structure of Serotonin

In 1956, a German anthropologist made his way to the upper reaches of the Amazon to study the Yanomami Indians, an isolated tribe living deep in the rain forest. There he discovered, and filmed, the ceremonial use of a snuff called by the Indians "epena." To prepare this material they must first locate a certain rare tree. Its bark is stripped, and the fibrous substance on the inner side of the bark is scraped. The scrapings are dried slowly over a fire, then crumbled to a fine dust by rubbing between the hands. Next, the bark of another tree (only a certain kind of tree) is burned to ashes, and these ashes are mixed in equal parts with the crumbled scrapings. The resulting snuff powder is then stored in a bamboo tube.

The snuff is used in the following curious way. With a special blowpipe about five feet long, one man blows a portion of the powder forcibly into another man's nostrils. The snuff produces severe headache, salivation, vomiting, and profuse sweating. The subject stares fixedly, and he begins a vigorous stamping dance accompanied by a chant. This is interrupted every few minutes by a fierce yell, while he spreads his arms toward the sky. The anthropologist learned that during the intoxication the Indians are convinced they have grown to an enormous size, big enough to converse face to face with the spirits in the sky—spirits that they report being able to see.

In contrast to the natural epena snuff, LSD is a highly potent synthetic hallucinogen, discovered entirely by accident in the laboratory. On Friday, April 16, 1943, a chemist working for the Swiss pharmaceutical firm Sandoz, in Basel, was engaged in a project to synthesize a large variety of compounds related chemically to lysergic acid. Lysergic acid is derived from chemicals in a fungus called ergot, which grows on spoiled rye grain. For many years, extracts of ergot—and more recently, pure compounds isolated from ergot—had been used in obstetrics to stop uterine bleeding after childbirth.

By systematically altering chemical groups on lysergic acid, the Sandoz chemists hoped to learn more about the relationship of chemical structure to biological activity. They were trying to find safer and more effective ergot drugs, because the existing ones had undesirable side effects, including the serious one of shutting off circulation to various parts of the body.

Ergot toxicity was well known in Europe since the Middle Ages, under the name "St. Anthony's Fire." When bread was made from rye flour contaminated with ergot, an entire village—all the villagers would have patronized a single bakery—would become seriously ill. Disturbances of the circulation were prominent, with terrible burning sensations (thus the name of the affliction) in the intestines and elsewhere in the body, and gangrene of the fingers and toes. The most severely affected victims also developed hallucinations and bizarre psychotic behaviors. An epidemic of ergotism was recorded as recently as 1951, in the little French village of Pont-Saint-Esprit, where several hundred people were affected. Some became delirious and confused, seeing imaginary animals and flames and other macabre visions, and a few of them died.

The Sandoz chemist had to leave his laboratory early that Friday afternoon because he felt oddly agitated and slightly dizzy. At home he lay down and tried to sleep, but weird things began to happen. Fantastic pictures appeared before his eyes, with a play of extraordinary, kaleidoscopic colors. He was clever enough to recognize that the toxic psychosis might be due to some chemical he had come in contact with in his laboratory. He was aware of the profound hallucinogenic effects of ergot, and one of the compounds he had made and crystallized that day was an ergot derivative, lysergic acid diethylamide (LSD). However, as the total amount he had worked with was only a few milligrams, it seemed to him most unlikely that enough could have gotten into his system to poison him.

He felt better the next morning, so to check out his suspicions about LSD he returned to the laboratory. He dissolved what he considered a tiny amount—250 micrograms—in water, and drank it. (We know now that this was ten times the effective hallucinogenic dose.) Forty minutes later, his notebook entry was:

Slight giddiness, anxiety, hard to focus my thoughts, disturbance of vision, impulse to laugh.

Here the notebook record stopped abruptly. A few days later he described why:

> Words could only be written down with great effort. I asked my laboratory assistant to accompany me home, for I expected the thing would run the same course as the disturbances of the previous Friday. But it was clear, even as I rode home by bicycle, that all the symptoms were worse than the first time. I had great difficulty speaking clearly, and my field of vision wavered like an image in a crooked mirror.

After he reached home, the visual disturbances became more vivid. Fantastic images appeared, colored bright blue and green. Most remarkable of all, sounds, as of passing cars, were somehow transmuted into optical sensations, "so that for each tone and each noise a corresponding kaleidoscopic form and color was produced." After a night's sleep, he felt completely normal again.

It turned out that LSD was by far the most potent hallucinogen ever discovered. Even the 250 micrograms taken deliberately by the chemist would be no bigger than a grain of salt, and the more typical dose of 25 micrograms would be practically invisible. Thus it was clear how, on that first Friday, the chemist might accidentally have contaminated himself, perhaps by merely touching a dirty finger to his lips.

It was the same chemist who first identified psilocybin, the psychoactive principle of a "magic mushroom." This chemical is also related to the neurotransmitter serotonin. Psychoactive mushrooms have been used since prehistoric times, especially in Aztec and other native religious rituals; in modern times they have entered the drug culture in the United States and Europe. When someone not too familiar with mushrooms mistakenly eats one of these, the effects can be quite alarming. A tingling numbness develops throughout the body, vision becomes blurred, and brilliantly colored images appear. Victims may panic, fearing they are going insane, especially when they experience feelings of disembodiment. In one reported case, a young woman "thought that she was a banana and that somebody was attempting to skin her." A three-year-old child was frightened by "seeing colored lights on the ceiling, seeing cats that were not there, and feeling that she was bigger than she really was."

Deliberate use of the mushrooms—as by cooking them into soups or omelettes—more often than not produces effects that are regarded as pleasant and interesting, since they are anticipated and desired. Colorful hallucinations are common, often accompanied by a sense of elation and uncontrollable laughing. However, the potency of psychoactive mushrooms varies unpredictably, as does the way different people react, so that "bad trips" are an ever-present threat. Panic attacks and "flashbacks" occur; these are psychotic reactions days or even weeks after the immediate drug effect has worn off.

In drug discrimination trials, laboratory animals trained to recognize LSD respond to psilocybin as if it were the same, and the effects in humans are much like those of LSD and other LSD-like drugs. For this reason, "psilocybin" sold on the street is almost always actually LSD, and ordinary mushrooms laced with LSD may be sold as "magic mushrooms."

Substances Related to the Structures of Dopamine and Amphetamine

The peyote cactus, native to the southwestern states and Mexico, has an ancient history of use for religious purposes among the North American Indians. Spanish explorers along the Rio Grande valley described the peyote rite in 1560, and archeological data obtained with carbon-14 dating now suggest a history that goes back 7,000 years. The peyote ceremony is today the central ritual of the Native American Church, founded about 1880. A meeting typically lasts all night, with chanting, drumming, prayers, and the eating of peyote "buttons" in strictly limited amount according to a prescribed ritual. The peyote experience was described by one participant as follows:

> The appearance of vision with closed eyes was very gradual. At first there was merely a vague play of light and shade, which suggested pictures, but never made them. Then the pictures became more definite, but too confused and crowded to be described, beyond saying that they were of the same character as the images of the kaleidoscope, symmetrical groupings of spiked objects. Then, in the course of the evening, they became distinct, but still indescribable—mostly a vast field of golden jewels, studded with red and green stones, ever changing. . . . All sorts of odd and grotesque images passed in succession through my mind. . . . Five or

six fish, the color of canaries, floating about in air in a gold wire cage.

According to anthropologists who have studied peyotism, frank hallucinations, like those described above, are the exception rather than the rule. The essential effect that is sought is rather the endowment of ordinary objects and events with profound significance. This subtle change in the way participants view their surroundings is considered to be an aid to introspection and to making prayers more efficacious. Except for people who are unusually sensitive to the psychoactive drug, hallucinations occur only at higher dosages than are normally used in the ceremony.

Mescaline is the active compound in peyote. Its molecular structure is nearly identical to that of amphetamine, which, in turn, is closely related to that of the neurotransmitter dopamine. The first experimental administration of pure mescaline to a human was conducted—on himself—by a German pharmacologist in 1897. The effects of hallucinogens are so modified by personal experience, and in today's drug-taking youth culture so exaggerated by subjective anticipation and shared mythologies, that it is interesting to read the discoverer's original account. He was reputed to be rather staid, stern, and objective, a no-nonsense scientist with a rigid personality and no preconceptions about what to expect.

> Violet and green spots appear on the paper during reading. When the eyes are kept shut there are visions of carpet patterns, ribbed vaulting, etc. . . . Landscapes, halls, architectural scenes (e.g., pillars decorated with flowers) also appear . . . Nausea and dizziness are at times very distressing. The appreciation of time is reduced. . . . Both mescaline and the crude drug (peyote) produced the characteristic visions.

He wondered whether peyote would "become popular amongst cultured people as an intoxicating drug," but thought it unlikely because the side effects were so pronounced that "they considerably spoil the appreciation of the beautiful visions."

Nutmeg contains a substance that is metabolized to a mescaline-like compound in the body. The seeds of a handsome East Indian tree, nutmeg had medicinal uses in ancient times, especially among Arab physicians. The neuroanatomist Johannes Purkinje tried some in 1829, and wrote: "My movements . . . were lost momentarily in dream pictures, from which I had to extricate myself with considerable force in order to keep on walking . . . dreams and physical activity battled one another." Distortions of space are especially common, described thus by one subject: "The kitchen was cathedral-like in its dimensions . . . and I was unusually tall, my feet were small and far away, it was like looking through the wrong end of binoculars." Often reported are sensations of floating, being transported aloft, or having one's limbs separated from one's body.

MDMA ("ecstasy") is a methamphetamine derivative that enjoys some popularity on college campuses. It is related chemically to dopamine and mescaline. For most people, the sense of disembodiment and the visual hallucinations are less extreme than with LSD or mescaline, and the feelings of elation are greater; but the effects are qualitatively very similar. In rats, MDMA causes massive destruction of serotonin neurons. That this alarming brain damage also occurs in humans has been demonstrated by PET imaging studies (chapter 3) using a positron-labeled ligand of the serotonin transporter as a way to measure the number of serotonergic neurons. This brain damage, in those with a long history of MDMA use, is very persistent; it may even be irreversible. In addition, deaths have been reported from acute failure of the cardiovascular system and temperature controls.

Phencyclidine (PCP, "Angel Dust")

This substance, although capable of producing hallucinations, is rather different from the hallucinogens discussed above. PCP acts consistently as a primary reinforcer in animal experiments: It is self-administered, whereas most other hallucinogens are not. This distinction is not absolute, however, for baboons will, indeed, self-administer a few compounds of the LSD group, even displaying what appears to be hallucinatory behavior, such as trying to catch imaginary objects. Drug discrimination experiments also set PCP apart. Animals trained to recognize one LSD-like hallucinogen usually cannot distinguish between it and others in the group, whereas they clearly perceive PCP as different. Human subjects seek euphoria from PCP and become truly addicted to it. It enjoys periodic popularity on the street, but unpredictable serious adverse reactions tend to limit its use.

Unlike the relaxed euphoria and emotional blunting caused by opiates, and unlike the euphoric stimulation caused by cocaine and amphetamines, the PCP "high" combines ecstatic pleasure with feelings of unreality, accompanied by distortions of time, space, and body image. Judgment and intellectual capacity are strongly impaired. Strange and bizarre behavior may occur, with thought disturbances, paranoia, and even violent (homicidal or suicidal) actions. At low doses, the balance between pleasant and unpleasant effects is unpredictable. Higher doses consistently produce restlessness, disorientation, panic, fear of impending death, obsession with trivial matters, paranoid thinking, belligerence, and impaired judgment. The full-blown PCP psychosis may include bizarre, violent, assaultive behavior, incoherent speech, blank stare, and compulsive repetitive movements. After recovery from the immediate drug psychosis, there is usually amnesia for the whole episode. An alarming feature is persistence of the delusional state for as long as a week or more, with recurrent panic attacks, hallucinations, and even the possibility of suicide during this period.

PCP resembles the opiates in producing a physical withdrawal syndrome in animals, but a less florid one than that of opiates. In humans, intense craving, depression, and extreme sleepiness are typical. Newborn infants of PCP-addicted mothers soon go into withdrawal; they become irritable, with a characteristic high-pitched cry, they are jittery, have hyperactive reflexes, feed poorly, and suffer from diarrhea. Major developmental deficits become evident in these children—trouble with adaptive behaviors, impaired learning, poor motor control, retarded acquisition of language skills, and problems in interpersonal relationships.

The chemical structure of PCP is unique and unrelated to that of any known neurotransmitter. It binds to opioid receptors, but its principal selective interaction is with a binding site on the NMDA receptor complex, an ion channel composed of several subunits (chapter 3). The natural ligand of this receptor is glutamate, a major excitatory neurotransmitter in the brain. PCP is an antagonist at this receptor, producing a long-persisting blockade of glutamate transmission. Just how blocking this ion channel leads to hallucinations and psychosis remains obscure. The identification of a PCP receptor initiated a search for an endogenous ligand, on the conceptual model of opioid receptors and endogenous opioids or cannabinoid receptors and anandamide. Intense interest attaches to this search because the behavioral disturbances caused by PCP resemble those of schizophrenia in so many ways. Thus, it has been proposed that schizophrenia itself might be due to a deficit in glutamate neurotransmission, possibly due to excessive production or defective removal of an endogenous PCP-like ligand.

Another Magic Mushroom

Fly agaric (Amanita muscaria) is a large, bright red mushroom with a long history of ceremonial use by shamans in Siberia and Northern Europe. Some anthropologists speculate that its history goes back to ancient times in India. The psychoactive principle of this mushroom, known as muscimol, is unrelated to serotonin or dopamine but, interestingly, is an agonist at the GABA receptor complex. It will be recalled that the GABA receptor is also thought to be a major site of action of alcohol and the benzodiazepines; yet muscimol intoxication presents a very different picture. There is a peculiar kind of half-sleep accompanied by colored visions and feelings of elation. Under the influence of this drug one has the impression of being able to perform amazing feats of physical effort, even to fly. One pharmacologist has described his own experience as follows:

> There was dizziness, speech was inarticulate, concentration was difficult. There were endlessly repeated echo-pictures of situations observed a few minutes before . . . hearing was noisy . . . there was confusion, disturbance of visual perception, illusions of color vision, disorientation in time and space, weariness, fatigue.

A curious property of the hallucinogenic substance in fly agaric is that it passes intact into the urine. Body metabolism removes various toxic impurities so that muscimol extracted from urine is actually more pure than it was in the mushroom. This unusual property (most drugs are destroyed as they pass through the body) was discovered in ancient times, so that drinking the shaman's urine and thus recycling the psychoactive substance became a part of the religious ritual. I am reminded of my days as an Army physician in 1944, when penicillin was first being introduced into medicine. This antibiotic is also excreted intact into urine. During those wartime years it was so scarce and precious that we actually recovered it routinely from patients' urine, purified it, and used it again.

Hallucinogens and Addiction

It is a remarkable fact that plant products have the power to alter the way the human mind functions. Like all the addictive drugs, the hallucinogens are closely related chemically to the natural neurotransmitters, and they act by disturbing the finely regulated chemical systems of the brain. Even the synthetic hallucinogens, by and large, are chemically modified natural plant products. How amazing it is that of the hundreds of thousands of plant species on the planet, humans should have discovered just those few that contain psychoactive substances!

Wherever anthropologists have gone, in whatever remote region of the world, they have found people using mind-altering drugs derived from natural sources. The great physician William Osler once said, jocularly, "The chief thing that distinguishes humans from other species is their desire to take medicines." A whole field of research, called ethnopharmacology, is devoted to searching out and studying natural drugs used by native cultures. In the story of epena snuff, it is noteworthy—and typical—that unschooled people were able to discover, and pass on from generation to generation, the kind of detailed knowledge that modern ethnopharmacologists now seek. Which rare tree was required? What part of the tree produced the psychoactive substance? How was the product to be prepared for use? Very likely the active material is destroyed when taken by mouth, so it has to be absorbed through the membranes of the nose. But this can only occur after a chemical treatment with alkali—a principle rediscovered by modern pharmacologists, and applied also in preparing crack cocaine from cocaine salt. But then, which other tree will produce an ash that is alkaline enough to be effective when mixed with epena ash? One is awestruck by the amount of experimentation that must have been needed, over the centuries, to develop this one hallucinogenic snuff for ritual use.

Does a chapter on hallucinogens belong in a book on drug addiction? Most would argue for including PCP, because it causes dependence and an opiatelike withdrawal syndrome. Some would argue for omitting the LSD-like and dopamine-related hallucinogens because animals, as a rule, will not self-administer them. However, clear-cut categories are difficult to establish because of the many overlapping actions of the psychoactive drugs. The brain is so complex, with so many subtypes of neurotransmitter receptors, that no single substance will ever have only a single biological effect. At the lowest dosages, for example of LSD, only visual hallucinations may occur. But as dosage increases, quite different mental and physical disturbances come into play. Thus, some drugs are primarily hallucinogenic at the lowest effective dosages, while others are primarily reinforcers at low dosage but may be hallucinogenic at higher dosage. Sometimes hallucinations at high dosage are part of a toxic psychosis, accompanied by serious thought disorders. Marijuana, for example, at low dosage produces only relaxation, altered mood, and some disturbance of time sense; but high dosage can produce frank hallucinations. Cocaine and amphetamines are powerful reinforcers, producing an intense "high" at ordinary dosages; but greater dosages and continuous binging cause outright paranoia, with hallucinations and manic behavior. Abrupt withdrawal from alcohol may produce vivid hallucinations with detailed content (for example, little men riding bicycles around the ceiling) rather than mere multicolored patterns.

Hallucinogens share with all addictive drugs the property that they are self-administered for the purpose of altering mood, perception, and emotions. But there are significant differences in the social context in which they are used. Among native peoples all over the world, hallucinogens are chiefly used ceremonially, on infrequent occasions, and under strict control of a shaman or other religious leaders. A similar mode of controlled drug use is seen in the way sacramental wine is used in the Jewish and Christian religions. These traditions seem to reflect an understanding, assimilated into human culture over the centuries, that unrestricted use of psychoactive drugs is dangerous.

In our own culture, on the other hand, hallucinogenic drugs are often used in an out-of-control fashion. Then craving may ensue between occasions of use; and panic reactions and toxic psychosis can be significant hazards, at least for some users. Long-term brain damage may be a real possibility with high dosage and repeated use, and "flashbacks" during periods of abstinence may reflect such irreversible disturbances of brain function. Fads in the use of one or another hallucinogen come and go. No one understands why LSD, for example, should have been so popular in the sixties, fallen off in popularity in the seventies, and made a partial comeback later.

Nor is it clear why drugs of this class can become popular in one geographic area but not at all in another.

Hallucinogens have been popularized as somehow being able to reveal mystical or symbolic aspects of the mind that are normally hidden from introspection—thus the term psychedelic, meaning "mind-revealing." The person on a "trip," as described by a knowledgeable psychiatrist, "passively watches as a range of novel emotional, perceptual, and cognitive events are intensely exposed." One subject, a scientist, described his own hallucinations as follows:

> What I was seeing was more clearly seen than anything I had seen before. At last I was seeing with the eye of the soul, not through the coarse lenses of my natural eyes. Moreover, what I was seeing was impregnated with weighty meaning. I was awe-struck.

Much as dreams are based on personal experience, the content of drug-induced hallucinations varies greatly from person to person. In the sixties, with the rise of the youth drug culture, some psychiatrists used hallucinogens to access what they considered to be aspects of a patient's mind that were otherwise inaccessible. Such therapeutic use has waned, perhaps because psychiatrists—like the rest of us—found it too difficult to draw valid conclusions from the productions of chemically disordered brains.

Summary

The hallucinogens, originally obtained from plants, and now synthesized in many varieties, have their roots in native cultures around the world. Historically, their use has been integrated into religious ceremonies, and surrounded by safeguards against rampant abuse for recreational purposes. In modern civilized societies, periodic epidemics of hallucinogen use occur. To alter one's perceptions of the objective world evidently is appealing to some people—especially to young people seeking new thrills.

Most hallucinogens act on one subtype of serotonin receptor, which is widely distributed in areas of the brain that process sensory inputs. Massive release of serotonin, with consequent serotonin deficiency leads—directly or indirectly—to the characteristic distortions of cognition, perception, and mood. Our understanding of the neurochemical mechanisms responsible for these psychoactive effects is still very incomplete.

The discovery of LSD is a classic study in serendipity. It was the extraordinarily high potency of this synthetic drug that allowed a remarkably tiny amount, ingested by accident, to cause bizarre symptoms in the chemist who had made it.

MDMA ("ecstasy") is probably the most dangerous of all the hallucinogens because—at least with chronic high dosage—it destroys serotonin neurons and thus may cause long-lasting, even irreversible, brain damage.

Phencyclidine (PCP) is extremely dangerous because of the violent paranoid behavior it provokes, which often leads to homicide or suicide. Because of the similarity of its effects to those seen in schizophrenia, it is hoped that research on its actions may reveal the causes of that psychotic condition. Newborns of women addicted to PCP suffer severe withdrawal symptoms after birth, and display many abnormalities of childhood development.

Part Three

Drugs and Society

15

Prevention:
Just Say No?

If you walked into a Kansas City sixth-grade classroom some years ago, you might have observed the following scene: Under a teacher's guidance, and with the whole class watching, a child pretends to offer a cigarette to a friend. The friend hesitates, uncertain what to do. The teacher intervenes. "Sally," she suggests, "you know that smoke makes people cough. Try saying that." The role-playing is repeated. The cigarette is offered. Sally says, boldly, "No thanks, I don't like the way smoke makes me cough." Then Sally turns her back and walks away with a determined air.

The slogan "Just say no!" expresses a valid goal, but by itself it is too simplistic. Although sometimes considered as a deterrent only for first use of drugs by children, this slogan really applies at all times of life—to occasional users, to those who have become addicted, to addicts in treatment, and to those who are in danger of relapse after treatment. Furthermore, in each of these situations a set of skills has to be taught in order to make "Just say no!" a reality. What has actually been learned about how to prevent children and adolescents from using addictive drugs in the first place? Obviously, without first use there could be no addiction, just as there could be no addiction if the particular drug were totally unavailable.

Drug Use by Children

Data on drug use by adults were presented in chapter 1 and the several chapters of Part Two. Caffeine, alcohol, and nicotine, in that descending order, are used most frequently, with marijuana in fourth place. Not surprisingly, these same drugs, in the same order, are typically used by children and adolescents, starting at about sixth grade (ages 11–12).

First use, in many children, occurs as an expression of natural curiosity, a desire to imitate grown-up behavior, or a daring venture into a forbidden realm. The degree of social deviance represented by first use is different for each drug and varies from one culture to another. In the United States and many other countries, first use of alcohol or tobacco usually signifies only a minor transgression of accepted social standards because these two drugs are so widely used in adult society. An exception is in families where these substances are strictly taboo on religious grounds; in that case first use may signify a more serious break with social convention. Even for alcohol and nicotine, which are legal for adults, the age of first use almost always precedes the legally sanctioned age; and therefore, use must be associated—to some extent at least—with a willingness to break the law.

Data from the most recent surveys of drug use by children will surprise most adults. In eighth grade, 52 percent of children have tried alcohol, and 25 percent have actually been drunk at least once. By twelfth grade, these numbers increase to 80 percent and 62 percent, respectively.

In eighth grade, 44 percent have tried cigarettes. By twelfth grade, 65 percent have smoked at least once, 23 percent smoke daily, and 13 percent smoke a half pack or more daily.

Marijuana was tried by 22 percent and 50 percent, respectively, of eighth-grade and 12th-grade children, with 10 percent and 23 percent having used within the past month. Although marijuana is a prohibited drug, its use is so widespread in some adult circles that first use by a child requires but little sociopathic behavior; and the route of administration—smoking—is already commonplace for tobacco.

Even by twelfth grade, fewer than 3 percent have ever used cocaine and fewer than 1 percent heroin in the prior month. First use of these drugs requires a high degree of deviance. Their illicit status forces the first-time user into criminal behavior at the outset. Just to "learn the ropes"—where and how to find the drug, how to prepare it for use, how to use it—requires experienced associates who are often already deeply involved in antisocial and frankly criminal behavior. Furthermore, if cocaine or heroin is to be used intravenously, the route of administration itself presupposes a high degree of social deviance; inserting a needle into one's own vein is for most people a strange, unnatural act not casually performed.

These figures come from the large-scale Monitoring the Future study for 1999, which includes the High School Seniors Survey. These surveys have been conducted annually for many years at the University of Michigan, with funding from the federal government's National Institute on Drug Abuse. We can summarize drug use by children as follows: Caffeine is used almost universally by very young children, typically in carbonated soft drinks (chapter 13). First use of any other drug, on a trial basis, can begin as early as sixth grade, and the drug is almost always alcohol and/or nicotine. Whatever the drug, use escalates sharply between eighth and twelfth grade. At all ages, the regular use of caffeine, alcohol, and nicotine is greater than of marijuana, and far greater than of cocaine or heroin. High-school dropouts are not included, so the true picture is even more bleak than the numbers cited above indicate.

Recruiting of new users to an addiction is made easier if the route of administration is socially acceptable. When tobacco was first introduced, people did not take to it readily because smoking seemed an unfamiliar and unpleasant behavior. Over the years, thanks to the tobacco industry's vigorous promotional efforts and improvements in cigarette technology, smoking became a normal custom in society. This process of acculturation of drug use will be recognized by older readers, who have seen, in their own lifetimes, how a habit that was socially unacceptable for women until World War II became as commonplace for them as for men. Today most people view intravenous drug self-administration as bizarre behavior and are reluctant to cross that line, but they have no such inhibitions about smoking. This probably accounts, at least in part, for the sharp increase in cocaine use when crack cocaine was introduced; cocaine for intravenous use or for "snorting" had been limited to a much smaller number of users.

Blatant advertising, as well as more subtle media messages extolling the virtues of drinking alcohol and smoking tobacco, contribute to making these dangerous addictive drugs seem acceptable to minors. A recent study of the 200 most popular video rentals and 1,000 most popular songs reveals how frequently tobacco, alcohol, and illicit drugs (usually marijuana) are referred to (in 98 percent of movies, 27 percent of popular songs). Unfortunately, drugs are often associated in these media with positive features like wealth, luxury, and sexual activity. In the majority of cases, no consequence to the user is shown or described.

In 1997, the federal Office of National Drug Control Policy (ONDCP) initiated a major campaign to use the mass media for discouraging drug use among youngsters. Heavily funded by Congress and by the advertising industry, this effort is focused on alcohol and tobacco (which are illegal for children) as well as on the drugs that are also illicit for adults. Developed in conjunction with experts in the drug abuse field, the program is based on substantial evidence that advertising can be effective in producing behavior change. The effort cannot be regarded as an experiment, however, because there can be no controls, no comparison groups. Only overall change with time can be assessed, and then the role of the specific program will be debatable. Thus, we are unlikely ever to know if it is cost-effective—indeed, if it is effective at all. This is a classic example of how efforts to change social customs and behavior may sometimes have to be mounted on a common-sense basis, without scientific proof of efficacy and without subsequent rigorous proof that any changes that did occur were due to the intervention.

Drug Education

Everyone would like to prevent children from using drugs, but how to accomplish that goal is not entirely obvious. In the sixties it was common practice for uniformed police officers to come into the classroom with untruthful or exaggerated stories about the evil effects of marijuana on the body and mind. Accounts of the criminal sanctions on marijuana possession and use, although more accurate, were also meant to terrify. And at a time when the use of cannabis was growing among adults, and when children learned from other sources that alcohol and tobacco were probably more harmful to health than marijuana, any positive effects of the teaching were undercut by the appearance of hypocrisy.

In the 1970s the pendulum swung, and an ambivalent message

about drugs was introduced into many classrooms. Some educators argued that the mere use of addictive drugs was not necessarily bad, that children had to be encouraged to learn all they could about the favorable and unfavorable effects of drugs in order to be able to "make their own decisions" about drug use. This view is no longer prevalent, in part at least because of outraged backlash from organized antidrug groups, especially parents' groups. Their position, grounded in a moral perspective, decries the failure of today's schools to teach "old-fashioned values," as schools used to do. So-called drug education, they complain, is not drug prevention education at all; it is simply telling children about drugs and then leaving them to make their own decisions. These groups argue that it is irresponsible to tell a youngster it is his or her decision, but not to give any guidance. What this does, they say, is to leave the child vulnerable to peer pressure and the drug peddler out on the street. There have been no experiments to test whether returning to earlier methods of education would be effective in reducing drug use by children.

Cigarettes and alcohol—because they are so easy to obtain—are often the first drugs that children use, and therefore they have been called "gateway drugs." Some might add caffeine, because it is the very first psychoactive drug used by small children (chapter 13). Blocking these first "gateways" might prevent progression to marijuana, which itself may be considered a gateway to the other addictive drugs. Systematic long-term studies have indeed shown that adolescents who become addicted to heroin or cocaine as they enter adulthood have almost always, when they were younger, used cigarettes and alcohol first, then marijuana. This progression is common (though by no means universal) and the reason is obvious—a child who decides to use any drug at all is likely to start with one that is readily available and legal in adult society, though illegal for minors.

The "gateway" concept is often misunderstood. It describes a statistical relationship, there being no evidence to suggest that using alcohol or nicotine causes any kind of inevitable craving for marijuana, cocaine, or heroin. And, as noted above, only a small fraction of children who do use alcohol or nicotine actually do go on to marijuana, cocaine, or heroin. Nevertheless, preventing young people from starting to drink or smoke, and reducing their drinking and smoking if they have already started, are important goals in their own right because of the major health hazards posed by the use of those two drugs. An additional benefit, then—though speculative—could be to reduce the likelihood of their progressing to the illicit drugs.

Attempts to Change Drug-related Behaviors

Much effort and many research dollars have been expended during the past decade to see what "works" and what doesn't work. Solid and rigorously controlled studies, as can be imagined, are very difficult, and the outcome criteria have to be evaluated for years. These studies are summarized in the excellent recent brochure published by the National Institute on Drug Abuse (NIDA). Target populations are considered, e.g., general community; children at special risk; various age groups and school-based approaches; geographic, ethnic, socioeconomic groups.

Social psychology research on ways of changing human behavior has revealed that many different influences have to be brought to bear in a prevention effort. According to modern social learning theory, behavior is shaped in a social context; and therefore changing children's behavior must involve teachers, peers, parents, indeed the whole community. Scare tactics alone are certainly not effective, and even in a diversified program are probably not very useful, given the striving of adolescents for independence and their natural tendency to rebel against adult authority. Three steps are necessary:

(1) Truthful information has to be imparted in order to generate motivation for behavior change. Only honest, straightforward, and full information about the health risks of the addictive drugs will meet this requirement.

(2) But it has been shown repeatedly that information alone is not sufficient; the means for behavior change have to be provided. Here many techniques have proven effective, especially teaching children how to resist peer pressure. It is important to promote a redefinition of drug-using peers as not "cool."

(3) Methods for reinforcing the new behaviors have to be employed. This means, in short, that children need recognition, praise, and other rewards for not using drugs. Emphasis on how drugs detract from a healthy body and an attractive appearance, for example, appeals to adolescents' interest in athletics as well as to

their developing sexuality and their striving for intimate peer relationships.

An important and relevant finding of social learning theory is the importance of self-efficacy. This quality, which is related to self-esteem, is the expression of people's belief that they are in charge of their own behavior, that they are capable of actually making a desired change. Those who have that self-confidence are more successful than those who doubt their own ability. If a child believes and asserts that he or she is capable of turning down a proposal to drink beer or smoke marijuana with a friend, that is likely to happen. Most important, self-efficacy can be enhanced through training and practice.

Self-efficacy has interesting neurobiological correlates. A rat can be taught that when a warning light comes on, an electric footshock will follow. If the rat is helpless to prevent the shock, the light itself becomes very stressful; and the rat's endogenous opioid (endorphin) pain-suppressing system is turned on, as though in anticipation of the painful shock. However, if the rat is taught that by pressing a lever when the light comes on, it can prevent the shock—in other words, that it has self-efficacy in this situation—stress is reduced and endogenous opioids are not activated.

Similar results have been obtained in humans. People who give themselves a high self-efficacy score have lower levels of stress-combatting hormones in their blood (as though they are not needed) than people who rate their self-efficacy as low. In chapter 5, experiments with the opioid antagonist naloxone in human volunteers were described, showing that stress activates the endorphin pain-suppressing system, as evidenced by the fact that stressful pain is made worse by naloxone. In an experiment with human volunteers, subjects were given mathematical problems to solve. Group A could regulate the level of difficulty of the problems, thus matching their self-efficacy to the task at hand. Members of Group B were given tough problems that frequently exceeded their capacities; this was evidently stressful, and they rated their own self-efficacy as low. Then, mild experimental pain was inflicted on both groups. In Group A, naloxone had no effect, indicating that no endogenous opioids had been mobilized. In Group B, naloxone made the pain worse, showing that the stress associated with feelings of low self-efficacy had activated the opioid system.

The Midwestern Prevention Project

Among the many programs aimed at modifying children's first use of drugs, this prevention program is one of the few carefully designed school-based experiments to be carried out on a very large scale, primarily in Kansas City. The skills of resisting peer pressure were taught through role-playing (as illustrated in the introduction to this chapter), and especially through the use of peers as group leaders. Parents were enlisted to reinforce the classroom experiences by participation in special homework assignments. Community organizations were involved, and the mass media were employed. The program was implemented in the sixth and seventh grades of 169 schools in 26 communities, altogether involving many thousands of students. Control schools and experimental schools were randomly matched.

The measure of success or failure was to be the rate of increase in the use of cigarettes, alcohol, and marijuana in the experimental schools as compared with the control schools. The study began with children who had barely begun drug use of any kind. From sixth grade on, as described earlier, drug use typically increases each year. Successful prevention in the experimental schools would mean reducing the rate of increase, compared with that in the control schools.

Self-reports by the children were used as the primary data; but how reliable would self-reports alone be? There was obviously no possibility here for double-blind design; children in the experimental schools were well aware that they were participants in a special program. They would know what was expected of them. Might they then fabricate or shade their reports to please the researchers? To address this problem, the investigators introduced breath testing for carbon monoxide and saliva testing for thiocyanate—these are reliable indicators of recent smoking. Very good agreement was found between the children's self-reports and the chemical measurements. Parents were also queried about their own and their children's drug use; but children are unlikely to confide illicit behavior to their parents. The important finding concerning parents was, not surprisingly, that a child's drug use (cigarettes, alcohol, marijuana) was likely to be similar to that of the parents.

At the outset, the experimental and control groups were comparable. One year later, as expected, more children in both groups had used drugs. However, the increase was less in the experimental schools than in the control schools. Smoking in the previous month, for example, nearly doubled from the initial 13 percent to 24 percent in the control schools but only to 17 percent in the experimental schools. For alcohol, the initial 8 percent increased to 16 percent (control), compared with 11 percent (experimental). For marijuana, the initial 1 percent had become 10 percent (control) compared with only 7 percent (experimental). On superficial examination, these effects, which are typical of what is seen with similar programs, may be considered small. However, for all three drugs, roughly half the children who would have started using were deterred from doing so. Moreover, several years later, although the school component of the program had not been continued, some effects of the experimental intervention did persist. If that beneficial effect were sustained as the children grew into adulthood, the benefit would indeed be great in terms of reducing the ultimate burden of drug use on the individuals and on society.

Even considering only the reduction in nicotine, alcohol, and marijuana use brought about during the intervention, cost-benefit calculations are encouraging, although they obviously must entail many speculative attempts to put dollar values on consequences of drug use. Once the program is up and running, the actual cost is about $22 per participant and the computed benefits are claimed to be many times that value. This research is ongoing; final estimates are not yet in print.

More than a dozen other prevention programs have been or are being carried out, like the one described above, on a scientific valid basis, allowing the conclusion that it is possible—depending on numerous factors, and with variable outcomes for different drugs—to reduce drug use to a meaningful extent.

Drug Abuse Resistance Education (DARE)

This curriculum originated in Los Angeles in 1983 as a joint effort of the police department and the school district. Since then it has been adopted by well over half of all school districts nationwide. The core curriculum consists of 17 weekly one-hour sessions in sixth grade, presented by police officers who have undergone intensive special training. The avowed aim is to "keep kids off drugs." Outcome measures include knowledge about drugs, attitudes toward drug use, social skills in resisting peer pressure, self-esteem, attitudes toward police, and of course actual drug use (as measured by self-report). The drugs that are used enough by children to permit statistical evaluations of outcome are alcohol, tobacco, and marijuana.

Well designed studies comparing schools randomly assigned to receive or not receive the DARE curriculum have revealed no differences in drug use one, five, or ten years afterward. However, there were modest improvements in the outcome measures that assess knowledge, self-esteem, and attitudes. One may conclude that 17 hours of instruction are not enough to cause significant behavior change in adolescence. Indeed, the trend of increasing drug use in adolescence may be a deep-rooted developmental behavior pattern that is refractory to change by any kind of adult-based instruction. Children may give "correct" answers to questions designed to assess their knowledge and attitudes, while nevertheless escalating their own drug use. One might hope that investing resources into a program demonstrated to be ineffective in achieving its stated goal would be reexamined. Modified versions of DARE are under study at several locations in the hope of identifying components that are useful.

Trends and Conclusions

The necessary first step in assessing trends is to have valid data. Fortunately, the official sources of information noted above—primarily the National Household Survey of adults and the Monitoring the Future study of secondary school children—have been collecting data annually for more than 25 years.

The number for prevalence of use "ever in lifetime" is not very useful; we want to know, for each drug, about ongoing regular use. The best indicator, for most drugs, is "past month use," implying a regular pattern of use, beyond an adolescent's initial experimentation. For alcohol, one wants also to know about frequent heavy drinking (defined as five or more drinks at a session) and especially about having been drunk.

In the whole population aged 12 and over, there has been a downward trend in drug use over the past decade or so. Past-month use of any illicit drug, for example, fell from 12 percent to 6 percent; from 6 percent to 3 percent for any illicit drug other than marijuana; and from 3 percent to 0.7 percent for cocaine. The reason for this

welcome trend is obscure, the history of drug abuse being characterized by mysterious upsurges and declines of popularity of one
drug or another. The downward trend for past-month use of alcohol
has been from 60 percent to 51 percent, and heavy use from 8 percent to 5 percent. Finally, cigarette smoking fell from 39 percent to
30 percent during this decade, most of those who were able to quit
having done so long before, in the two decades following the Surgeon General's 1964 report.

Not surprisingly, perhaps, the trends for adolescents have been
generally similar to those for adults. Trend data for illicit drug use
(chiefly marijuana) over the years were encouraging from 1978 to
1992, but then, for reasons that are unclear, the trend reversed. For
alcohol and tobacco, the high use rates cited above remained essentially unchanged over the past decade. In twelfth grade, past-month
use of any illicit drug fell dramatically from a peak of 39 percent in
1979 to 14 percent in 1992, but then rose again to 26 percent by
1998. The corresponding figures for cocaine were 12 percent, falling
to 3 percent, then rising to 5 percent. Paralleling the adult trend,
improvements were much more modest for past-month alcohol
use—87 percent, falling and stabilizing at 75 percent; heavy use 41
percent to 30 percent, and having been drunk 52 percent and not
decreasing at all. Past-month smokers fell from 38 percent to 30
percent, then rose to 37 percent; daily smokers from 29 percent to
18 percent, then up to 23 percent. PCP, LSD, and all other drugs
showed similar trends. Heroin has never been used by more than a
fraction of a percent of the high school population.

A striking feature of the annual surveys on children was the finding of a strong inverse relationship between perceived risk and drug
use (Fig. 15.1). For all drugs, over this same 13-year period, although
there was no evident change in drug availability, when more students
perceived use as harmful, fewer students actually used. At the same
time, the overwhelming majority of students reported having seen
or heard antidrug commercials in the previous month, and about
three-quarters of them stated that the commercials had to some extent made them less likely to use drugs.

All these results can be interpreted as meaning that large-scale
educational efforts on the community or national level can bring
about behavior change by tapping into the health concerns of young
people. Such change occurs gradually but steadily—often with temporary reversals—and it affects the whole population (though with

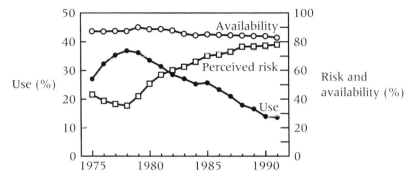

Fig. 15.1: *Past-month marijuana use, high school seniors. Perceived risk and availability, 1975–1991. (From L. D. Johnston et al: National Institute on Drug Abuse, publication no. 93-3480, Washington, D.C., Fig. 23.)*

some ethnic, class, and geographic differences). Cigarette smoking is the prototypic example. At the peak of its popularity, in 1964, when the first Surgeon General's report focused public attention on the health risks, 53 percent of adult males in the United States were smoking, and 32 percent of adult females. Over the next 35 years of public education, reinforced by regulations about where and when smoking is permissible, these figures had fallen, by 1998, to 29 percent and 26 percent, respectively.

What about the cost-effectiveness of prevention education for the young? Several excellent research studies have taught us that it is possible, through appropriate methods of prevention education in the schools, to reduce drug use. However, whether the extent of reduction obtainable is worth the extra effort and expenditure for special programs is a difficult question to answer. Consider cigarette smoking. As noted above for high school seniors, fewer than one-quarter now become daily smokers. Thus, in terms of health benefit, special smoking prevention programs for the early grades may be unnecessary for three-quarters of the children, who will not become smokers anyway. Moreover, much prevention education is already being done, routinely, at low cost, by regular teachers, in most schools, and at all grade levels.

In order to prove anything conclusively, prevention research projects have to be planned with meticulous care and carried out on a massive scale. While that kind of research design is necessary to learn what actually does and does not work, it is also extremely costly. Society would certainly not be willing to pay for special programs on that scale in all the nation's schools. Yet all the data from trials suggest that there is a "dosage" effect even for studies that do not employ medications, that the number of contact hours in the classroom does make a difference. The key question, therefore, is whether the procedures that work in successful research projects can be implemented on a national basis by regular teachers within the regular curriculum. To find out will presumably be the next practical step in prevention research.

Some experts have suggested that actions such as enforcing bans on cigarette sales to minors and raising taxes on cigarettes and alcohol might be more cost-effective than across-the-board prevention education in the schools. The laws prohibiting sales of cigarettes to minors are rarely enforced. In studies conducted in the San Francisco Bay Area and in Washington, D.C., it was found that when obviously underage children were sent around to supermarkets and small stores they were able to purchase cigarettes in over 80 percent of the cases. An informational campaign directed at the store owners and clerks, and posting prominent signs at the checkout counters, reduced the number of violations; but when children were sent out again, they were still able to buy cigarettes 30 percent of the time.

Summary

The good news: Drug use of all kinds has declined substantially from historic highs around 1979 and before. The bad news: Since 1992, the downward trend has reversed, though not nearly to the earlier high levels. The very bad news: With respect to alcohol and tobacco, the trend data for young people are worse than for adults. This discouraging fact has driven the massive media campaign mounted by the Office of National Drug Control Policy (ONDCP) since 1997, and heavily funded by Congress.

Thus, drug use by children, starting at a very young age, presents a major challenge to prevention efforts. The main lesson to be had from research on drug abuse during the critical years of childhood and adolescence, when curiosity is a driving force and drugs are first tried and then used increasingly, is this: Classroom education to teach children why to say no and how to say no is essential, but it is not enough. Nor can it have more than marginal effects unless it is supplemented by broad parental and community-wide efforts. Drug prevention education in the schools has to be viewed as an integral part of bringing about a pervasive change in societal attitudes toward all addictive drugs.

We can hardly expect to prevent children from using drugs unless they can actually see that adults are willing to set a consistent example in their own behavior and are prepared to enforce the laws that are supposed to restrict access of minors to addictive drugs. Banning cigarette machines would be an obvious step in the right direction; but this has proved to be extraordinarily difficult, perhaps because of tobacco industry money corrupting state and federal legislatures. Selling cigarettes and alcohol at supermarkets and other retail markets increases availability to underage minors; restricting sales of both drugs to licensed liquor stores might provide better controls.

16

Treating Addiction, Preventing Relapse

One of my patients (let's call him Charlie T.) was an accomplished musician. His career had been wrecked by heroin, and now he had been on methadone for three years. For all that time he had participated in group counseling sessions. His therapist had helped him find a job with a local opera company. Marital counseling had helped him reunite with his wife. He belonged to a neighborhood bowling club and had recently won a trophy. He had used no heroin or other illicit drug for two whole years, as proved by regular urine testing. A year ago, as he was doing so well by all the indicators, his therapist had agreed that he might be ready to discontinue methadone, and he had been reducing dosage very, very gradually since then.

One day, to my great surprise, his urine test showed that he had used heroin. He admitted the truth, but he was at a loss to understand why. Suddenly overwhelmed by an irresistible craving, he had rushed out of his house to find some heroin. As he described the event, it was as though he were driven by some external force he was powerless to resist, even though he knew while it was happening that it was a disastrous course of action for him. I asked what he was doing just before he rushed out of the house. "I guess I was watching

TV," he said. "And what, exactly, were you watching, Charlie?" There was a long silence before he replied. "Oh, yes," he said, "now I remember. It was a program about addiction. They showed an addict fixing, putting the needle into his vein. And suddenly I felt sick, just like needing heroin. I got that craving. I broke out in a sweat. I had that old feeling that only a fix would cure me." An all too familiar story—successful treatment followed by relapse.

Treatment

The challenge is to move addicts from an addicted to a drug-free state, if possible, or at least to free them from the compulsion of drug use, which dominates their lives. Changing established addictive behavior is a complicated business, and removing the addictive drug is only one part of an overall treatment plan. Moreover, speaking of "the addictive drug" is an oversimplification because a pattern of using several drugs simultaneously (polydrug abuse) is so common. Fads in drug combinations come and go; currently, mixing heroin and cocaine is popular. Treatment then requires not only addressing each drug appropriately, but also dealing with the many ways that the drugs affect each other. And because people vary so in the total circumstances of their addiction, what works well for one may not work at all for another. Therefore, the skilled therapist is flexible, nondogmatic, understanding, supportive yet demanding, with long-suffering patience, and willing to discover by trial and error what is best for the individual addict. A central theme of treatment is expressed in the slogan "Different strokes for different folks."

The National Institute on Drug Abuse (NIDA) has produced a research-based guide to treatment. This brochure describes 13 principles of treatment, a catalogue of what works and what is essential, especially what has been learned from systematic research in the field over the years. Following is the list, taken verbatim from the NIDA brochure, Principles of Drug Addiction Treatment (see Some Suggestions for Further Reading):

1. No single treatment is appropriate for all individuals.
2. Treatment needs to be readily available.
3. Effective treatment attends to multiple needs of the individual, not just his or her drug use.

4. An individual's treatment and services plan must be assessed continually and modified as necessary to ensure that the plan meets the person's changing needs.
5. Remaining in treatment for an adequate period of time is critical for treatment effectiveness.
6. Counseling (individual and/or group) and other behavioral therapies are critical components of effective treatment for addiction.
7. Medications are an important element of treatment for many patients, especially when combined with counseling and other behavioral therapies.
8. Addicted or drug-abusing individuals with coexisting mental disorders should have both disorders treated in an integrated way.
9. Medical detoxification is only the first stage of addiction treatment and by itself does little to change long-term drug use.
10. Treatment does not need to be voluntary to be effective.
11. Possible drug use during treatment must be monitored continuously.
12. Treatment programs should provide assessment for HIV/ AIDS, hepatitis B and C, tuberculosis, and other infectious diseases, and counseling to help patients modify or change behaviors that place themselves or others at risk of infection.
13. Recovery from drug addiction can be a long-term process and frequently requires multiple episodes of treatment.

Treatment programs are residential, hospital inpatient (rarely), and outpatient. Programs may be publicly or privately funded. For budgetary reasons, residential programs (the most costly) are usually reserved for the most recalcitrant addicts, who cannot deal effectively with their addiction in the same setting that nourished their drug use in the first place. Some programs insist on immediate total abstinence, others encourage slow reduction of drug use with ample counseling support. For addicts to heroin or other opiates, methadone may be used for short or long periods. Some programs make use of pharmacological agents to allay withdrawal discomfort, while others absolutely reject drugs of any kind. A nationwide network of groups dealing with various drug addictions by the 12-step Alcoholics Anonymous model (chapter 9) accepts no public funds and uses no professional counselors. Self-directed residential therapeutic communities for rehabilitation of drug addicts include Phoenix House in New York and elsewhere, and the Delancey Street Foundation in San Francisco. According to official U.S. government sources, more than five million drug users need and would probably benefit from treatment; but fewer than two million actually receive treatment, and fewer than half of those are in "slots" funded by public sources. The need is especially great for a sophisticated and comprehensive treatment system, inasmuch as nearly half of those in need of treatment suffer from comorbidity, i.e., another mental illness along with the drug addiction. Many addicts are unemployed and cannot afford the treatment they need so desperately, so for the good of society treatment ought to be subsidized.

"Cold turkey" withdrawal is unlikely to be accomplished successfully without extraordinarily strong motivation, strong external support, and—again, as for prevention—strong self-efficacy. Virtually all addicts have tried to discontinue use on their own, but the discomfort of the withdrawal syndrome, with its accompanying intense craving, makes success rare. If there is a solid supportive environment, some argue, the best treatment approach begins with "cold turkey." Even addiction to heroin or other opiates, in which the withdrawal syndrome is reputed to be intolerable, is often treated this way in residential facilities devoted to self-help with intensive peer support.

The most widely used treatment methods employ slow detoxification combined with pharmacotherapy to reduce withdrawal distress. For nicotine addiction, this may include the temporary use of nicotine skin patches. For heroin addiction, it may include short-term administration of methadone, followed by slow dosage reduction (but do not confuse this use of methadone with methadone maintenance!). To make withdrawal syndromes characterized by agitation and anxiety more tolerable, clonidine or mild tranquilizers may be used. Benzodiazepine tranquilizers (e.g., Valium) are traditional mainstays for managing alcohol withdrawal. Antidepressant medication is effective where depression is part of the withdrawal syndrome, as with amphetamines, cocaine, and sometimes nicotine. Whatever the addictive drug, the first step in treatment is to remove it, with pharmacological and social support—rapidly or gradually, according to the particular treatment philosophy and the response of the individual patient.

Powerful Jekyll-and-Hyde forces are struggling within the addict. If there is no motivation to give up the drug, it is extremely difficult to begin treatment; but even then, compulsory treatment is by no means useless. And if an addict does present for treatment voluntarily, it is usually with ambivalent feelings. Typically, some kind of pressure brings them to the treatment facility—perhaps insistent urging by family, or the cost of a drug escalating out of control, or the prospect of losing a job, or trouble with the law, or health concerns, or—at long last—dissatisfaction with self. But counterpressures are also hard at work—craving the next smoke, injection, snort, or drink; wanting to remain a member of an addict peer group; feeling despondent about a future with never another taste of the drug. As long as the addict can just walk away and fail to keep the next clinic appointment, the negative forces often win out. Treatment personnel have to anticipate this self-defeating behavior and be prepared to start treatment over and over again.

Compulsory treatment is often proposed as a solution. In fact, we already have such a system for the illicit drugs. When an addict engages in criminal activity, the criminal justice system requires abstinence as a condition of probation in lieu of incarceration, or as a condition of parole after early release from prison; and then continuous participation in treatment is obligatory. Alcohol addicts who are habitually arrested for driving while intoxicated are typically required to attend Alcoholics Anonymous or some other treatment program. Legally mandated supervision has been found, in several research studies, to be an extremely effective method of ensuring abstinence. However, it is hard to see how compulsory treatment could be instituted, in our free society, in the absence of a court conviction and sentence.

A special problem is presented by the extraordinary numbers of drug offenders who are incarcerated. More than five million adults are under some form of correctional supervision (incarceration, probation, parole), with one-quarter of the state prison population and 60 percent of the federal having drug problems. The average cost to incarcerate an inmate is about $25,000 a year, so that many billions are expended for this purpose. Treatment in prison, to break the cycle of addiction, would be cost-effective; yet fewer than one-fifth of inmates who enter prison as addicts actually receive treatment there. Ample data show that those who are treated in prison are far less likely to be rearrested after discharge, and less likely also to return to drug use. Interpretation is clouded by the fact that there is no random assignment to treatment or no-treatment, and obviously, those who choose treatment are better motivated than those who do not. However, this is another instance in which common sense should prevail, in the absence of rigorous scientific proof. Clearly, offering treatment instead of incarceration for nonviolent drug offenders (for example through drug courts), and providing treatment in prison for all who wish it, makes good social and fiscal sense.

The same principles that guide prevention education in the classroom (chapter 15) are also relevant to treatment. To be motivated is not enough. The addict has to be taught, explicitly, the many day-to-day techniques of living without drugs. A system of contracts is established, whereby the addict agrees to comply with a step-by-step program of progress, worked out jointly with the therapist. For many heroin or cocaine addicts, a major part of counseling is to teach the practical skills that are needed for rehabilitation after a life of crime. These include job training and education, legal assistance, counseling to restore disrupted family life, attention to neglected medical conditions, advice about HIV risks, and prenatal care for pregnant women.

Objective measures of drug use—saliva, urine, or breath tests—are absolutely essential. Their purpose is to confront the addicts with reality, for the experienced therapist never accepts self-reports as the truth. People with organic or mental disease are usually eager to communicate accurate information to their physician or other therapist. But with Jekyll-and-Hyde drug addicts, of whatever socio-economic class, of whatever educational level, and whatever the drug of addiction, this straightforward honesty cannot be assumed. I have been asked repeatedly, often angrily, by heroin addicts, "Don't you believe me when I tell you I haven't used heroin in the past week?" My answer is, "No! Why should anyone believe you at this point? The record of your recent life doesn't exactly inspire trust. Let's work together to change that situation, but it takes time and effort to earn trust." The need for objective evidence is not limited to the illicit drugs; drug use is always likely to be underreported because the addict is in denial about drugs, or habitually shades the truth about all antisocial behaviors. Self-reports become remarkably more truthful when saliva, urine, or breath samples are taken randomly for testing!

The general approach to addiction treatment can be described as breaking a big task into manageable bits, each tailored to the needs of the individual patient. If a suitable medication is available, total abstinence may be put off to a later time, when the addict will have better support systems and greater self-efficacy. In that case, the first step is to break the cycle of repeated spiking of drug levels in the brain. For heroin addicts, methadone (also LAAM and buprenorphine) does this, and since the medications are taken by mouth once daily or even less often, they allow the addict to discontinue intravenous injections, to stop seeking and using heroin several times daily. In the maintenance mode, these medications cannot even be rightly described as heroin substitutes; the pleasurable, reinforcing effect of spiking heroin levels in the brain—the "rush," the "high"—is not obtained at all, but instead, a stabilizing and normalizing of neurochemical and hormonal systems that were chaotically disordered by the pattern of repeated heroin self-injections. After personal and social rehabilitation is well under way, and when absolutely no heroin has been used for many months, one can think about tapering off the medication. At that point some people will be able to give it up quickly and easily; but others may take a very long time, and some may actually require it indefinitely (see chapter 10).

The same principles apply in treating nicotine addiction. Many people can quit, cold turkey, and never smoke again. Others find it harder. Substituting a nicotine patch for cigarettes maintains a stable blood and brain nicotine level and permits addicts to discontinue the repeated spiking of nicotine levels in brain. But there are some hard-core, heavily addicted smokers who are not yet ready to face life without smoking; they can at least be helped to reduce their intake. This is a "harm reduction" approach. After all, smokers who cut down from two packs a day to one reduce all their tobacco-related health risks by half. The principles of behavior modification dictate that the conditioned cues that control the lighting of every cigarette (see chapter 8), have to be recognized and then extinguished, one by one.

Central to these treatment approaches is the goal of breaking the hold of the addictive drug. Another approach defines "harm reduction" differently; it does not seek to terminate the addiction, but focuses entirely on "harm reduction." Advocates of this position argue that, at least for addicts who can not or will not discontinue drug use, it is better for them to go on using under supervised and safer conditions. Large-scale attempts to furnish pure heroin and clean injection equipment to addicts are under way in Switzerland and some other European countries (see chapter 18). Limited data obtained thus far in controlled clinical trials do show a substantial reduction in overdose deaths and in HIV transmission. It is also argued that bringing addicts off the street and into a well-run clinic opens the way for other helpful interventions. This approach—some would hesitate to call it addiction treatment—could, in principle, be tested with other drugs. A nicotine inhaler, for example, could provide the pleasure sought by a smoker, without the risks of lung cancer, bronchitis, and emphysema caused by smoke from burning tobacco leaves.

Twenty-five years ago, I suggested a scheme for letting heroin addicts inject pure heroin in a clinic environment. This was to be the first step in a series of treatments aimed at eventual total abstinence. Called Sequential Treatment Employing Pharmacologic Supports (STEPS) (see Some Suggestions for Further Reading), it proposed offering heroin as a means of attracting addicts into the treatment environment, but anticipated an early transition to methadone maintenance. A hostile political climate in the United States prevented STEPS from ever being tested. The aim of heroin maintenance in Switzerland, the UK, and elsewhere is quite different in that terminating the addiction does not seem to be a goal at all.

Relapse Prevention

There is some truth in the saying "Once an addict, always an addict." The formerly addicted person has drug-related memories and experiences not shared by those who have never been addicted. And these—under the right conditions—can trigger a relapse. Recognizing this vulnerability is important for protecting the once-addicted person after abstinence has been achieved—a view emphasized by Alcoholics Anonymous in their insistence on calling their members "recovering alcoholics," never "former alcoholics." If we knew how to prevent relapse reliably, it would be a great deal easier to solve the drug addiction problem once and for all.

Relapse is, of course, always preceded by a decision to use, however vague and inchoate that decision may be. It is an impulsive decision, not a rational one, and it is provoked by (or at least associated with) craving—the intense and overwhelming desire to use the drug. Although craving is a constant feature of early withdrawal, it may also occur even years after the last drug dose. That kind of craving, which is obviously not part of a withdrawal syndrome, is poorly understood but enormously important, for it can drive the ex-addict into relapse even after long-sustained successful abstinence. Animal and human experiments reveal a "priming effect" of a drug to which a subject was previously addicted. This means that a small dose of the drug, administered to an abstinent ex-addict, can immediately initiate self-administration behavior—the very phenomenon that AA warns of, that abstinent alcoholics can not resume occasional drinking without losing control.

Conditioned withdrawal plays an important role in provoking relapse. For the abstinent ex-addict, any of the circumstances and environments surrounding former drug use can provoke craving. These may have become conditioned stimuli for the rewarding effects of the drugs, and certainly they are stored as long-term memories—conscious or subconscious. It is thought that such stimuli, by activating the reward systems, can mimic drug action and thus produce what is tantamount to a "priming effect" even though no drug was taken. And as though the brain needs its next dose, the symptoms of withdrawal are experienced. The case of Charlie T., which began this chapter, is a good illustration. Conditioned withdrawal has also been demonstrated in the laboratory. Ex-addict volunteers who had not used opiates for months or years were shown a video of someone using heroin. They displayed many of the signs of withdrawal—sweating, chills, a running nose, and goose bumps. They felt that they were undergoing actual opiate withdrawal, and they experienced intense craving for heroin. Such observations help us understand why addicts so often relapse when they are returned, immediately after detoxification, to their previous environment, with all its drug-related associations.

The medical management of withdrawal can be so smooth and painless that all addicts, whatever their drug, can be brought readily and relatively painlessly to a drug-free state. But then a sudden attack of craving can start the whole cycle over again. Therefore, the therapist has to teach the techniques for eliminating conditioned craving by desensitization—by extinction of the conditioned cues. That requires being exposed repeatedly to situations that were formerly associated with drug use, but without drugs being available. Watch a smoker as she gets into her car in the morning to drive to work. She reaches into her purse, takes out a cigarette, lights up, and inhales deeply. Before long, getting into the car becomes a conditioned cue for smoking that cigarette. Getting into the car provokes immediate craving for nicotine; and with cigarettes available, the craving leads to nicotine use. To desensitize, to break the conditioned association to that cue, means regularly and consistently getting into the car without smoking that particular cigarette.

I heard the following account from a colleague who had been a nicotine addict but had not smoked for years. He had abstained from cigarettes in a variety of situations where he had smoked in the past, and thus he had desensitized himself to a variety of conditioned associations—cigarettes at parties, cigarettes at morning coffee, cigarettes at the desk, and so on. One day he went to the beach and suddenly experienced an intense craving for a cigarette. He found this beyond understanding, until he realized that smoking on the beach had been an important pattern at one time in his life, and that he had not had the opportunity to extinguish that particular conditioned association.

Contrary to what most people might think, craving is not provoked by the absence of the drug to which a person was addicted, but by its presence—that is, by its availability. This is illustrated by the nicotine addict who goes skiing for a whole day, leaving cigarettes behind. No thought is given to cigarettes—they are simply unavailable. Then back at the lodge, where nicotine is available again, intense craving strikes, and the addict lights up. With nicotine, someone else's smoking is a potent conditioned cue for lighting up; that is why regulations that establish smoke-free environments are so helpful to nicotine addicts and ex-addicts in reducing their consumption or maintaining their abstinence. In the story of Charlie T., even the conditioned craving would soon have passed, were it not for his knowledge that he could actually go out and find heroin.

Antagonists can play a role in preventing relapse. They abolish the psychoactive effects of a drug in either of two ways—by blocking the receptors or by directly neutralizing the drug as it circulates in the blood stream. Receptor blockade is exemplified by naltrexone, used for opiate addicts; but experience with it has not been encouraging (see chapter 10). Naltrexone cannot be started until no opiate dependence remains, else a severe precipitated withdrawal syndrome would result; therefore, slow withdrawal followed by a period of successful abstinence is a precondition for its use. This is very difficult to accomplish, most addicts relapse to heroin use even before the state of dependence has dissipated. Then, although highly effective in blocking the rewarding actions of heroin—and perhaps for that very reason—naltrexone is dropped quickly by most addicts who try it. Successful exceptions are those who are under some strong external compulsion, as by law enforcement or the need to maintain professional licensure. For most addicts, part of the problem seems to be poor motivation; but in addition, blocking the normal functions of the opioid receptors may cause subtle negative mood changes, as suggested by research on normal volunteers.

Antibodies have been developed to neutralize cocaine, and some of these are catalytic antibodies, which accelerate the degradation of cocaine in the body. Antibodies, in general, are induced by a vaccination procedure (active immunization) or by direct administration into the blood stream (passive immunization); effects on reducing cocaine self-administration by rats have been encouraging. Unfortunately, typical doses in a cocaine binge are very large (hundreds of milligrams), easily exceeding the binding capacity of the antibodies. Thus, it is not difficult for the addict to use enough drug to override the antibody protection. Nevertheless, cocaine antibodies are able to rapidly reduce the drug level in the circulation, and this can be life-saving in the emergency treatment of toxic reactions to cocaine—especially the adverse effects on the heart. A nontoxic small molecule to bind cocaine directly and inactivate it might be useful, but none has yet been found. Finally, the antibody approach may prove useful for discouraging the use of drugs that are highly potent (e.g., LSD) and therefore are used in tiny amounts that can be bound effectively to antibody molecules.

Aversive medication is illustrated by disulfiram (Antabuse, chapter 9). Alcoholics who take disulfiram regularly are deterred from drinking because of the knowledge that they will become very ill if they do drink. Disulfiram is an important tool in the therapist's kit; but as with antagonists, compliance is a major problem. For reasons that are not clear, disulfiram (and recently acamprosate) is more often prescribed and used in Europe than in the United States.

Relapses will occur; there is no perfect preventive. The important thing is for a relapse to be contained. A relapse from successful abstinence is just a mistake. Some people panic, taking it as a sign that they cannot remain abstinent after all. They let the relapse destroy their self-efficacy. Then, instead of a single episode of drug use, which would have done no great harm, they end up with a total relapse, severely addicted again. That pattern of successful abstinence, a single relapse, and then reversion to full-blown addiction is all too common. Training in the skills of handling relapses when they occur is, therefore, an important part of drug addiction treatment.

Summary

This chapter has explored the many ways that a determination to "Just say no!" has to be implemented in successful treatment and in relapse prevention. What stands out is the great diversity of treatment approaches that are available, recognizing the importance of flexibility in providing "different strokes for different folks." Treatment is certainly effective, and it is highly cost-effective as compared with no treatment or with incarceration. Yet the availability of treatment, for all who need and want it, leaves much to be desired. For street addicts, who often have no financial resources whatsoever, free treatment on demand should be available. Every addict in jail or prison should be treated, to reduce the likelihood of relapse after release.

Relapse, usually provoked by conditioned cues, presents the greatest challenge. A fast-acting pharmacological agent to block the rapid progression from craving to relapse—perhaps administered by inhalation for instantaneous effect—would be extremely useful. None has been discovered, and none is likely to be developed until we learn more about the neurochemical basis of relapse.

17

Three Lessons from the Street

The stereotyped drug addict whose image fills the newspapers, magazines, TV screens, and politicians' speeches is only part—and a small part at that—of our addiction problem, as I have pointed out throughout this book. Drug addiction afflicts all economic classes, all educational levels, and all ethnic groups. But although nicotine and alcohol, rather than cocaine and heroin, affect society on the largest scale, it must be acknowledged that the street addict (the "junkie") is a conspicuous reality, one whose very existence frightens and disgusts many citizens. This chapter focuses on some of the problems street addicts present to the larger society. These include the addicts' criminal activities, difficulties encountered by health professionals in establishing treatment facilities, and intravenous drug use as a major factor in the epidemic spread of AIDS.

Crime and Punishment

Addicts commit two kinds of crime. One kind is crime by definition, since buying, selling, or possessing an illicit drug is illegal. Every year there are about a million and a half arrests for drug violations; approximately one-third of these are for trafficking, the remainder for possession. We could think of these as crimes against society but without direct and identifiable victims. Sometimes they are called "victimless crimes"; but there are frequently innocent victims such as members of the addict's family and others who are affected by the addict's behavior or by the health consequences of the addiction. The other kind of crime is not uniquely related to drugs, but it is often committed to obtain money for drugs, as well as for other purposes. The common crimes in this category are theft (especially shoplifting), burglary, robbery (often with personal violence), and homicide (incident either to robbery or to battles over trafficking), as well as prostitution.

Are street addicts criminals first, so that the use of illicit drugs is essentially a part of their antisocial behavior pattern? Or are they addicts first, who innocently became enmeshed deeper and deeper in the drug scene, and then become criminals to raise the ever-increasing sums needed to support an addiction? There is no simple answer, but studies of those addicted to the illicit street drugs do reveal a pattern. Most inner-city street addicts belong to the lower socioeconomic class, so it is not surprising that there is a high proportion of ethnic minorities. Most street addicts were juvenile delinquents first, with records of truancy, gang activities, fighting, stealing cars for joy rides, petty shoplifting—even before their first contact with an illicit addictive drug. Most had a juvenile criminal record before the age of 16 and were unemployed when not in custody. Often they are victims of child abuse, products of broken families, and dropouts from school at an early age. Leading lives without apparent goals, they frequently become members of street gangs. Nearly all of them have used alcohol and smoked cigarettes—the two classic gateway drugs—at a very early age, before it was legal for them to do so. Next came marijuana, and then heroin and either cocaine or amphetamines. The addict-to-be was typically introduced to each new drug by a friend, rarely by a "pusher."

Middle-class and wealthy addicts go through the same progression of drug use, beginning, usually in high school, with the same two gateway drugs, nicotine and alcohol, then graduating to marijuana and finally to cocaine and heroin. Gross antisocial behavior is not so evident in this group before they begin using drugs, but a troubled psychiatric history and severe personality problems are common. Then, as the use of illicit drugs becomes more intense, drugs come to occupy more and more of such a person's time at the expense of educational or employment activities. With these addicts, serious criminality starts when the cost of supporting an addiction escalates and becomes a real burden. Then one often sees a pattern of white-collar crimes, not burglaries and street muggings. Typical they are embezzlement, theft from a family member or employer, writing bad checks, and running up enormous credit card and other debts.

For all the illicit addictive drugs there is a common pattern of progression from experimental use to increasingly frequent use, and finally to full-blown addiction. Fewer and fewer people move to each successive step, so that by and large only the most sociopathic, the most mentally disturbed, the least educated, the habitual losers, go all the way. Consider the most recent (1997) statistics on the use of marijuana in the 18–25 age group. Forty-two percent had tried it at some time in the past, 22 percent had smoked it during the previous year, 13 percent during the previous month, and only 8 percent during the previous week. Contrary to a widely held belief, these numbers do not differ substantially between ethnic groups. The same general pattern also applies to the progression from licit to illicit, from nicotine and alcohol to marijuana, and then to heroin and cocaine (or amphetamine); and likewise from the socially acceptable smoking or drinking route of administration to the intravenous route.

A major issue, concerning which there is uncertainty in the court system, is to what extent addiction exculpates crimes committed either under the influence of a drug or in the course of obtaining the drug. I sat on a jury once, in an open-and-shut case of drunk driving. After the defendant was found guilty, the public defender argued for leniency on the ground that her client was an alcoholic and therefore could not help drinking. True, no one had been injured by this defendant's irresponsible actions, but many innocent people had been placed in jeopardy. Fortunately, the judge was not persuaded by the defense attorney's peculiar logic. Fortunately, too, it is becoming increasingly common to hold drunk drivers fully responsible for the consequences of their behavior. Thus, the idea that alcoholism exculpates crime is being rejected, and the same principle should apply to all the drug addictions.

A few years ago I was asked to meet with a committee of the Santa Clara County (California) Bar Association to discuss drugs and crime. These lawyers were deeply interested in the problem, and they had plenty of firsthand experience defending drug addicts. I was astonished to hear them express the naive notion that an addict who "needed" a drug had no alternative to criminal activity. "He had no choice," they told me in effect, "he had to mug the old lady for her money, else he would have gone into withdrawal." In other words, these lawyers had actually come to believe the exaggerated and self-serving accounts of their clients. A less kindly way to put it would be that the addicts had "conned" their attorneys.

I pointed out that although cold-turkey withdrawal from heroin is very unpleasant, it is by no means intolerable; and it is almost never life-threatening. Indeed, cold-turkey withdrawal is actually the method preferred by certain ex-addict groups (for example, Synanon and some other therapeutic communities) that try to help addicts become abstinent. And although cocaine withdrawal is unpleasant and is associated with intense craving, its physiological symptoms are milder than those of heroin withdrawal. Thus, there is no medical reason that could justify doing physical harm to other human beings or depriving them of their property in order to obtain funds to purchase an addictive drug. Addicts certainly know right from wrong!

I explained to the lawyers that addicts should be expected to bear full responsibility for their crimes, whether they are in treatment or whether they have chosen to reject treatment. What I was saying was pretty simple—that the alternative to committing crimes is not to commit crimes, that addiction does not force a person to be a criminal. Moreover, if treatment were available to all who want it, even the weak defense of "needing" the drug would collapse. Studies in Baltimore and other cities have shown that criminal activities decline substantially while heroin addicts are enrolled in a methadone maintenance program but increase again if they leave the program. Those studies, incidentally, make a strong case for the cost-effectiveness of addiction treatment: It costs a lot less to keep an addict in treatment than society loses—not only directly but also through the expensive arrest, prosecution, and incarceration process—when that addict, left untreated, continues to engage in criminal activities.

"Not in My Back Yard"

It is one thing to say, as a statement of principle, that addiction should be treated like any other disease. It is quite another to put the principle into effect. Negative societal attitudes toward certain kinds of addicts create real obstacles. And the antisocial attitudes of some addicts make matters worse. The story of my own research clinic is an instructive example of how the NIMBY ("Not in my back yard") syndrome operates.

Picture the neighborhood. Stanford Medical Center with its medical school and hospital occupies a large area on the edge of the Stanford University campus. A stone's throw from the hospital is Welch Road, attractively manicured, with trees and green lawns, a quiet and refined suburban street. Here you find physicians' and dentists' offices and many kinds of up-scale businesses, but no private residences.

In the 1970s my clinic occupied one of the Welch Road office buildings. The purpose of our clinical research was to test the efficacy of two maintenance drugs for heroin addicts—LAAM, the long-acting methadone, and the opiate antagonist naltrexone. The clinic was supported by federal grants, and treatment was free. Even then, at the height of federal funding, it was the experience everywhere that demand for treatment exceeded the capacity of treatment programs. Thus, within weeks of opening our doors, addicts were coming to us from as far as 10 or 20 miles away, and we soon reached our limit. Every Monday, Wednesday, and Friday, 120 patients attended the clinic. As both LAAM and naltrexone need to be taken (by mouth) only three times a week, all medication was consumed on the premises. This eliminated any possibility of diversion into illicit channels, of nearby trafficking in these drugs, or of accidental poisoning of addicts' children or others—all major problems with "take-home" methadone.

Almost at once, the landlord began complaining. He said that we were bringing "unsavory characters" into the neighborhood, that his other tenants were frightened, that the comings and goings of our patients were inappropriate to the Welch Road environment. Of course, many more people came and went every day at the hospital next door, at the bank across the street, at the ice cream parlor, at the doctors' and dentists' offices. So the problem was not the numbers. Our patients were the "wrong kind of people"—Latino, Oriental, and African American, as well as Caucasian. This was unusual enough for Welch Road. But far more upsetting, our patients came from the lower socioeconomic classes. Most did not follow the Welch Road dress code, and some wore tattered clothing and presented an unkempt appearance. Without a doubt, it must be admitted, some also behaved in an offensive manner, without consideration for others. The vernacular of the streets, not typically heard in this neighborhood, was used freely and loudly. Occasionally a fistfight would break out between patients.

The landlord sought an injunction to close the clinic, alleging it was a nuisance to his tenants. In addition, he sued my research foundation for compensatory damages (because of the alleged effect on the value of his property) in the amount of a million dollars—considerably more than our total endowment. I refused to take all this seriously. It seemed so unjust, so obviously motivated by class and racist biases. Surely we had a right to conduct a humane and socially useful treatment program, especially right next door to a hospital. Surely the law would uphold our good deeds against the crass position of the landlord. Or so I thought.

Unfortunately, some of our patients played right into the landlord's hands. A few of them, with criminal records and deft fingers, wandered the halls of the buildings; and wallets and purses began to disappear. Some patients, despite our earnest explanations and warnings, began to loiter in the parking lot. In one memorable confrontation, a patient urinated against a car—the landlord's car, no less! When the landlord objected, the patient swore at him, using obscenities. This particular episode was described in lurid detail in the depositions that initiated the legal proceedings.

Soon I began to get advice from colleagues throughout the country. What was happening, they told me, was not at all unusual. Moreover, in every case that had actually gone to trial, injunctions were indeed issued; and clinics had to shut down or move. I had better take this seriously, they warned. And I had to admit that the antisocial attitudes of some street addicts—although I could understand that some of their hostility was a reaction to the way they were treated by society—would make it nearly impossible to operate a clinic in harmony with this neighborhood.

Reluctantly, I closed the clinic. In the four years we were able to operate, we had accomplished a great deal, both in treatment research and in humane services to heroin addicts. The main lesson I learned was that even a compassionate recognition that addiction should be treated as a disease leaves unchanged the deep gulfs that separate the middle class from the underclass in our society and that divide ethnic minorities from the white majority. Well-to-do Silicon

Valley addicts, coming for treatment to physicians on Welch Road, attract no attention. If one wishes to treat typical street addicts, one had better do it in a large public health facility, preferably located in a run-down part of town, where the residents and proprietors of small businesses are too powerless to object. This is a depressing reality, but it is hard to envision a practical alternative, given the present atmosphere.

Clean Needles, Safe Sex

Tacoma, Washington—the first needle exchange program in North America. Started privately by a citizen concerned about the spread of AIDS, this program was taken over in 1988 by the Tacoma County Department of Health. At five locations throughout the county, hundreds of addicts who use heroin or cocaine intravenously come to exchange their used syringes and needles for a fresh supply and also to get free condoms. Similar programs have now come into being at many locations throughout the United States and Canada. Even before 1988, needle and syringe distribution schemes had been established in the Netherlands, the United Kingdom, and elsewhere in Europe.

Most needle exchanges operate by initially giving an intravenous drug user a supply of clean sterile syringes with attached needles. Thereafter, a one-for-one exchange of used paraphernalia for new is typically (though not always) required in order to prevent reuse or discard in public places. Return rates vary between 50 percent and 90 percent. Condom distribution is always free.

The idea of distributing the very equipment that is needed for intravenous drug use aroused bitter opposition at first, opposition that persists in some circles today. In New York City for example, although more than half of intravenous drug users were known to be infected with HIV, the mayor responded to strong public pressures by canceling a newly instituted needle exchange program. Two years later it was reinstated. Opposition arguments centered about the fear that such official programs would legitimize drug addiction, would "give the wrong message," would attract naive young people to become intravenous drug users.

The rationale for needle exchange (the term always implies syringe exchange as well) is straightforward. Intravenous drug users typically share syringes and needles, and the AIDS virus (HIV) is spread readily by this route. If addicts have sterile needles and syringes—so the argument goes—they will stop sharing, and the transmission of HIV will be interrupted. At the same time, the other mode of transmission, sexual contact, which can spread the virus to sexual partners (homosexual or heterosexual) of intravenous drug users, will be blocked if condoms are made freely available and are used regularly.

The basic question is whether the exchange programs actually do reduce the spread of HIV. That is not easy to answer. As with so much social science research, controlled experiments, the kind one could do in the laboratory, may not be practical. Ideally, here is what one would want to do. Find two comparable groups of addicts, perhaps in different cities but of the same age, gender, ethnic composition, socioeconomic status, educational level, and so on. Ascertain that the HIV seropositivity rate (the percent of people testing positive for the virus) is substantially the same, and low, among addicts in the two cities. An initially low rate is essential in order to have a large range of possible rates of conversion from seronegative to seropositive. Flip a coin, and establish a needle exchange in one city, keeping the other city as a control for comparison.

Even if the needle exchange were effective, it would take years to accumulate the data to prove it. Meanwhile, the addicts in the control city are by no means isolated from the many sources of public-health information; so their behavior may well change, based on that information. Quite unrelated to the needle exchange, then, we are likely to find that the rate of new HIV infection decreases in both groups.

Another difficulty arises from the fact that the needle exchanges have to be voluntary. This raises a serious question of whether addicts who decide to participate are representative of addicts in general. They are not. In one study that examined this question, it was found—not surprisingly—that participants had a lower infection rate initially than those who allowed themselves to be tested but then declined to participate. Participants presumably had a less chaotic lifestyle, engaged in less risk-taking behavior, and had more concern for personal health. Thus, the value of a needle exchange could well be greatest for those who need it least, and least for those who need it most.

Natural epidemiology—as opposed to controlled experiment—offers some fascinating information, but few firm conclusions. Let's look at a famous specific case, in which the lack of equivalence of two cities frustrates any scientifically valid interpretation. In Glasgow in 1989, the HIV seropositivity rate among addicts who came into contact with a treatment facility or the criminal justice system was only about 3 percent, approximately the same as for other British cities at that time. In Edinburgh, however, only 40 miles away, the rate was over 50 percent, and by 1990 had reached 85 percent. In Glasgow, a municipally sanctioned needle exchange had been operating for several years. In Edinburgh, the city fathers and police took a different line. Their policy was not only opposed to needle exchanges, they forbade the sale of injection equipment entirely, in the hope of thus stemming the increase in intravenous drug use. As the HIV infection rate climbed, a few needle exchanges were belatedly established, but even these operated in so half-hearted a manner as not to attract and hold many clients.

Enthusiasts for needle exchange schemes have pointed to these two cities as evidence in favor of their position. One article states categorically: "If needles and syringes had been readily and legitimately available in Edinburgh during the 1980s, the rate of HIV infection would be substantially lower than that found today." However, deeper analysis reveals that addict behavior in the two cities was quite different; moreover, the difference existed before 1983, when HIV first appeared on the scene. Edinburgh (but not Glasgow) had a tradition of "shooting galleries," communal gathering spots for addicts, where needle sharing was routine. A large new group of intravenous drug users, mostly youngsters, came onto the drug scene in Edinburgh, into this fertile field for epidemic spread of bloodborne infection, just at the moment when HIV first arrived. We have no idea how the virus was introduced into this discrete pool of intravenous drug users already sharing needles and sex promiscuously; presumably, one infected intravenous drug user came to Edinburgh from somewhere else. Therefore, although the contrast between Edinburgh and Glasgow is interesting, the complicated differences in history and addict culture between them frustrate any attempt to draw firm conclusions about the effectiveness of needle exchanges.

During the first few decades of a novel disease that is transmitted by sex and body fluids, pockets of high and low infection rates are to be expected. It may be, for example, that the difference between Edinburgh and Glasgow was simply due to relative lack of mobility— thus relative isolation of each pool of infection—with the high rate in Edinburgh due to the accident of early introduction of the virus. Albuquerque, New Mexico is a city of over half a million in an isolated location on the desert, with a tradition of low population mobility. At the present writing, when one-third of intravenous drug users in New York City are HIV seropositive, only a few percent in Albuquerque carry the virus; and this number seems to be growing extremely slowly. Yet, at the same time, in both cities, the same groups of intravenous drug users are infected with hepatitis B and C at rates approaching 100 percent. The reasons for the curious paradox are unclear, but it may be that the virus first appeared in Albuquerque only after education had brought about relevant behavior changes.

There is not a shred of credible evidence that needle exchanges promote intravenous drug use by those who would not otherwise become addicts. In many programs that have been in operation for years, the average age of new applicants, which would be expected to decrease if young people were being recruited to intravenous drug use by the needle exchange, has not done so.

Sophisticated research is not needed to tell us that behavior change is the key to stopping the spread of AIDS—in all segments of society, not only in the addict group. Behavior change requires that new information be disseminated and—most important—accepted. In the gay community, AIDS education brought about early changes in sexual behavior (less promiscuity, more use of condoms), which resulted in a dramatic reduction of new HIV infections. These gains, unfortunately, do not seem to be sustained among a new generation of gay men, nor could addicts be expected to sustain a similar behavior change with respect to either sexual behavior or needle sharing. In the state of intense craving provoked by having heroin or cocaine in hand, how many addicts will stop to take precautions? For some addicts, needle sharing has a ritual significance as a token of intimacy; how many will give it up willingly? And when about to engage in sex under the stimulatory influence of cocaine, will a man stop to put on a condom, even if he has one? Are addicts too impulsive, too prone to take risks, too undisciplined? After all, hepatitis B, other life-threatening blood-borne infections, fatal overdoses, and lethal adulterants are nothing new to addicts—yet they continue to inject themselves intravenously with unsterile needles and syringes. Ironically, HIV is not even a robust virus; it is easily killed by even the most perfunctory methods. Rinsing a syringe and needle with readily available household bleach would take only a few seconds and would be highly effective. If addicts will not take the trouble to do that, argue the pessimists, why would they bother to use fresh sterile syringes and needles even if they had them?

The optimists, while agreeing with these characterizations of addict behavior, argue that many addicts are indeed amenable to behavior change, that addicts as a group are not suicidal. The optimists see the needle exchange as a vehicle for reaching out—carrying an educational message about AIDS, raising consciousness about health risks, offering counseling and other services—and thus leading addicts to take the first step toward treatment. Solid data are showing that active intravenous drug users can, indeed, be brought into treatment and reduce their HIV risk behaviors through such outreach. Ideally, treatment would also reduce the addict's intravenous drug use. The response to the worry that needle exchanges will "send the wrong message" is—they argue—that the real message of the needle exchange is "We care about you here."

Are needle exchanges worth the cost and the effort? In Britain, the rationale in their favor has been formulated by the official Advisory Council on Misuse of Drugs as follows:

> We have no hesitation in concluding that the spread of HIV is a greater danger to individual and public health than drug misuse. Accordingly, services which aim to minimize HIV risk behaviour by all available means should take precedence in development plans. . . . The containment of the spread of the virus is a higher priority in management than the prevention of drug misuse.

In 1995, a panel established by the Institute of Medicine of the National Academy of Sciences attempted an analysis of what data could be found concerning needle exchanges and the use of disinfectant bleach in several programs throughout the United States and Canada. The panel concluded that household bleach was certainly effective in killing the AIDS virus, but that much education was required to persuade intravenous drug users to employ bleach. It also concluded (though not very strongly) that needle exchange programs seemed to be effective in reducing the number of contaminated needles in circulation, and therefore in reducing the transmission of HIV. The panel noted the value of needle exchanges in bringing addicts into treatment, and the unlikelihood of recruiting those who were not already intravenous drug users.

Common sense tells us that all possible means are in order to try to check the worldwide AIDS epidemic. In this desperate situation, even though a scientifically valid cost-benefit analysis will probably never be possible, the chance of needle exchanges reducing existing harm is substantially greater than of their causing harm. Thus, they are a legitimate weapon in the public-health approach to the drug addiction problem. Recent studies suggest that when (and only when) a needle exchange operates as an integral component of a full treatment system, it can, indeed, draw some of the most difficult cases into treatment. Whether or not needle exchanges are in operation, a wide range of other services can play a key role in bringing about the necessary behavior change for stemming the spread of HIV. In this regard, well-run methadone maintenance programs are especially important, because heroin addicts substantially reduce or discontinue intravenous heroin use while they are taking oral methadone.

Summary

Three social consequences of addiction "on the streets" were examined in this chapter—crime and how we deal with it, negative societal attitudes that impede treatment, and the role of street addicts in the spread of AIDS. These have something in common; all three call for policies that reduce the damage addicts do to themselves and others. At the same time, humane treatment of addicts, and respect for their human rights have to be balanced against the rights of other members of society. This theme will be developed further in the final chapters, first by examining some innovative drug policies in other countries, then by focusing sharply on drug policies in the United States.

18

Three Lessons
from Abroad

Drug addiction is unbounded by geography, form of government, politics, ethnicity, economic status, or degree of formal education. In other words, it is a problem of the human condition. Three European nations—Great Britain, the Netherlands, and Switzerland—stand out as having special ways of dealing with some aspects of drug addiction. In particular, their governmental policies are based solidly on public-health considerations—on pragmatic attempts to reduce harm wherever possible, without the moralistic crusading that has typified our own "war on drugs." This chapter explores the similarities and differences between their approaches and our own, with a view to seeing what we can learn from them.

Great Britain: Myths and Realities

Proponents of legalizing addictive drugs often point to Britain as an example that we should follow. They usually put forward one or more of the following assertions about the British:

> That they have brought their drug problem under control. That they have legalized the drugs that are prohibited in the United States.

That by legalizing these drugs, they have broken the connection between addiction and crime, virtually eliminating drug-related crimes.

That by letting addicts have their drugs of choice under hygienic conditions they have greatly improved the addicts' health.

That they have rehabilitated the addicts in a social and economic sense, integrating them into society as productive citizens, by treating them as patients rather than as criminals.

A lovely picture! But unfortunately, although there are elements of truth here, the assertions are—by and large—false. Since the myth of the successful British system is repeated so often, we need to examine it, point by point, get the facts straight, and then see what useful lessons we can learn.

Addictive drugs have not been legalized in Great Britain. It is true that heroin, which is totally prohibited in the United States, is approved for medical use there. However, double-blind studies have shown repeatedly that for the control of pain in hospitalized patients, heroin has no advantage over morphine. The American medical profession accepts this evidence-based conclusion; the British medical profession disputes it and continues to prescribe heroin for relief of severe pain. But whether heroin is or is not approved for medical use has no bearing whatsoever on the problem of heroin addiction.

Great Britain is signatory to the same United Nations Single Convention on Narcotic Drugs as is the United States. This is the uniform international treaty with which drug laws in the signatory nations are required to comply. In Great Britain, law enforcement is vigorous, not only on trafficking, but also on possession. There are customs seizures at the ports and airports, and special narcotics squads in every local police force. Penalties have increased significantly over the past decades, so that trafficking now carries a sentence of 14 years to life; and even for simple possession, the penalty is five years. Marijuana seizures exceed those of all the other illicit drugs, while convictions for marijuana possession represent three-quarters of all convictions for drug possession. In all these respects the British and American policies are alike.

Despite the formal similarities in the drug laws, history has shaped attitudes differently in the two countries. In the United States, in the nineteenth century, drug addiction was regarded as an unfortunate disease requiring medical attention, and addicts were objects of sympathy. Many of the addicts were middle-class women, for whom physicians furnished morphine on prescription. Radical changes in public perception and in U.S. government policy began in the first decades of the twentieth century. This coincided with the height of the temperance movement and the adoption of a nationwide prohibition of alcohol. It also coincided with a spread of marijuana and heroin to inner-city populations, to lower socioeconomic classes, and to ethnic minorities. This demographic change provoked a panic reaction, which was exacerbated by government agencies. Harry Anslinger, head of the Federal Bureau of Narcotics, conducted a propaganda campaign to persuade the public that heroin, cocaine, and especially marijuana (which he dubbed the "killer weed") were corrupting youth and threatening the very foundations of society.

In the wake of this onslaught, politicians responded by enacting and enforcing stronger prohibitions. Especially troubling to them were the maintenance clinics, at which opiate addicts were being given morphine; these were summarily shut down. New federal statutes and legal interpretations, and a few well-publicized prosecutions, made physicians fear to treat addicts. Thus, responsibility for dealing with the addiction problem was shifted from the medical profession to the law enforcement agencies, where it remained, exclusively, until the 1960s. Then, methadone maintenance had a strong impact in redefining the drug addictions—especially heroin addiction—as medical disorders (see chapter 10).

Although British urban life after World War II was transformed by the immigration of large numbers of ethnic minorities from all over the former British Empire, drug addiction was (and remains) less common in those groups than among the Anglo-Saxon majority. The medical profession resisted attempts by the Home Office (the law enforcement branch of the national government) to criminalize prescribing of opiates to addicts. A balanced system evolved, with good cooperation between the public health and law enforcement authorities. Physicians retained their right to treat addicts according to their best medical judgment, even if treatment included longterm prescribing of the addict's drug of choice. At the same time, physicians were required to notify the Home Office of the identity of addicts under their care. In consequence, an official statistical database was maintained, a resource for following national trends and for tracking drug traffickers. In practice, the local police exer-

cised discretion in not arresting addicts for simple possession, provided they were not involved in trafficking. As addicts were prescribed their drugs of choice, there would presumably be no reason
for them to resort to the black market.

It did not quite work out that way. Until about 1960, the total
number of users of heroin, cocaine, amphetamines, and all the other
illicit drugs was so small that it was claimed, with some justification,
that Britain really had no significant problem. For example, according to official estimates for 1960—amazing as it sounds now—the
total number of known heroin addicts in the entire British Isles was
94, and of addicts to all illicit drugs only 437. The few heroin addicts,
most of them in London, were managed well enough by physicians
in ordinary medical practice, who often prescribed heroin, syringes,
and needles. In the late sixties, however, there was a sharp increase
in the number of heroin addicts. Clusters of new users were appearing, owing their existence to a few unscrupulous or gullible physicians who were prescribing heroin willy-nilly to all who asked for
it. Then, as black-market heroin became increasingly available, addicts under treatment, who could not get all the drugs they wanted
from physicians, began to supplement their prescribed heroin or
amphetamines with drugs purchased on the street. Then, with increasing demand on the street, some were selling off portions of
their prescribed drugs. The government responded, in 1968, by restricting the right to prescribe addictive drugs for addicts to a small
number of physician experts based at specially authorized clinics.

By the 1980s, the epidemic of heroin addiction had continued to
escalate, and it spread beyond London to other parts of the country.
As illicit imports rose, a significant black market in heroin developed. The attempt to maintain addicts on heroin was deemed a
failure. At the clinics, which were operated in good faith by health
workers devoted to the welfare of the addicts—and despite the provision of psychiatric and counseling services—true rehabilitation was
a rare event. Criminal activities continued, as did the chaotic, antisocial lifestyles of a large fraction of the addict population, and the
spread of diseases by needle sharing. Some British clinics switched
from injectable heroin to injectable methadone, failing to grasp the
therapeutic importance of the oral route in helping break the needle habit. But most of the clinics—as one option in a menu of diverse treatment procedures—did eventually adopt oral methadone

maintenance, following the path pioneered in the United States (see chapter 10).

All estimates of how many addicts there really are in any country have to be taken with many grains of salt. If one recalls the raging arguments about undercounting after the 1990 U.S. census, where it was simply a matter of counting heads, it is easy to appreciate how difficult it must be to count accurately those engaged in an illicit activity like heroin use. In Britain, the centralized registry known as the Addicts Index has been abolished in favor of even less statistically valid regional databases, which depend largely on reporting by physicians and health services. Confidential surveys reveal that only about one-quarter of addicts in treatment are actually reported. And addicts who have not yet sought treatment are missed entirely—especially young people just embarking on an addiction career. In the United States, estimates come from national questionnaire surveys, clinic attendance, emergency room admissions for adverse drug reactions and overdoses, and arrests, each of which is certain to produce underestimates.

Given all those caveats, the best information available indicates that Britain is no longer very different from the United States in the magnitude of its addiction problem. With a population of 59 million, the United Kingdom is thought to have about 150,000 heroin addicts, approximately two per thousand population, and clustered in the large cities. In the United States, with a population of 272 million, and around 800,000 heroin addicts, the ratio is nearly the same. The dismal outlook for heroin addicts is no different from that in the United States. Two out of every hundred die each year—60 percent by drug overdoses, and the remainder from blood and heart valve infections due to unsterile syringes and needles, AIDS, suicide, homicide, and complications of alcoholism.

Recent developments in the British drug scene have followed a pattern much like that in the United States except that at the moment, heroin—rather than a diverse variety of drugs—is overwhelmingly popular. Nevertheless, "party drugs" like MDMA ("ecstasy") and GHB (gamma-hydroxy-butyrate) are on the increase. The relatively small amount of serious violence related to drugs probably reflects a long history of cultural difference between the two countries, including a major difference in the prevalence of guns in private hands.

Contrary to what is often asserted in the media, what we can learn from British policies has nothing to do with legalizing drugs—that never happened there. It has everything to do with regarding addiction as a disease. This unambiguous position, which is held by all branches of the British government, contrasts with the view still prevalent in many influential circles in the United States that drug addicts deserve punishment more than they do sympathetic treatment. The British medical orientation is reflected in the composition of the several government commissions that, from time to time, examine the drug addiction problem and offer recommendations; medical and public health experts have always played a prominent role. Moreover, there has been an official permanent expert group, the Advisory Council on Misuse of Drugs (and now a special cabinet office for drugs) upon which the government relies for continuous monitoring, analysis, and recommendations for changes in policy.

An important difference from the American drug addiction scene is the existence of the National Health Service in Great Britain. Established 50 years ago, this system guarantees free and unlimited medical care to everyone, and therefore provides—as a right—universally available treatment for addicts. By informal agreement between the local police and the local treatment facilities, addicts tend not to be criminalized for their addiction, but are held fully responsible for crimes against persons or property. With free treatment available, the addict has no excuse for trafficking in drugs, or for other criminal activities. Without such universal access to treatment, addicts in the United States can claim a defense (however unconvincing) for their property crimes—that they wanted treatment but it was unavailable.

An important similarity to the United States is the recent greatly increased government concern about drug abuse, especially among youth. Like the well-organized and well-funded strategic plans of our own Office of National Drug Control Policy (ONDCP), the British government is implementing a comprehensive program of demand reduction activities to supplement the traditional supply reduction efforts by law enforcement agencies. Drug Action Teams, for example, consist of local and regional groups that cooperate in formulating and carrying out programs tailored to local needs. Data on the incidence and prevalence of drug use are published regularly by the nongovernmental Institute for the Study of Drug Dependence as well as by government agencies.

The details of treatment in Britain are left to the clinic medical staff and the addicted patient to work out. Treatment comprises a large umbrella, including psychiatric services, practical assistance in job training and job finding, marital counseling, advice about AIDS prevention, and help in settling problems with law enforcement, among other services. Detoxification may be a part of this treatment (especially for young addicts), followed by a plan for sustaining abstinence through hospitalization, placement in a halfway house, peer group attendance on the 12-step model, or other approaches, including methadone maintenance.

Especially for older people who have been heroin addicts for many years, it is recognized that abstinence without supportive medication may be an unrealistic goal. For such patients, the treatment plan may include drug maintenance—occasionally (even now, in some clinics) on intravenous heroin, but more typically on oral methadone. In response to the AIDS epidemic among intravenous drug users, a deliberate change of emphasis has been recommended at the highest levels of drug policy making. The aim of keeping addicts in treatment with a view to preventing the spread of HIV is now perceived as having higher priority than just stopping the addictive behavior. Thus, confrontational approaches (such as pressing for detoxification and abstinence) are being modified in favor of more permissive ones.

The present medical consensus concerning the prescription of heroin for heroin addicts is that if included at all in a treatment plan, it should be restricted to those who fail every other treatment approach. One of Britain's leading experts on addiction, who had played an important role in the early trials of heroin maintenance, put it this way: Perhaps it is justified, he said, for "a very small proportion of very chaotic and disturbed addicts. . . . But the last thing that I would recommend anybody should do is to say right, all you have to do is give heroin, give all the drugs you want to an addict, and everything will be fine. That would indeed, in my view, be a recipe for catastrophe."

The Netherlands: "Soft Drugs, Hard Drugs"

Utrecht is an ancient university city in the center of Holland, less than an hour from Amsterdam on those amazing Dutch trains that run precisely on time. The old windmills are gone, but the city cen-

ter is full of lovely seventeenth-century buildings on picturesque canals. My guide was a professor of social psychology with a special
interest in drug policy. We entered a little coffee shop. On the
counter was a surprising menu featuring cannabis products. On one
side were listed four brands of hashish, on the facing page five
brands of marijuana leaf. A young man sitting at the counter was
sipping coffee, and a sweet aroma made it obvious what he was smoking. The scene seemed very strange; but I had to admit, it didn't
look like a den of iniquity.

The Dutch are proud of what they call their "pragmatic" policy
on drugs, which differs significantly from both the American and
the British approaches. "Drug use is neither favored nor encouraged," wrote a key government official in the Ministry of Welfare,
Health, and Cultural Affairs, "but if people take drugs, the least we
can do is to limit the hazardous effects. . . . We hold the view that
drug use is not primarily a problem for police and the courts, but
rather a matter of public health and social well-being." An official
government document states that "criminal law plays only a minor
part in preventing individual drug abuse. Although the risks to society must, of course, be taken into account, every possible effort
must be made to ensure that drug users are not caused more harm
by criminal proceedings than by the use of the drug itself."

I had heard and read many journalistic accounts about the supposed legalization of marijuana in the Netherlands, but what I
learned on the spot was quite different from what I had expected.
Beginning in 1976, a very sharp distinction was made in the law
between "hard drugs" (heroin, cocaine, amphetamines) and "soft
drugs" (cannabis). I use the terms "hard drug" and "soft drug" for
convenience, but government policy actually speaks of "drugs presenting an unacceptable risk," on the one hand, and "cannabis products" on the other.

Alcohol and nicotine are not included in these classifications at
all. The main Dutch innovation was not to change the laws substantially, but to enforce them— with respect to cannabis—in a discretionary manner. Thus, on the one hand, importing, manufacturing,
possessing for sale, and selling cocaine, amphetamines, and heroin
or other opiates remains illegal and subject to heavy penalties. Possession of small amounts of these "hard" drugs for personal use is a
felony, but subject to lighter penalties. Sale or possession of can-

nabis, on the other hand, is a mere misdemeanor, punishable by a fine. Here is where discretionary enforcement enters the picture. While I was studying the cannabis menu, a police officer entered, chatted a bit with the proprietor and the customer, and departed. I was puzzled, for the coffee-shop manager was selling marijuana and hashish in flagrant violation of the law. What was going on here? My host explained the system, and the chief of police later verified what I had heard.

The Dutch argue that enforcing a strict prohibition on "soft drugs" would merely drive the users underground and bring them into contact with criminal elements trafficking in more dangerous drugs. The specially designated coffee shops are licensed to operate, but only under strict rules—no advertising, no minors under age 16 allowed on the premises, no "hard" drugs in or near the shop, and no breaches of decorum. In addition, these places are allowed only in certain specified areas of the city. As long as the rules are observed, the police do not enforce the law; but if they are broken, the proprietor not only can lose his license but also faces criminal charges.

Has this policy led to an expansion of the pool of cannabis users? As with so much data from real life, the answers are not clear. It all depends on how the sampling is done, on whether one believes self-reports, and on which trends in drug use are actually consequences of policy changes. Dutch government sources claim (and some independent surveys confirm) that although there are certainly more cannabis users than before, there has not been a major increase in cannabis use. For example, across the whole country and all ages, past-month use in 1998 was 2.5 percent, compared with 5.1 percent in the United States. Among Amsterdam youth aged 16–19, the youngest permitted in the coffee shops, past-month use in 1997 was 15.2 percent, up modestly from 11.6 percent a decade earlier. In 1995, among 15-year-old youth nationwide, past-month use was 15 percent, compared with 16 percent in the United States. Even opponents of the policy have to admit that it has not led to a massive recruitment of young people to the use of marijuana and hashish. Moreover, the statistics on cannabis use are remarkably similar to those for the United States, despite the major difference in law enforcement policy. There is, of course, the possibility that legitimizing cannabis (even though it is not actually legalized) will eventually lead to wider use, that changes in social acceptance of a drug occur slowly, possibly requiring generations rather than a few years to come about.

I spent a most interesting half hour with Utrecht's commissioner of police. He was an extraordinary man, with a doctoral degree in law, and a humane attitude toward the drug problem. He epitomized, for me, a major difference in law enforcement attitudes between Holland and the United States. Of course, there are educated and humane police chiefs in the United States, too, but such qualities in our law enforcement community are not always given adequate recognition. And the Dutch have nothing like our tradition of Wild-West shootouts, rampant "macho" attitudes, disrespect for ethnic minorities, disdain for drug addicts, and—too often—corruption. These differences could well make it impossible to transplant Dutch drug policies, even if we regarded them as enlightened. The commissioner of police saw no problems in the practical workings of the cannabis policy. Toward heroin, cocaine, and amphetamines he was ambivalent. While enforcing those prohibitions strictly, he expressed the same frustrations heard from police in the United States concerning the apparent failure of prohibition to ameliorate the hard-drug situation.

I accompanied a couple of narcotics officers on their daily sweep of the large shopping mall next to the main railway station. This police action could just as well have taken place in any U.S. city; the main aim was to harass the intravenous drug users and alcoholics, most of them homeless derelicts. The storekeepers and their customers (often upright citizens from farming communities) considered the "junkies" to be a nuisance and wanted them removed. The merchants' association had even provided the police with a special fund to hire additional narcotics officers. As we made the rounds, the officer in charge, an energetic and intelligent young woman, would stop and question drug users, seeking information about a recent burglary. Perhaps because of stringent and effective enforcement, the cost of hard drugs throughout the Netherlands is very high, and many addicts engage in property crime as their principal livelihood. Unlike the drug scene in American cities, there is relatively little serious violence—no doubt reflecting the major difference in violent behavior and ownership of firearms in the two countries. In 1996, for example, the homicide rate (adjusted for the large population difference) was only one-fifth that of the United States.

The next day found me in Amsterdam, the "big city," waiting on the stoop in front of Binninkant No. 46, one of those charming old three-story attached buildings that line the canals. Across the little street were houseboats tied up along the bank. A lovely old brick church on the other side had a clock tower, and the chimes were just striking half past the hour. The man I was waiting for was late, but my patience was soon rewarded. A group of young people strode up the street with a businesslike air. Their leader introduced himself, and I followed him up the steep steps into the building. I had come to find out what a "junkie union" was, an unimaginable concept in the United States.

Angelique was a former heroin addict, who had become a full-time employee of this union. A few others sat around a table with us and joined the discussion as she recounted the history and purpose of the union. Actually called the Medical Social Service for Heroin Users, it had been organized by parents of heroin addicts. Its aim was to ameliorate conditions of life for "junkies." I was astonished to learn that the city government provided a subsidy sufficient to pay the salaries of three staff members. The union, in turn, represented the interests of drug users to various municipal agencies. Currently, they were attempting to secure improved housing for prostitutes addicted to heroin. The Dutch welfare system provides a minimum stipend for anyone with a regular address. This creates a special problem for homeless addicts, a problem that the union was also trying to grapple with.

I was curious to find out the attitude of this union—so devoted to the welfare of intravenous drug users—to drug use itself. About hard drugs the answer was clear—they were absolutely opposed to their use, and sought to encourage addicts to become abstinent. At the same time, the union saw the addicts as victims, whose rights and welfare required protection. Moreover, they believed that giving up hard drugs had to be a voluntary action, not something compelled by the government. Meanwhile—again the pragmatic approach—the union tried to promote harm reduction policies. They carried out educational programs about AIDS prevention; the walls were covered with posters urging the use of condoms and clean needles. In these health-related matters, the union and the government reinforced each other's efforts.

A striking difference between Dutch and American policies was the openness of the AIDS prevention campaign. The United States has now at last caught up with European realism about informing the public on how to prevent the spread of this epidemic. But in 1991, at the time of my visit to Holland, the difference was striking. Intravenous drug users constitute a large pool of infection, which is spread both by needle sharing and by sexual activity. The addict group includes many prostitutes, who become a major channel for spread of the epidemic into the heterosexual population. Addicts, with their impulsive and compulsive drug seeking and drug using, are not easily influenced to change their behavior. The Dutch health authorities recognized very early that heroic efforts may be required, including open and widespread dissemination of information. Thus, government policy in the Netherlands rests on intensive, explicit education—directed at the general public, including schoolchildren—on how AIDS is spread and how the spread can be prevented. For heroin users, in addition to well-disciplined methadone programs of the kind one sees in other countries, a few of the larger cities operate a system of "methadone buses"—an innovative solution to the "NIMBY" problem described in chapter 17. These buses tour the city, stopping in the neighborhoods for an hour at a time and dispensing methadone to all addicts. There are no onerous requirements, no tedious paperwork, and no waiting lists. There are no urine tests, and continued heroin use is not cause for expulsion. Addicts drink their methadone on the spot; they are never given any to carry away with them. The harm-reduction principle behind the liberal dispensing policy is obvious—every dose of methadone an addict takes by mouth is better than a dose of heroin by vein. The bus also dispenses free sterile needles and syringes, as well as free condoms. Personnel on the bus offer counseling services and referral to definitive treatment facilities.

Could such a policy be instituted in America, perhaps on a trial basis in one state? Alaska, Oregon, California, and eight other states began to move in that direction in the 1970s, adopting more lenient laws concerning possession of small amounts of marijuana for personal use; but that trend was reversed by voters and legislatures before long-term results could be evaluated. However, in the few instances in which adequate data were obtained, there was clearly an increase in consumption during those few years of relaxed prohibition. Unfortunately, much that is attractive about the innovative approach to the drug problem in Holland would probably not be applicable to the United States. Holland is a small, heavily industrialized country, only the size of Vermont and New Hampshire, with a population of 16 million. Although ethnic minorities (chiefly from Surinam and the East Indies) have immigrated in recent years, the country as a whole, historically and culturally, remains quite homogeneous, in contrast to the United States. It seems to me that their policy of discretionary enforcement of drug prohibitions could not work in a society ridden with racism, as ours is; inner-city ethnic minorities would surely be targeted unfairly, while drug use by other segments of the population would be tolerated. However, we could well adopt the humane Dutch attitude toward addicts, regarding them as victims of a disease, and providing treatment for all who desire it. The recent positions expounded by our Office of National Drug Control Policy (ONDCP) strongly support this view, and stress the importance of universal treatment availability.

Switzerland: "Needle Park" and Its Aftermath

January, 1991. Switzerland was cold and raw. If you were not on the ski slopes, it was best to be indoors. But here I was, standing in a park in the middle of Zurich, a cold wind chilling my face, and the pervasive dampness numbing my feet. The fame of this "needle park" had spread worldwide to all who despair over the epidemic of intravenous drug use. I had heard this novel Swiss project praised by journalists and politicians. I had heard it put forward as a model approach to dealing with drug addicts. I had to see it for myself, study its history, and learn how well it really worked.

Around me, in the little park, were about a hundred young people, some still teenagers, some more mature, huddled together against the cold. I watched the scene intently. Money changed hands in exchange for drugs. A little kiosk, once a public lavatory, housed a first-aid station, with a young doctor in attendance. At a window of the kiosk, brand-new syringes and needles, as well as condoms, were being dispensed, free.

I watched as a shabbily dressed young woman nearby rolled up the sleeve of her overcoat. Holding a filled syringe between her teeth in order to free both hands, she improvised a tourniquet by hanging a shopping bag over her arm, spinning it to twist the rope handle tightly. She tried impatiently to find a vein with the needle, poking herself again and again until she could draw blood back into the syringe. I judged by her ineptness that she was still a novice. When she found the vein, she let the shopping bag spin free, releasing the tourniquet; and with a deep sigh of satisfaction she injected the heroin. A few minutes later she was overcome by nausea. Walking onto the nearby grass, she bent over double, retching and vomiting—a textbook example of heroin's effect on the novice user, an unpleasant side effect that wears off with repeated use.

A couple of police officers in uniform strolled by, casually surveying the scene. The young doctor, assigned to the first-aid station by the Department of Social Welfare of the municipality, told me how he resuscitates one or two overdose victims every day. As in some surrealistic film, while addicts bought, sold, and self-injected all around us, we held a professional medical discussion about the use of naloxone for heroin overdose. Here is an example, the doctor explained, of a situation in which this opiate antagonist is inappropriate because of its short duration of action. Naloxone can certainly revive people with lethal doses of heroin in their systems; but then a victim, who feels quite normal, may go off and die somewhere else when the naloxone wears off before the heroin is eliminated from the circulation. So the doctor used naloxone only in the most extreme cases, depending usually on conservative methods—artificial respiration, sensory stimulation, exercise, and close observation for long enough to make sure that recovery is complete. He was nearly at the end of a six-month rotation in this job. Eager to return to the practice of medicine in a more favorable clinical environment, he expressed frustration and irritation at what he saw as a mere pretense of providing needed clinical services to these unfortunate young people.

A few paces away was a group of tables under a quaint rotunda that had once served as an open-air bandstand. The ground was littered with paper syringe wrappers. Here entrepeneurs sold drugs openly—chiefly heroin and cocaine. Also for sale was the traditional equipment, such as bent spoons and spirit lamps for dissolving the powdered drugs. One man was extracting cocaine with a solvent to make free-base crack suitable for smoking; crack, I learned from the doctor, was not yet on the market here as a regular commodity. As I took in this strange scene, the same two police officers walked over for a friendly discussion with one of the dealers. I learned later that although the police were under orders not to interfere with drug sales or drug use, they were permitted to seek information in the course of investigating personal or property crimes. Earlier that day, a commissioner of police had showed me a map of Zurich with a red dot for each property crime committed in the past year. Right in the center of the cloud of red dots was—you guessed it—"needle park."

An ancient green school bus stood nearby, and I followed some of the addicts inside. Here a potbelly stove radiated warmth, hot tea and coffee and cookies were available, and two social workers were in attendance. Operated by the Department of Social Welfare, the bus provided shelter from the cold, but the crude facilities and lack of privacy were hardly conducive to serious counseling. Around a long table, near the stove, sat a couple of dozen addicts, many of them "nodding off" under the influence of heroin, some just sitting quietly and sipping a hot drink.

I wanted to know how this remarkable place had come into being. So the next day found me sitting with the woman who was primarily responsible for the park's establishment. An economist and politician, a member of the City Council, and director of the Department of Social Welfare, she viewed the park as the embodiment of a harm-reduction policy. Intravenous drug use goes on anyway, she argued, and law enforcement is ineffective in stopping it, so why not recognize it and give it a place to operate? Distributing syringes and needles and condoms was meant to help reduce the spread of AIDS, the green bus was a statement to addicts that someone cared about them, the social workers available for counseling might help with some urgent problems such as homelessness, and the presence of a physician could save lives.

The humanitarian motive was certainly there. But a more pragmatic (and misanthropic) motive could not escape one's notice. Concentrating illicit drug use in "needle park" cleared addicts out of the rest of the city—the shopping malls, railroad stations, and other public facilities—where merchants and other upright citizens had objected strongly to their presence. The leniency of the police in "needle park" contrasted sharply with their energetic hounding of addicts out of the "respectable" parts of the city.

Later that day I spoke at length with the surgeon general of the canton of Zurich. He was vituperative in his opposition to "needle park." Centralizing intravenous drug use was exactly the wrong policy, he argued; it should be decentralized by sending addicts back to their hometowns and villages, where they were known, where they had family, where they could get individual help, where they could be hospitalized if necessary, where someone truly cared about them. In addition, he argued, "needle park" acted as a magnet, attracting addicts from elsewhere in Europe, especially from Germany, where drug prohibitions are rigorously enforced. Worst of all, in his opinion, the park served to attract unstable young people to the drug scene, and thus to recruit new addicts from among the most vulnerable youths. Finally, he argued, the existence of open and visible drug trafficking and self-injection, under the auspices of the city government and under the eyes of the police, conferred an undesirable cloak of legitimacy on intravenous drug use itself.

As my Boeing 747 climbed away over the city, I could look down on the little park, situated on a tiny island in the river, right in the center of the city. From this remote vantage point in the sky it seemed a picturesque spot. Who would imagine the human misery concentrated down there? It seemed to me that the needle park was a wrong way to deal with the problem of intravenous drug use. I mused over the fact that an economist-politician had advocated and actually managed to establish it, while expert medical opinion opposed it. In much the same way, in the United States, the chief advocacy for legalizing the presently illicit drugs comes from people without medical training, who are uninformed about the actual physical, psychological, and societal dangers of the drugs and of drug addiction.

A year after my visit, "needle park" was closed. According to the newspaper reports, it had gotten "completely out of hand." Addicts from all over Europe had poured into the city, crime had soared. The noble (if naive) experiment had failed. But how could it have succeeded? Surely no addicts could have been cured in this park. Following the closing of the park, the city officials returned to the punitive police policy of hounding addicts and driving them underground or to jail or to some other city. But then, an interesting shift of national policy occurred. In 1992, the Swiss government authorized the establishment of a network of clinics at which heroin addicts could inject pure heroin or other opiates with sterile equipment under medical supervision. A very complex study was carried out at 18 treatment centers throughout this little country (population 7.3 million) over the three-year period 1994–1996, during which 1,151 patients were admitted to the program.

Perhaps so radical an experiment could have been carried out as a controlled clinical trial on a very large scale, to obtain decisive answers to a few well-chosen questions. Unfortunately, as so often happens, politics seems to have trumped science. With the disastrous "needle park" fresh in their memory, the citizens evidently wanted fast action to get heroin addicts off their streets. Consequently, what developed in this unusual trial allowed few decisive conclusions; but given the circumstances, it was probably the best that could be accomplished. In 1999, a report was published by the Swiss program managers, detailing methods and results.

"The designated target group of subjects," according to the report, had "chronic heroin addiction, failed previous treatments, and marked deficiencies in terms of health and social integration . . ." It was noted, especially, that patients "coming from methadone substitution treatment had continued to use illicit heroin to a large extent while being maintained on oral methadone." The report concludes that heroin-assisted treatment is useful for the designated target group and can be carried out with sufficient safety; as a result of good retention rates, significant improvements can be obtained in terms of health and lifestyle, and these persist even after the end of treatment; the mortality rate of 1 percent per year is relatively low, being up to two times higher in methadone substitution treatment; the economic benefit of heroin-assisted treatment is considerable, particularly as a result of the reduction in the costs of criminal procedures and imprisonment and in terms of healthcare costs.

The data show, not surprisingly, that heroin addicts avail themselves of free heroin if it is offered, that there were few significant side effects, that infections related to unsterile injection procedures decreased, and that fewer criminal activities were noted. No objective measures could determine (as in a urine test) the difference between heroin injected in the clinic and heroin secured on the street, so it remains uncertain to what extent the participants abstained from illicit heroin. Finally, over the three-year period, there were improvements in general health and social rehabilitation. These results support the harm-reduction principle—that addicts are better off getting pure than impure heroin.

No firm conclusion could be drawn about whether receiving intravenous heroin in a clinic environment for three years would encourage a commitment to recovery from addiction, nor was that outcome defined as a goal of the program. Since other treatment modalities are available, are results better with supervised heroin injection in a clinic than in drug-free therapeutic communities or

with oral methadone? Comparison with oral methadone maintenance at adequate dosage is important, not only because an orally
active long-acting opiate is pharmacologically superior in principle,
but because methadone stabilizes the neurochemical disruptions
caused by brain spikes of intravenous heroin (see chapter 10). If
abstinence is considered to be the only worthwhile goal, then the
Swiss project, thus far, contributes little or nothing to that.
Needed—but not yet available—are convincing data that long-term
retention in treatment, social rehabilitation, and employment are
better than with oral methadone maintenance. Especially important
would be comparisons of long-term abstinence rates for matched
groups entering heroin maintenance and therapeutic communities.

At the present writing, only one well-controlled trial has been
reported in the peer-reviewed literature—a small one in Geneva.
Heroin addicts who had failed repeatedly in standard treatment
were permitted to enter a short-term heroin maintenance program.
Two groups of about 25 were randomly assigned to immediate intravenous heroin maintenance (experimental group) or to a waiting
list (control group). The control subjects continued whatever treatment they were receiving (usually oral methadone maintenance).
After six months, only one experimental subject but 10 control subjects were—by self-report—still using street heroin; a highly significant difference, but as noted above, such information cannot be
verified objectively. Benefits were seen for health status, social functioning, and property crimes. On the other hand, there were no
differences between groups with respect to gainful employment or
use of other drugs. Surprisingly, when—after six months—the group
on the waiting list was given an opportunity to enter the heroin
maintenance program, only one-third chose to do so. In other
words, six months on methadone had apparently benefitted these
addicts sufficiently that they no longer saw an advantage in receiving
free heroin.

Finally, on the other side of the planet, we now have seen yet
another example of politics overriding science. In Australia, a small
test of heroin maintenance was proposed. Devised by medical addiction experts and social scientists, the clinical trial design called
for a mere 40 heroin addicts to be given heroin under close supervision. After the trial design had been approved by the health authorities, it was abruptly forbidden by the federal government.

Summary

In this chapter I have tried to draw some lessons from addiction policies in three European countries—Great Britain, the Netherlands, and Switzerland. Much of the chapter is based on my own visits in January 1991, brought up to date by study of the published research of the past nine years. What seems to work reasonably well are pragmatic harm-reduction policies based on the disease concept of drug addiction. There is no indication that relaxing prohibitions on the most dangerous addictive drugs (and therefore making them more available) would be useful. The Dutch policy of distinguishing between "soft" and "hard" drugs (and the quasi-legalization of cannabis) seems to work reasonably well there, but it is unclear how effective it would be in America. The short-lived "needle park" experience in Zurich suggests that simply adopting a laissez-faire attitude toward use of the presently illicit addictive drugs would not solve any drug addiction problems—least of all the problems that afflict the addicts themselves. Because of the paucity of controlled research, the jury is still out on the aftermath of "needle park"—the network of Swiss clinics where addicts can legally inject pure heroin under medical supervision.

In my opinion, humane treatment—perhaps even starting with heroin in a clinic environment, as in the Swiss project—could be offered to all addicts who desire it, even while the prohibitions on dangerous drugs remain in effect and are strongly enforced. It seems to me that citizens have a right not to be confronted with addicts using drugs in their streets and public places; but then they also have an obligation to offer treatment services to those who are victimized by the addictive drugs. Heroin could be provided as a short-term initial step in treatment, as I suggested 25 years ago in my "STEPS" proposal (see chapter 16). The question to be answered by rigorous research is how the harm-reduction benefits of providing heroin to heroin addicts on a long-term basis would compare with alternatives (like methadone, LAAM, or buprenorphine) that offer a more stable lifestyle through maintenance on an orally administered long-acting medication.

19

Prohibition vs. Legalization

—A False Dichotomy

Frustration with our present drug policies has fueled well-meaning suggestions that the illicit drugs should be legalized. If the "drug problem" is defined as a crime problem, then there is a certain simplistic logic to making the drugs legal. On the other hand, if addiction is basically a brain disease, then legalizing the drugs would be the very opposite of treating the addicts. To analyze the arguments for legalization, we need to know what, exactly, is meant by the word. Is cocaine to be sold to minors in supermarkets? Except for the most extreme libertarians, even those who advocate legalization agree that there have to be some legal restrictions after all. So we must ask, which drugs, what restrictions, and why? This chapter examines the dual strategy of supply reduction and demand reduction, draws lessons from the history of alcohol prohibition in the United States, and addresses directly the principal arguments for and against legalization. It concludes—as explained further in chapter 20—that neither blanket prohibition nor blanket legalization is appropriate, but that each drug requires its own appropriate level of regulatory control.

Supply Reduction, Demand Reduction

There are two ways to wage a "war on drugs." Most forceful, most visible, and therefore most appealing politically, is to attempt to cut off illicit drugs at the source and at every lower level of the distribution chain. All such activities are described as supply reduction. The other—and less dramatic—way is by demand reduction, comprising all the methods of reducing people's desire to obtain addictive drugs. These include prevention education, targeting especially vulnerable groups, ameliorating conditions of life that are associated with drug-seeking behavior, and above all providing adequate treatment and social rehabilitation services for addicts. Demand is also reduced effectively by closely monitoring their abstinence when addicts are on probation (as an alternative to jail) or parole (following early release from incarceration).

Supply reduction and demand reduction are not mutually exclusive alternatives. Both strategies have the same goal, to reduce the total consumption of addictive drugs. Supply reduction seeks to accomplish this by reducing the availability of the drugs to the would-be consumer. With ideal success of a supply-reduction strategy, the drug would no longer be available at all; but this goal is only occasionally and partially and slowly attained. Nevertheless, drug demand is clearly elastic enough to respond to price changes, so successful supply reduction, resulting in price increases, can reduce demand.

The demand-reduction strategy also produces results slowly. The frustrating pace of demand reduction is illustrated by the nicotine experience. The educational campaign about the health hazards of smoking has now been in effect for more than a generation, since the mid-1960s. And it has, indeed, resulted in a substantial change in smoking behavior. This change is pervasive, it cuts through the whole society, and it is being reinforced year after year by new statutory regulations at the federal, state, and local levels. Nevertheless, there remains a very large group of hard-core nicotine addicts who are unwilling or unable to alter their behavior. More discouraging, the impact on recruitment of youngsters to this addiction, especially in the past five years, has been disappointing. With illicit drugs, we must expect a similar slow change. First, the uncommitted occasional users will get the educational message, then little by little the more heavily addicted will follow suit, eventually leaving a hard-core group untouched. How easily educational messages will affect the recruiting of youngsters to the use of cannabis, heroin, cocaine, amphetamines, and other illicit drugs is uncertain. Many who are addicted to them already—in contrast to cigarette smokers—are alienated from mainstream society, are often school dropouts, lead chaotic lives, and are not reached easily by educational messages. In 1997, Congress appropriated $197 million for a major advertising campaign—the National Youth Anti-Drug Media Campaign, which the Office of National Drug Control Policy (ONDCP) is currently implementing, in partnership with nongovernmental organizations. How effective this massive educational effort will be remains to be seen.

Demand reduction by offering free and readily available treatment is a way to reach the hard-core addicts; and research findings show clearly that treatment is an effective means of demand reduction. Every addict reaches a point where life is so out of control (or rather, so controlled by a drug) that some remedy is sought. With some drugs, dosage may have escalated so that obtaining sufficient drug is simply beyond the addict's means. Sometimes a serious adverse drug effect provokes a decision to seek treatment—a toxic reaction, a near-lethal overdose, a serious infection requiring hospitalization. Often law enforcement pressure forces the addict to seek treatment. Sometimes a religious conversion or similar experience changes the addict's whole outlook on life, and drugs are rejected. The big unsolved problem is how best to sustain the benefits of treatment and prevent relapse.

Was Prohibition a Failure?

The main premise of the argument for total prohibition is that it actually can reduce the consumption of addictive drugs. But the social cost of such a policy may not be acceptable. The Chinese experience is relevant. Opium addiction was widespread in China in the first half of the 20th century and there were many millions of addicts. Although opium was nominally prohibited, enforcement was lax, corruption was rife, and government officials as well as warlords benefited from the opium traffic. The Communist government, when it came to power in 1949, made eradication of opium addiction a major and well-advertised national goal. Although at that time the methods were not publicized abroad, it is clear now that they were truly draconian. Apparently, traffickers were summarily executed by the thousands. Addicts were sent to the countryside for rehabilitation through hard labor and reeducation after undergoing "cold-turkey" withdrawal. Subsequently their state of abstinence was closely monitored. Experts visiting China in the 1980s, after the Cultural Revolution, reported with astonishment that neither drug addicts nor addictive drugs could be found anywhere.

That harsh policy was not an aberration of the early days of the revolutionary regime. While I was teaching a course at Beijing Medical University in 1991, I was told that after a drug-free quarter century, opiate addiction was reappearing because of importation of heroin across the southern border. The government's reaction had not softened with the passage of time. I read a newspaper account and personally watched the TV coverage of a public hanging of 52 alleged heroin traffickers in a public square. Thousands watched, and the governor of the province gave a rousing speech, saying, "This is how we deal with drug traffickers!" Such methods are incompatible with our concepts of personal liberty, and I abhor them. My point here is simply that harsh methods can, without doubt, be effective in reducing the incidence of drug addiction.

Another example comes from Japan. Immediately after World War II, a large supply of amphetamines, which had been stocked by the military, found its way onto the civilian market. A serious epidemic of amphetamine addiction ensued. The government stepped in with strong, unambiguous, and well-publicized law enforcement measures. Supplies were seized, traffickers and users were jailed. In short order the epidemic was terminated.

Drastic measures are most effective when they command public support. That was true in China, where revolutionary fervor created consensus for the many policies instituted to build the new society. It was true in Japan, where the national will was being mobilized to build a new nation on the ashes of defeat. It is true today in Saudi Arabia and other Moslem countries dominated by Islamic law, where the prohibition of alcohol is enforced with severe penalties.

American history is relevant, too- -our national prohibition of alcohol. The temperance movement at the turn of the century led first to state-by-state prohibition laws. By 1916 alcohol was effectively illegal in most states, and this status was codified in federal law by the Eighteenth Amendment and the Volstead Act in the years just after World War I. Everyone knows that Prohibition caused serious problems. There was widespread bootlegging, new criminal gangs got a foothold, and spectacular violence sometimes erupted as rival traffickers fought for market share. Furthermore, many ordinary citizens violated the law, fostering disrespect for law in general. Those consequences weigh in heavily on the cost side of the ledger. But on the benefit side, it is clear that Prohibition did result in a major reduction in the consumption of alcohol and a concomitant major decrease in the harm caused by alcohol. To say that "Prohibition failed" is simply wrong without close examination of its effects on alcohol consumption.

Deaths from alcoholic liver cirrhosis dropped very sharply after the institution of Prohibition, remained at a low level, then climbed again after repeal in 1933 (Figure 19.1). An important virtue of liver cirrhosis as an indicator is that it is due chiefly to alcohol, and that it is serious enough to bring its victim to a hospital; thus it is an objective measure of heavy drinking, which cannot easily be concealed. Accurate consumption figures are impossible to obtain for the period when alcohol was illegal, but research in several countries has demonstrated that cirrhosis is a good indicator of total consumption of alcohol by a population. Those who drink most heavily are in the "tail of the distribution curve" (in statistical terms). When everyone drinks more, there are more people in that tail of the curve; when everyone drinks less, there are fewer heavy drinkers. One might have guessed that even when the population as a whole reduces its average consumption, alcohol addicts do not—that their demand for alcohol is inflexible. The data, however, refute that idea; the response to reduced availability is that all groups drink less.

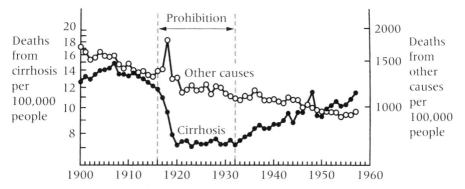

Fig. 19.1: Death rates from alcoholic cirrhosis and all other causes, United States. Vertical scales are logarithmic. (From H. Kalant and O. J. Kalant: *Drugs, Society, and Personal Choice*, Addiction Research Foundation, Toronto, 1971, Fig. 5.)

A similar picture, even more dramatic, is seen for the death rate from cirrhosis in Paris. Deaths from all other causes declined slowly over the 30-year period studied, 1935–1965, with a brief increase during the years of World War II. The death rate from cirrhosis remained stable until World War II came to French soil, when strict alcohol rationing was instituted. Then, it fell precipitously, from 35 to 6 per 100,000 population. When rationing was abolished, the rate rose again, over the next seven years, to prewar levels.

A remarkable experiment was carried out in 1951–1953 in several villages of rural Finland that had been "dry" for many years. The farmers residing in these villages could obtain alcohol legally only by travelling some 15–30 miles to a large town with a government monopoly liquor store. Some argued that if the weaker alcoholic beverages (wine and beer) were made easier to obtain, people would substitute those for the more dangerous distilled spirits. So beer and wine stores were opened in selected experimental villages while no change was made in matched control villages. Careful interviewing yielded baseline information about consumption of the various kinds of alcoholic beverage before the experiment began. Then the same subjects were interviewed a year or two later. The experiment showed that total beer and wine consumption rose dramatically in the villages where the new beer and wine stores were opened. However, these increases were not accompanied by a corresponding decrease in the drinking of hard liquor. Thus, making it easier to get beer and wine resulted in a substantial increase in total alcohol consumption. At the same time there was little or no change in the control villages.

Finally, the heroin epidemic among U.S. troops in Vietnam confirms the general rule that drug availability strongly influences drug consumption. There, where heroin was pure, cheap, and readily available, many thousands of American young men became addicted who would never have even experimented with heroin at home. Moreover, when they returned home, the great majority of them never used heroin again.

In summary, the consumption of addictive drugs is responsive to availability, and availability is affected by legal status. These are not absolutes, of course. Even when an addictive drug is prohibited—as alcohol was from about 1916 to 1933, or as cannabis, heroin, cocaine, and amphetamines are today—some people break the law and obtain it anyway. But during Prohibition a person could not walk into the nearest supermarket and buy liquor, nor drop into the corner bar, nor readily order a couple of martinis at a business lunch, nor partake of beer at an athletic event, nor have a drink or two on an airplane, nor drink wine or champagne openly at a public reception, nor be influenced by liquor advertisements on billboards and in magazines or beer advertisements on television and radio. Yes, some folks did drop into a speakeasy once in a while, and some laid in stocks of bootleg liquor. But all in all, under Prohibition, it was much less a drinking culture than we live in today.

Some Costs of Supply Reduction Strategies

Drug business is, of course, no mom-and-pop affair. Although an exact figure obviously cannot be obtained, its annual volume, worldwide, amounts to hundreds of billions of dollars, without even considering tobacco and alcohol. According to U.S. government statistics, Americans spend $57 billion a year on illicit drugs. The illicit drug business is run by huge cartels, with resources adequate to ensure the flow of goods to the market and the flow of cash through an organized international system of "money laundering." It is big business, run on a colossal scale. The cartels have their own armies and their own means of transport by land, sea, and air. Banks under their control, in sheltered spots around the world, manage their finances. They openly challenge governments, conducting their operations by a combination of bribery and terror. The brazen way they assassinate judges, prosecutors, and elected officials startles the world. In Colombia, where much of the world's cocaine is produced, whole regions of the country are no longer under effective control of the government. Similar situations exist, to some extent, in other drug-producing countries such as Peru, Afghanistan, and Thailand. When it comes to interfering with the operations of the drug cartels, "war on drugs" is no longer a metaphor but a reality; the situation calls for actual military force. At times, in the past, corrupt elements within our own government agencies were part of the problem rather than of the solution. This unsavory history is reviewed in detail by A. W. McCoy in *The Politics of Heroin* (Lawrence Hill Books, New York, 1991), and by P. D. Scott and J. Marshall in *Cocaine Politics* (University of California Press, Berkeley, 1991) and in other well documented studies, including the official 1989 Kerry Committee report to the U.S. Senate, *Drugs, Law Enforcement and Foreign Policy* (U.S. Government Printing Office, Washington, D.C., 1989).

Today, the stated mission of our Office of National Drug Control Policy (ONDCP) is to deal forcefully with sources of supply by supporting democratic governments in their attempts to suppress the production and export of addictive drugs. Much effort is also devoted to interdiction at our borders, but this seems an unrealistic—indeed, hopeless—exercise. As an illustration of the basic futility of interdiction, it may be noted that the world production of illicit opium is 30 times what the United States consumes as heroin. Moreover, whenever production of any illicit drug is reduced in one country, another takes up the slack; for example, when coca cultivation was successfully reduced in Peru and Bolivia in recent years, the major source of cocaine shifted to Colombia.

To reduce corruption in drug law enforcement within the United States is also not an easy task. The newspapers regularly carry accounts of agents of the Drug Enforcement Administration or of local police drug squads being arrested, charged, and convicted of accepting bribes or even of participating in the drug distribution network. At the lowest level of enforcement—the cop on the beat—newspaper photos of drug markets conducted openly, with police standing by, tell us that something is radically wrong. When money is the carrot, and coercion—including the real threat of death by traffickers—is the stick, it may be difficult for police officers, bureaucrats in the law enforcement system, or customs inspectors to resist. And when nothing seems to make a serious dent in drug availability, it is little wonder that law enforcement agents can become cynical.

The situation I describe here—locally, nationally, and internationally—fuels the arguments in favor of legalizing all addictive drugs. According to these arguments, if the presently illicit drugs were legal, the market price would drop drastically, drug quality controls could be implemented, tax revenues could be collected, gun battles for market share would cease, respect for the law would be restored, and corruption would be ended. No doubt some of these desirable things would happen—but at what cost to the public health? Legalization means increased availability, which would certainly increase the number of first users (especially young people) and consequently the number who would become addicted.

No Person is an Island

Among the many definitions of legalization is one that is based on the principle that government has no right to limit people's freedom to do what they wish to their own bodies, and therefore to use whatever drugs they wish. This position is easy to understand, and its total consistency makes it attractive. It is usually called libertarian, but I would characterize it as selfishly anarchistic. It is important to recognize its full implications.

Modern societies, especially those with representative governments, try, by means of appropriate laws, to protect their citizens against harm. In our technically advanced civilization, there are many hazards that the ordinary person is not equipped to understand and recognize or is powerless to avoid. Familiar examples are air and water pollution, toxicity due to lead in gasoline or paint, radioactive waste, inadequately treated sewage, electric shock risks in household appliances, fire hazards in public accommodations, toxic substances in foods or cosmetics, and dangerous medications prescribed by physicians or sold over the counter. Protecting consumers against these is the proper and necessary function of government through the Environmental Protection Agency, the Food and Drug Administration, the National Transportation Safety Board, the Department of Energy, and numerous other federal, state, county, and municipal agencies.

In addition, there are obvious hazards, against which prudent people protect themselves. Here risk-taking behavior by some is a proper concern of society because the adverse consequences may harm others, or because the harm that risk takers do to themselves will place an additional burden on the rest of us. Classic examples of the latter rationale are laws mandating seat belts and motorcycle helmets. The truth is—and fortunately so—we are, on the whole, a compassionate society. If you came upon a motorcycle accident in which the helmetless rider was lying by the side of the road with severe head injuries, you would not ignore the victim and drive away, thinking, "Rider, it's your problem, not mine; you failed to take sensible precautions." Like it or not, we are—and ought to be— concerned about our fellow human beings. And so, we have a vested interest in risk avoidance by others. No person is an island, and there are few if any truly "victimless" crimes.

As it is a universally accepted principle that the law should protect one person from being harmed by another, we should be especially concerned about the effect of maternal drug use on fetal health and the future development of the child. Every civilized society takes collective responsibility for the mental development of its new citizens, a commitment that is expressed in the fact that we support universal education through taxation, even if we have no children ourselves. The tragedy of a child born malformed or mentally retarded as a result of unknown causes has always been accepted as a responsibility that a humane society willingly accepts. But what if that tragedy results predictably from maternal drug use? Is not the drug-using behavior of the pregnant woman a legitimate concern for everyone?

If we deny the right of government to be involved in any of these matters, it will follow, of course, that government has no right to be in the business of regulating addictive drugs. However, if we accept any role of government in reducing the harmful effects of addictive drugs, we will have to get past philosophical generalizations and come to grips with details; what degree of regulation is appropriate for which drugs, and for what reason?

The propensity of experimental animals to self-inject addictive drugs, and to become truly addicted, is universal. However, it can be modified by environmental factors, so it is not permissible to conclude by analogy that all humans would become addicts if there were no legal controls. We do have to infer, however, that if all addictive drugs were easily available to everyone, and if there were no social pressures to discourage their use, a very large number of people would become addicted, probably many times the current number. Alcohol and nicotine give us some insight into what can happen when addictive drugs are freely available—we have more than 50 million cigarette smokers and 15 million severely impaired alcohol addicts. Since heroin, cocaine, and amphetamines are no less powerfully addictive than nicotine or alcohol, free availability might well bring us many times more than the few million cocaine, amphetamine, and heroin addicts we have now. Is that a price we are willing, as a society, to pay?

Harm Reduction, Not Legalization

A warning: The term "harm reduction" is sometimes used to camouflage a quite different aim—the legalization of some or all addictive drugs that are currently illicit. Chapter 18 presented examples of different ways the United Kingdom, the Netherlands, and Switzerland have implemented true harm-reduction policies. The status of certain drugs may have been modified, as by limited decriminalization of possession for personal use, or by furnishing specific drugs to some addicts under tightly controlled conditions. But in none of those countries (or elsewhere) have any illicit drugs been legalized.

Without making the presently illicit drugs available to everyone, young and old, might we nevertheless provide the drugs to bona fide confirmed addicts? The argument for doing this is that they are already using anyway, and that they are the main source of society's drug problems. The hope is that we might thereby undercut the black market and eliminate drug-related crime. In addition, it is argued, furnishing addicts with pure drugs of reliable quality instead of the uncontrolled illicit ones they use now would improve their health and longevity. In addition, fed up with urban crime, many believe that if we give the addicts heroin and cocaine and whatever other drugs they want, they will stop stealing and stop shooting each other and innocent passersby. This seems logical, but the actual evidence is conflicting. As noted in chapter 18, when London addicts were legally furnished pure heroin at very low cost, they nonetheless continued their criminal activities. Frequently, illicit drug use and criminality are not cause and effect but parallel forms of antisocial behavior. On the other hand, the current Swiss project (chapter 18) does suggest a reduction in crimes committed by heroin addicts.

This harm reduction approach would not be easy to implement. First, we would have to decide who qualifies as an addict; and that is not so simple. We could test for dependence on heroin, for example, and then make the drug available only to those who pass the test. But what about the 18-year-old who uses heroin occasionally but has not yet become dependent? When we refuse that person heroin, would we not be saying, "Go out and use more, and when you become dependent and can pass our test, we'll give you the heroin you want?"

Perhaps dependence is a poor criterion. We might instead say, very simply, that anyone who is already using an illicit drug should be able to get it at a clinic. We could test a sample of urine and know with certainty if a person had used an opiate or cocaine or amphetamine or marijuana in the previous few days. But what about youngsters who have smoked crack once or twice and liked it, but are not using enough (or using frequently enough) to test positive? In order to qualify for legal and cheap supplies, they would first have to use crack more heavily on the street. Would we then be complicit in their addictive behavior?

There would presumably have to be some ceiling—however high—on dosage dispensed. We can predict with fair confidence, on the basis of research studies, that heroin and cocaine addicts will escalate their dosage to that ceiling. Then, when their demands for more are rejected, they are likely to look to the street (this happened in Britain), and thus sustain an illicit market after all. Ironically, the addict would then have to spend even more for the illicit drugs because tolerance to the increased dosage would greatly increase the amount of supplemental drug needed to produce the desired hedonic effect.

A complex set of deterrents—and not least the legal prohibitions—is presently discouraging all but a few children and adolescents from trying the most dangerous illicit drugs. To some degree, the existence of clinics or dispensaries where cocaine and heroin are distributed would tend to legitimize the drugs. "If a government clinic dispenses it," a youngster may well think, "it is probably not too dangerous. Maybe I can find some and try it—just once." All addicts used their drug "just once" the first time.

Many prominent politicians and thoughtful people from other walks of life, who are fed up with crime in the streets, think that abolishing drug prohibitions entirely—or at least giving addicts their drugs of choice on demand—will solve the drug problem. But they define the drug problem as crime in the streets rather than as drug addiction itself. According to the medical and public health perspective presented in this book, the extreme course of legalizing the drugs for everyone would certainly have serious adverse consequences for society. Even the more limited option of giving their drugs of choice to addicts on demand, while it might reduce criminality, could hardly be called treatment for their addiction. Whether, on balance, addicts who have proved refractory to all available treatments might benefit from carefully monitored drug administration in a clinic—as in the Swiss model—should continue to be the subject of research. Some problems have no perfect solutions, and some "solutions" can be worse than the problems they are meant to solve.

Summary

Supply reduction, by assisting source countries to reduce production, by interdiction at our borders, and by domestic law enforcement aimed at major traffickers is worth some effort—if only for its symbolism—but is very unlikely to have a major impact. Therefore, the primary aim of drug policy should be to reduce the prevalence of drug addiction and the recruitment of new addicts, i.e., demand reduction. Every policy has its costs, both monetary and human. Prohibitions cause harm, but this harm has to be weighed against the damage that is caused by the drug being prohibited. Chapter 20 proposes concrete policies based on what we know about each family of addictive drugs. Whatever the drug, our general aim should be to strike the right balance—to achieve the greatest degree of harm reduction by means of the least necessary degree of regulation.

20

New Strategies for
Rational Drug Policy

What should be the purpose of government policy on addictive drugs? What should we be trying to accomplish, and why? It is certainly in the interest of society as a whole to reduce the amount of damage done by drug addiction. This means preventing youngsters from being drawn into using addictive drugs in the first place. It means cutting down the amount of drug use by people already addicted, improving their physical and mental health, and trying to free them of their addiction. It also means reducing the harm caused to others as a result of drug use by addicts. At the same time, we have to take care that implementing drug policy does not cause more harm to individuals and society than do the drugs themselves. To strike the right balance requires careful, thoughtful analysis, with a recognition that changes come slowly, that there are no quick fixes.

In this chapter, I first propose general policies that apply to the drug addiction problem as a whole. Then, since each drug calls for a different approach according to the specific dangers it presents to the individual and to society, I suggest detailed drug-by-drug policies. Many of the proposals offered herein were developed in a lengthy scholarly article coauthored with my Canadian colleague Dr. Harold

Kalant and published in the 28 September 1990 issue of the journal *Science* (vol. 249, pp. 1513–1521).

General Policies

1. Consider drug addiction to be primarily a public health problem. Drug policies have too often been driven by public panic and media hysteria, to which politicians respond by whatever actions they think will be reassuring in the immediate crisis. This pattern does not address the real need. It is time to return the drug problem to the domain of medicine and public health, where it belongs. For many reasons (see chapter 1), it is logical to approach drug addiction as if it were an infectious disease. Such concepts as incidence, prevalence, relative immunity, and genetic and environmental influences on susceptibility can be applied to both. Attempts at prevention, eradication, education, treatment, relapse prevention, and containment are comparable. And important for preventing the spread of drug addiction is the fact that—as with infectious diseases—it is primarily the newly infected who transmit the condition to their peers. Quarantine, which has sometimes been used in severe and life-threatening epidemics, can be an effective tool (especially for diseases that are transmitted readily by casual contact); but it always raises ethical and legal issues concerning the degree to which it is permissible to restrict the personal liberties of those who are infected in order to protect those who are not.

The argument that the analogy of addiction to infectious disease is false because people are passive victims of infectious disease but actively seek out addictive drugs was discussed at length in chapter 1. There it was pointed out that in both cases human behavior is responsible, at least in part. The person who gets AIDS or hepatitis through promiscuous unprotected sex and the person who gets lung cancer through addictive smoking are both responsible for the public health burden they place on society.

The public health approach rests on the philosophy of harm reduction. This is an attitude, a way of approaching difficult and sometimes intractable problems, which is commonplace in public health and medical practice. It is the very opposite of rigid, judgmental attitudes based on concepts of morality. The reorientation of thinking that is proposed here would counter the kind of simplistic "drug war" mentality that has been so unproductive in the past. The slogan "war on drugs," however, has much to recommend it. It is appropriate in the same way that we might speak of a war on AIDS, a war on cancer, or a war on poverty. The metaphor implies that there is a serious threat to our society, that national resources need to be mobilized, that a united nation can best accomplish what is called for, that large investments of money and energy will be required, that the effort commands a high priority, that the best minds need to be tapped for solutions, that "business as usual" will not do.

Bearing in mind the warning in chapter 19 about misuse of the term, true "harm reduction" should be the central strategy in the war on drugs. Physicians recognize that some diseases can neither be eradicated nor cured. They simply do the best they can to minimize the harm, acknowledging that not every problem has a totally satisfactory solution. Illustrative is the physician's approach to a chronic disabling disease like rheumatoid arthritis. No cure is yet known, but the pain and disability can be managed moderately well with appropriate medications. The condition is subject to relapses, even after long periods of remission—a noteworthy similarity to the drug addictions.

The key to treating such conditions is to avoid unrealistic expectations and to accept small victories gratefully. It is important not to regard relapse as failure, but rather as a challenge to reinstitute and improve the treatment. Although it would be lovely if by some magical means we could wipe out all drug addictions, that is just not going to happen. Once we recognize and accept that reality, we can go forward to craft realistic policies for reducing the harm done by each addictive drug to the addicts and to society.

In recognition of the importance of the drug addiction problem to the nation's health, a special agency was established in the executive branch of government—the Office of National Drug Control Policy (ONDCP). An important role of this office is to coordinate the activities of the many federal agencies with responsibilities related to drug abuse and addiction. The annual National Drug Control Strategy document and other ONDCP publications are invaluable sources of data on all aspects of our drug problem and the activities being pursued to bring it under control. ONDCP also provides an important pulpit for educating the public; and positions expounded by ONDCP have often coincided with those advocated in this book. Especially significant have been repeated pronouncements by General Barry McCaffrey, director of ONDCP, to the effect that national drug policy must be driven by science, not by ideology. But a weakness imposed by Congress is distinctly unscientific and needs to be remedied; conspicuously absent from the authorized mission of ONDCP are nicotine and alcohol (except as concerns children, for whom these drugs are illegal). Finally, ONDCP is playing a leadership role in drawing up specific recommendations for rational and consistent harm-reduction policies through legislative, executive, and judicial actions at federal, state, and local levels of government.

The principal improvement needed, overall, is a shift in emphasis from supply reduction to demand reduction activities. With more than $18 billion federal dollars now (in the 2000 budget) expended annually on the drug problem, a way needs to be found more quickly to reverse the overall imbalance of expenditures, which continues to be nearly 70 to 30 in favor of supply reduction over demand reduction.

2. Make demand reduction the primary strategy. Throughout history, societies have attempted to eliminate one addictive drug or another (whichever was most abhorrent to the dominant culture) by harsh punitive measures—even capital punishment for the users. Sometimes such measures have been effective (see chapter 19), but whether truly draconian policies might work is really an academic question for Americans. American society is built on respect for human rights, as enshrined in the U.S. Constitution's Bill of Rights. To sacrifice those principles for the sake of reducing or even eliminating (if it were possible) drug addiction would not—I hope and trust—be acceptable to the majority of citizens. Without infringing on constitutional liberties, the best hope of making a significant impact on the drug problem is to reduce demand, and to do so patiently and systematically, through two approaches.

First, expand prevention education, continuing and accelerating the current trend toward honest, health-based, elementary and secondary education about all addictive drugs. Get rid of the misleading terms "alcohol and drugs" and "nicotine and drugs," which imply that alcohol and nicotine are not drugs, whereas they are actually the ones that cause the greatest harm to public health. Moreover, they are the gateway drugs, the ones that children and adolescents use first, after which some progress to marijuana, then to cocaine and heroin. Educate in an evenhanded manner about the effects of all the addictive drugs. "Just say no!" is useful and necessary, but by no means sufficient. Teach why saying no is a wise policy. Teach that children should not use any addictive drugs because—whatever their legal status—they are harmful to health and can lead to uncontrolled use and all the consequences of the addicted state. Concerning those drugs that are illicit, every child, at the appropriate grade level, should be taught respect for the law in a context of learning the history and basis of the drug laws and the political processes for debating and changing the laws in a democratic society.

Second, make treatment readily and universally available. This is one of the most reliable and cost-effective ways of reducing demand for drugs. The number of funded treatment "slots" presently falls far short of meeting the demand. Every day an addict spends in treatment is a day of reduced drug use and of reduced crime (to the extent that criminal activity was motivated by the need to support the addiction). As discussed in preceding chapters, research has confirmed this socially beneficial effect of treatment on drug-related crime. In addition, since the addict's motivation to enter treatment is often weak, finding a treatment facility and being admitted rapidly to treatment must be made easy. The Dutch have set a good example of how to do this (see chapter 18).

3. Address the spread of AIDS and other infectious diseases by intravenous drug users. We need to continue dealing with the role of intravenous drug use (primarily of cocaine, amphetamines, and heroin) in the spread of AIDS and hepatitis. The AIDS virus (HIV) accidentally found a foothold nearly 20 years ago in the community of gay men in the United States; but it soon spread, through heterosexual contacts, to an increasing number of women. The spread of HIV among intravenous drug users affects all of society, for the virus will not confine itself to the addict group any more than it has to the gay community. Prostitutes, especially, play a role in the spread of HIV and other sexually transmitted diseases, and prostitution is a common means of financial support for addicts. Providing sterile needles and condoms to all addicts is a policy already instituted in many communities, and it ought to be implemented everywhere. The data show convincingly that providing sterile needles and syringes does not recruit new users.

It is true that there is still no strong scientific proof that needle exchanges and condom distribution will stop the spread of HIV among intravenous drug users. However, the public health approach to a death-dealing virus must be based on whatever partial evidence is available, on common sense, and on the need to teach the facts about intravenous drug use, AIDS, and hepatitis. Unfortunately, powerful forces are opposed to this simple public health measure because of worry about "sending the wrong kind of message." It seems to me that the wrong kind of message would be, "We don't care whether these diseases continue to spread or not." With respect to needle exchanges, as for some other aspects of drug policy, we have much to learn from countries like the United Kingdom and the Netherlands.

Even more important than needle exchanges in stemming the spread of AIDS and hepatitis is expansion of methadone maintenance programs to accommodate all heroin addicts who are willing to enroll. It is a well established fact that when addicts are stabilized on an adequate dosage of methadone in a well-run program with ancillary services, they drastically reduce or discontinue their intravenous drug use and thus their sharing of needles.

4. Address the problem of fetal damage caused by addictive drugs. The special problem of addictive drug use by pregnant women will need urgent and very careful consideration. This issue is of major concern to society for both humanitarian and economic reasons. Drugs used by a pregnant woman affect in several ways how her fetus will develop and thus how much of a burden that child may ultimately be on society. First, there are the obvious congenital malformations, such as are seen in fetal alcohol syndrome. Second, evidence (though still inconclusive) from both animal and human studies suggests the possibility of permanent damage to the developing brain, resulting in mental retardation and behavioral abnormalities that may only be evident years later. Third, both because of drug effects and because the addicted woman is unlikely to maintain her own health during pregnancy, the infant is likely to be born prematurely and of low birth weight, causing an array of adverse health consequences. Fourth, the newborn baby is likely to be dependent on the addictive drug and require special detoxification treatment.

What to do about this problem is a thorny question. Pregnant addicts ought to be afforded free treatment for their drug addiction, coupled with free prenatal care; those are good cost-effective investments for society. But should we do more? Can a case be made for compulsion—for allowing the interests of society to override the civil liberties of the pregnant woman? Long-acting injectable contraceptives could be made available; some argue that court-ordered compulsory contraception may be appropriate in some cases. Mandatory diagnostic procedures could provide findings that might justify abortion of a severely damaged fetus. Public debate is needed about how to develop disincentives to pregnancy in untreated addicts, and about the degree to which the interest of society in healthy babies justifies government intervention. The birth of a drug-damaged child is not only a tragedy; it can also be considered a crime against humanity—provided, of course, that effective alternatives to drug use are made universally available to female addicts of childbearing age.

5. Enact and implement laws that support social norms. Advocates of drug legalization often argue as though legal restrictions and drug education were mutually exclusive. They point to the salutory progress in the United States in reducing the prevalence of nicotine addiction. "See," they say, "the harmful use of an addictive drug is best reduced through education, through health consciousness, in short, through voluntary actions rather than through governmental intrusions." But "rather than" implies a false dichotomy (see chapters 8 and 19), which distorts what actually happened with tobacco smoking.

The historic decline in smoking over the last 25 years illustrates how laws and education complement each other. Biomedical science led the way in providing irrefutable evidence of the damage to health—evidence summarized in the 1964 Surgeon General's Report. Then, as education made people more aware of the health hazards, and made nonsmokers more aware of their rights, people gradually became more accepting of increased regulation. As an example, the ban on smoking in commercial air travel was first instituted on flights of two hours or less, then later extended to all domestic flights. Regulation of smoking in restaurants began with establishment of smoking and nonsmoking sections, but now, in many places, has given way to a total prohibition. As awareness grew, and with more nonsmokers and former smokers in the population, tougher regulations became acceptable, such as prohibition of smoking in all public facilities and in the workplace. Increased taxation as a means of reducing consumption has also gained acceptability. Much more needs to be done, but we see here a working model of how regulations can promote attitudinal change, and how attitudinal change, in turn, can make ever tougher regulations more acceptable. These examples also illustrate how regulations short of complete prohibition can be effective without significantly criminalizing an addictive behavior. At the same time, educational efforts emphasizing harm reduction should be directed at hard-core addicts who continue to resist total abstinence.

6. Consider actual crime—whether or not drug-related—to be primarily a law enforcement problem. For the purpose of this discussion I exclude the "crime" of drug possession for personal use. By actual crime I mean burglary, robbery, theft, shoplifting, and embezzlement, as well as large-scale drug trafficking, gun battles over turf, and all manner of other violent offenses. These should be dealt with on their own terms and not be allowed to detract from the public health approach to the majority of addicts. Violent crime and property crime, whatever their causes, must be dealt with so that innocent citizens can enjoy the right to live in a safe neighborhood, to go about their peaceful pursuits without fear. In short, we should deal with drug-related crime as we deal with any criminal activity. Being addicted does not exculpate actual crime.

A constructive policy will distinguish between the victims and the predators, between the addicts on the one hand and the traffickers who are the real criminals on the other. And the law can distinguish easily between the health problems of addicts and the serious criminal actions associated with addictive drugs. There is a precedent in the way we handle a legally available drug, alcohol. Numerous control measures are directed principally at the traffickers—the manufacturers, advertisers, and distributors. For example, those who manufacture alcohol illicitly, who distribute it without paying the taxes, or who sell it to minors, are subject to criminal sanctions. But users are affected by the law only to the extent that their drug use results in rowdy behavior, drunk driving, assault, or other violations of the rights of others—behaviors that are in themselves criminal.

The objection is often raised that on the street it is impossible to make a clear distinction between users and traffickers because so many users of illicit drugs are also sellers. I find this a specious argument. The major traffickers deal in such large quantities that their status is unambiguous. The fact is, however, that major traffickers are difficult to apprehend; it is much easier to expend police efforts on street addicts, who typically divide and sell some of their own heroin, cocaine, or marijuana. Admittedly, going after the "big fish" is easier said than done, and to do it effectively will require tackling the pervasive problem of corruption at all levels of the law enforcement system.

The laws on possession of illicit drugs ought to be modified so that we stop filling the jails and prisons with hapless users, as in our present revolving-door system. This applies especially to youngsters, experimenting for the first time, who only need a firm slap on the wrist, not criminal sanctions or treatment. In this regard, one of the unfortunate consequences of the panic-driven policies of recent years has been the establishment of mandatory minimum sentences for drug offenders. This misguided approach has deprived judges of the discretionary power to distinguish, in the case of illicit drugs, between major and minor crimes, between significant and trivial offenses. A great many judges have urged restoring judicial discretion in sentencing. In short, the common sense principle of letting the punishment fit the crime needs to be reestablished in the field of drug offenses. The system of drug courts should be expanded quickly, so that first offenders can be offered the option of closely monitored treatment instead of jail.

7. Increase funding for basic and applied research. This recommendation may be discounted as self-serving, coming as it does from a researcher. History teaches us, however, that investment in biomedical research pays off handsomely. The more we know, the better we can apply our knowledge to solve problems. Basic research yields the understanding that permits us to fashion novel practical solutions, without which there would be only guesswork and superstition. Applied research teaches us how best to develop and implement novel practical solutions.

Consider the development of methadone maintenance. Many years of basic research on the biological actions of opiates were needed before—in Germany before World War II—methadone could be synthesized as a morphine substitute for pain relief. As the chemical structure of methadone is not even close to that of morphine, it never would have been developed were it not for the deep understanding, generated over many years of basic research, of those special properties of the morphine molecule that are responsible for its biological effects. The idea of using methadone for maintenance treatment because of its long duration of action depended on much prior research concerning how drugs are metabolized and eliminated from the body. Finally, rigorous applied research was needed to demonstrate that methadone really works in heroin addicts, that it is both safe and efficacious.

Both basic and applied research deserve support as part of any coordinated attack on drug addiction. The mechanisms of research funding should be reviewed, to see if there is need for greater leadership at the federal level to ensure that the most important problems in addiction are attacked as promptly as new knowledge and new technology permit. Numerous unsolved problems call for solution. For example, we are desperately in need of treatment for cocaine addiction. Why is no satisfactory pharmacotherapy yet available? Because it is only recently that basic neurobiology research is showing us where and how cocaine acts in the brain. We might soon be able to learn how to prevent the paranoid psychosis that results from heavy binge use of cocaine or amphetamines. If we understood more about the neurochemistry of craving, we might be able to develop anticraving medications, and thus address the all-important relapse problem. If we knew more about the brain damage caused by chronic use of addictive drugs, we might learn how to prevent or repair that damage. We might even learn how to prevent or reverse the destructive effects of alcohol or cocaine on brain development in the unborn child.

Finally, the Human Genome Project opens the way to learning why some people are so much more vulnerable than others to addiction. That knowledge may prove useful in targeting prevention measures toward children who are at high risk. Even more important, whenever we discover a previously unknown gene that influences vulnerability to addiction, we will find out that gene's normal function in the brain. That means discovering receptors, neurotransmitters, regulatory proteins, and brain pathways that play a role in drug addiction, that can become novel targets for pharmacotherapy.

Drug-by-drug Policies

Each of the addictive drugs calls for a different degree and kind of regulation. The sensible policy for each one will lie somewhere between total legalization and total prohibition. Some of the drugs need tighter regulation than we have now, some need a relaxation of prohibitions, and some need no major policy change at all. Policies ought to be flexible enough to adapt to changing conditions.

Therefore drug-by-drug policies should be reexamined continuously by ONDCP and its science and health advisors.

1. Nicotine. Here we have a powerfully addictive drug that is too easily available at too low a cost, and that consequently causes enormous harm to individuals and society. The chief public health hazard of nicotine addiction consists of the chronic diseases and deaths—especially lung cancer and emphysema—caused by the tar in tobacco smoke. Other hazards are damage to the fetus of pregnant heavily addicted smokers, and the minor health effects of secondhand smoke. In an ideal world, tobacco products would be banned entirely, would not be manufactured, would not be sold. Possibly, had the health costs been recognized a century ago, total prohibition of nicotine products might have saved millions of lives. To institute prohibition now, when so many people are already addicted, would pose new and significant costs of many kinds. Nevertheless, many positive steps short of outright prohibition could be taken. Specifically, I would propose several types of action, as outlined in the following paragraphs.

First, make it harder for minors to get cigarettes. Most states do have laws forbidding sales to minors, but they are not well enforced. Banning cigarette machines would surely have a beneficial impact, as indicated by how fiercely the tobacco industry resists every attempt to pass such a law in the state legislatures. A useful measure, in my opinion, would be to restrict the sale of tobacco products to liquor stores, where effective means of preventing sales to minors have long been in effect. At the same time, no adults would be denied the right to purchase tobacco products, albeit less conveniently.

Second, regulate cigarette advertising more strictly, and invest public funds in counteradvertising, as in the ONDCP's Youth Anti-Drug Media Campaign, and as was mandated not long ago in California by a voter initiative. As cigarette advertising is already banned from radio and television, there is precedent for attempting to ban it also from the print and billboard media. An interesting legal challenge for consumer advocates will be to discover how to prohibit incidental background advertising in motion pictures or television, such as showing a cigarette brand name in the background at a sports event, or emblazoned on the T-shirts of athletes. Blatant propaganda directed to children, such as the notorious "Joe Camel" advertisements, should be banned; such advertising could also be challenged through class action law suits against the tobacco companies, brought by parents with support from the government. The spurious claim of First Amendment rights raised by the tobacco interests should be pursued through the courts until a clarification of constitutional law is achieved. It may be noted in this connection that the First Amendment has not been construed to prevent FDA or other consumer protection agencies from prohibiting false product labeling and false advertising.

Third, increase taxes on tobacco products in order to reduce consumption, but without raising the price so high as to promote a significant black market; this can only be effective if neighbor states cooperate to levy equivalent taxes. Earmark the tax revenues exclusively for prevention education (including antismoking advertisements), treatment of hard-core smokers, and research on nicotine addiction. Current policy, both at the federal and state levels, usually treats tobacco (and alcohol) taxes as general revenue. The proposed change would have only a small impact on total tax revenues—1 percent for the federal government, 2 percent on average for the states. The chief reasons for earmarking in this way are to get rid of the present immoral arrangement in which the government profits from sales of this truly destructive substance, and also to avoid any ambivalence (however subconscious) on the part of government agencies about the desirability of reducing tobacco consumption. In addition, substantial incremental sums would become available for prevention education, treatment, and research—sums that would decrease appropriately in proportion to decreased need as consumption decreases.

Fourth, continue to institute new restrictive regulations about where and when smoking is permitted. As the number of nicotine addicts continues to decline, such restrictions become more and more socially acceptable; indeed, they are demanded by the majority. Ordinary citizens can play a constructive role by helping to create an antismoking climate in their own communities, and withholding their patronage from businesses that promote, advertise, or glamorize smoking.

Fifth, bring economic policies of the federal government with respect to tobacco into line with its status as a product that causes illness and death. Enact legislation to block tobacco exports. A first step could be to abrogate the present government policy of actively promoting such exports, especially to developing countries, where demand is very high and antismoking campaigns are only just being initiated. At the same time, abolish all domestic subsidies to tobacco growers, coupling that with active steps to promote (and subsidize, if necessary) alternative crops.

2. Alcohol and related drugs. Like tobacco, these dangerous addictive drugs, especially alcohol itself, are responsible for huge social costs. Alcohol is directly responsible for an enormous number of accidental deaths, homicides, and chronic illnesses with fatal outcome (see chapter 9). From the public health standpoint, alcohol is as dangerous to the addicted user as is tobacco, and it is clearly more dangerous to the fetus. Moreover, unlike nicotine, its direct effects on behavior (especially in promoting violence) are dangerous to society as a whole. The present degree of regulation varies greatly among the states. One example of this unscientific ambiguity is the definition of the blood alcohol level considered to be presumptive evidence of "driving while intoxicated." Another example is the restriction of sales to state monopoly liquor stores—only Canada and a few U.S. states now do this. Greater uniformity would be desirable to convey a clear message to the public about the dangers of this addictive drug. And much could be done to discourage consumption without returning to outright prohibition, as suggested in the following paragraphs.

First, remove alcohol, in all its forms, from supermarket shelves, and restrict its sale to licensed liquor stores. This recommendation is supported by the Canadian experience, which showed increased consumption when service by clerks was supplanted by self-service in the government monopoly liquor stores. Consider the further step of permitting only such state-operated liquor stores, making it less convenient but still possible to purchase liquor, and at the same time removing some commercial pressures on the public to buy. As noted for tobacco, this restriction to licensed liquor stores will also help prevent sales to minors.

Second, as with tobacco, increase taxation to a degree that would discourage consumption without unduly encouraging a black market. The optimum level could be found experimentally by keeping accurate records of sales and hiking the tax from time to time or from place to place over a long period. As proposed for tobacco, earmark the tax revenues for prevention education, treatment, and research.

Third, find a legally acceptable formula for abolishing "happy hours" and all other reduced-price gimmicks that are intended to increase consumption of alcohol. Establish alcohol-free times and places; a working model already exists in the British policy of forcing pubs to close during certain hours of every day. Ban alcohol on college campuses and at sports events and other public entertainments and ceremonies, and make it unavailable under as many circumstances as possible—for example, in all forms of public transportation. Make all official federal, state, and local government social functions alcohol-free, thus setting a model for alcohol-free office parties and private receptions. Measures like these help, albeit slowly, to change the present societal acceptance of alcohol as a natural, virtually indispensable accompaniment to so many social activities. Happily, this cultural shift in the social norm is already in progress, with decreased consumption of hard liquor, substitution of wine and beer, and increasing acceptance of nondrinking as a valid option on social occasions.

Fourth, forbid all advertising of alcoholic beverages, including beer and wine, in all the media; and find a way also to restrict background advertising, as with tobacco products. Citizen pressure on the motion picture and television industries to eliminate favorable depictions of drinking (as of smoking) could be highly effective. ONDCP, as well as private organizations, should continue to promote public educational media campaigns with respect to all the addictive drugs.

Fifth, continue the present trend toward tougher law enforcement on "driving while intoxicated." Establish the uniform low blood level of 0.05 percent in all the states as presumptive evidence of intoxication; in some people this level may be attained after only one or two drinks, and research has established that it causes definite behavioral impairment. Make penalties for drunk driving more severe, as in countries like Sweden—for example, loss of driver's license for a year at the first offense, jail time for the second offense. Effective law enforcement does, indeed, alter behavior, as evidenced by the "designated driver" procedure that has long been in effect in Sweden and has been adopted increasingly in the United States. I strongly favor random roadblocks with compulsory Breathalyzer testing on the highways, despite the arguments of civil libertarians. As long as the stops are truly random, without selective ethnic or other profiling, and provided the highway police are not permitted to use the occasion for irrelevant vehicle searches, it seems to me that protection of the public from dangerous drivers far outweighs the inconvenience and alleged invasion of privacy.

ONDCP, in consultation with the medical profession, should study the controversy over the prescribing of Valium and other benzodiazepines. These drugs are much like alcohol in their neurochemical, behavioral, and addictive properties; and they are therefore classified with alcohol in this book. Reckless overprescribing has sometimes produced a significant addiction problem. Although these drugs are intended to allay anxiety and promote sleep, their effects tend to dissipate on regular long-term use, and then dependence (especially on high dosages) makes discontinuance difficult. When New York state instituted a system of triplicate prescriptions with centralized record keeping, the number of prescriptions fell dramatically. More impressive, the street price of illicit benzodiazepines rose, indicating that there had been significant diversion under the old and less tightly controlled system. Critics claim, however, that psychiatrists and other physicians are now fearful of prescribing these drugs even when their patients would benefit. Furthermore, more dangerous antianxiety and sleep-promoting drugs are sometimes being prescribed instead. The question—which requires more solid research evidence before it can be answered—is whether benzodiazepines should be more tightly regulated on a national basis.

Inhalants, used primarily by children, are extremely toxic. They cannot be banned because they are ordinarily articles of commerce like gasoline, paint thinner, erasing fluid, and the like. Some laws now make it illegal to sell some of these volatile substances to children; but intensive prevention education would seem to have the best chance of reducing the toll of brain damage and death.

3. Opiates. Retain the present total prohibition on heroin (which is not needed in medical practice) and the present restriction of other opiates to medical use; I see no compelling reason to modify the current legal status. The immediate need is for expansion of methadone treatment so that all who wish treatment can obtain it easily. This is especially important as an effective means of preventing the transmission of HIV and other infections by needle sharing. The Dutch system of "low-threshold" treatment programs has much to recommend, based on the reality that when motivation to seek treatment is weak, it is in society's best interest to "go the extra mile" to bring addicts into treatment. "Going the extra mile" may even be taken literally, with methadone dispensed from a mobile van to reg-

istered addicts in their own neighborhoods—an approach that might circumvent the NIMBY problem (chapter 17). Another alternative would be to permit specially trained and certified physicians to administer or prescribe methadone in their own offices.

Expedite FDA approval of newer maintenance medications for heroin addiction as they are developed, so as to give physicians a full range of pharmacologic options. The historic record shows that heroin addiction is a serious life-threatening disease, that the life expectancy of heroin addicts is radically shortened because of suicide, violence, infections, associated alcoholism, and overdoses. This poor prognosis places heroin addiction in the same category as cancers and other lethal diseases that have required FDA to reconsider its caution over the possible toxicity of proposed medications, in view of the urgent need for treatment. The rigorous scientific criteria for proof of safety and efficacy, appropriate in most contexts, may have to be relaxed somewhat in recognition of the known high probability of a fatal outcome in heroin addiction.

Proper medical practice entails determining, by an appropriate diagnostic test, that an applicant for treatment is a bona fide confirmed opiate addict, already dependent on the drug. Therefore, make diagnosis and treatment of opiate addiction the exclusive business of physicians and health workers, without bureaucratic interference by state and federal government agencies. Establish medical (not governmental) criteria for admission to treatment, for dosage, and for duration of treatment. The legitimate role of government is to ensure that methadone and similar opiates, which can be lethal to nontolerant people (especially children), are administered under strictest supervision. Allow patients to take their medication home only after they have demonstrated by their behavior and by urine testing that they have stopped using illicit drugs and are responsible enough to exercise due caution. Finally, with treatment universally available, hold to account for their crimes any addicts who continue to engage in criminal activities.

4. Cocaine and amphetamines. Because of the dangerous behaviors induced by these drugs—more disruptive to the user and more threatening to society than the effects of opiates—and because of the intensity of the addiction, leave in place the present prohibitions.

More research is needed, both basic and applied, that could lead to effective pharmacotherapy for this addiction. More research is also needed, both in animals and humans, to establish conclusively if, under what conditions, and to what extent cocaine and amphetamines are harmful to fetal development, especially as regards the long-term intellectual development of a child born to an addicted mother. Addiction to cocaine (especially to crack), although far from our most important problem in terms of numbers of people affected, is certainly, together with alcohol, the most serious in terms of disruptive effects on society.

5. Cannabis. Although this drug cannot be described as harmless, the present degree of regulation seems excessive; the laws barely differentiate cannabis from opiates or cocaine. The key question is whether relaxing the prohibition on marijuana would lead to a major increase in the number of users. The Dutch experiment suggests that this might not happen. There may, indeed, be advantages (as the Dutch argue) in making cannabis available through mechanisms that do not bring users into contact with traffickers in the "hard" drugs (heroin and cocaine). On the principle that weak forms of an addictive drug are safer than concentrated forms, any modification of the present prohibition on a trial basis should apply only to marijuana leaf, not to hashish.

ONDCP should study this issue with a view to implementing a few controlled trials of penalty reductions or even discretionary enforcement of the laws. The key phrase here is "controlled trials." Before making any change at all in the legal status of cannabis, ensure that data systems are in place for following the outcome systematically. Then allow the modified regulations (perhaps limited to a few states) to operate for long enough to establish clearly what happens. As social changes occur only slowly, "long enough" could mean many years. Finally, by appropriate use of pardons or parole, rectify the injustices being suffered right now by many unfortunates who posed no serious threat to society but are nevertheless serving prison terms for mere possession of modest amounts of marijuana for personal use. Let the punishment fit the crime!

On the other hand, stricter enforcement is required, with adequate testing, to ensure that cannabis is not used in sensitive professions (for example, transportation) where public safety is at stake. Likewise, the public deserves to be protected from impaired motorists "driving while stoned"—just as it is now protected from those who drive while intoxicated. When technology permits rapid non-intrusive testing for marijuana (perhaps by a saliva test), random stops on the highway will be appropriate, as for alcohol by Breath-alyzer at present.

More animal research is needed to clarify whether irreversible brain damage can be caused by heavy chronic use of cannabis. A few research reports have indicated truly alarming toxic effects on the brain; but remarkably, government agencies have not taken the lead to ensure adequate replications of the critical animal experiments.

Finally, prevention education is especially important in blocking the progression, in young people, from the gateway drugs—nicotine and alcohol—to cannabis. ONDCP, the Substance Abuse and Mental Health Services Administration (SAMHSA), and the National Institute on Drug Abuse (NIDA) should continue to study the cost-effectiveness of prevention education techniques, so that whatever works and can be afforded is quickly implemented in classrooms nationwide. Equally important, what does not work (see chapter 15), or works only marginally, or is absurdly expensive, should be eliminated. When advocates make a heavy investment of research funds and energy and emotion in a particular education project, it is easy to understand their bias in its favor. But research on prevention education, because such large numbers of students have to be studied over such a long time, is necessarily very, very expensive, and therefore requires stringent, objective evaluation in the public interest.

"Medical marijuana" initiatives continue to be passed in state after state, undercutting the essential role of FDA in approving and monitoring medications based on scientific evidence of efficacy and safety. This complicated issue was discussed at length in chapter 12; it needs to be removed from the political and legal arenas and dealt with on the same basis as any other pharmacotherapy.

6. Caffeine. Caffeine is the least harmful of the addictive drugs. It is also the most widely used, and there is increasing concern that it may not be entirely harmless after all. Medical experts worry about the large amounts of caffeine taken freely by children in the form of soft drinks. More research is needed to determine what adverse effects this known addictive psychostimulant may have on developing brains, whether caffeine-induced sleep disturbance affects daytime learning in the classroom, to what extent caffeine may contribute to (or ameliorate) attention deficits, and so on.

An educational campaign to reduce caffeine consumption would be in order, complemented by the commercial manufacturers' production of caffeine-free products for an expanding market. Indeed, the consumption of decaffeinated coffee and caffeine-free herb tea has been increasing steadily. Could caffeine be removed entirely as a food additive, and retained only in natural products like coffee and tea? The Food and Drug Administration (FDA) can mandate this and other measures, such as requiring a warning label or discouraging sales to children. At this writing, FDA requires disclosure of the presence of added caffeine in manufactured food and drink, but not the amount. With many scientists and physicians, however, I believe that parents have a right to know how much caffeine their children are consuming, and therefore that FDA should mandate a statement of amount on the label. Beyond this, and although there would surely be no harm in promoting a caffeine-free diet for children, I do not think sufficient evidence is yet in hand to make any firm recommendations for government action.

7. Hallucinogens. The hallucinogenic drugs constitute a vanishingly small part of the total drug addiction problem. Nevertheless, their unpredictable and sometimes truly dangerous effects on behavior, as well as acute fatalities, justify the present prohibition on their use. The popularity of hallucinogens waxes and wanes, and with the passage of time one or another comes into and goes out of fashion. As they appeal primarily to youngsters looking for new sensations, intensive education is desirable to warn of the true hazards. Illustrative of the problem is the frequent use of MDMA ("ecstasy") and other "party drugs" (see chapter 14) on college campuses despite evidence of potential brain damage. There seems to be a widespread lack of understanding of the danger—in principle—of exposing the brain to any substance that grossly alters its function. This carelessness about chemical maltreatment of the brain is probably in large measure a consequence of the inadequate teaching of biological science at all levels of our educational system.

A specific issue concerning hallucinogens calls for clarification; that is the legal status of peyote, as used in the religious services of the Native American Church (see chapter 14). Federal laws and those of many states exempt this practice from the general prohibitions on hallucinogens. Some states, however, maintain a total ban on peyote, and in 1990 the Supreme Court ruled in their favor, despite the religious freedom clause of the First Amendment.

Summary

In this book I have taken you on a long journey through familiar and unfamiliar territory. The rationale for writing it was my conviction that by learning more about drug addiction, in all its complexity, the intelligent citizens of a democracy would be better equipped to understand and evaluate the way we, as a society, deal with the addictive drugs and the addicts.

Part One explored similarities and differences among the seven families of addictive drugs—their actions in the brain, their addictiveness, and the way they induce tolerance and dependence. The basis was laid for considering drug addiction to be primarily a brain disease, a public health problem. An important goal of future research will be to work out all the chemical steps between the binding of an addictive drug to its receptor and the ultimate effect of the drug on reward systems and behavior. Another research aim is to learn about genetic predisposition to addiction in order to clarify why it is that only a fraction of all the people who try an addictive drug find it attractive enough to use repeatedly and thus to become addicts. Research accomplishments will inevitably lead to novel methods of prevention and treatment, as they always have in the field of biomedicine.

Part Two expanded on the theme—drug by drug—that addicts (as stated explicitly by Dr. Alan Leshner, director of NIDA) are victims of a brain disease. For each of the seven drug families we saw how the disease typically develops and how it can be treated. These chapters laid the basis for the later discussions of what degree of regulation is appropriate for each drug. Future research will focus on establishing, in rigorous trials, what treatments are best for each addiction, and what better treatments can be developed.

Part Three examined some major societal issues concerning prevention education, treatment, and relapse. We noted that although criminality is associated with addiction, blaming the criminal behavior wholly on the addiction is entirely too simplistic. The major role of intravenous drug use in the epidemic spread of AIDS and hepatitis was analyzed. Some novel British, Dutch, and Swiss approaches were examined to see what lessons might be learned for U.S. drug policy. The debate over legalizing addictive drugs was analyzed, recognizing that most people agree that drugs need some degree of regulation. I have suggested that the degree of regulation ought to be different for each drug, tailored to the danger posed by that drug to individual and societal health and well-being. In the present chapter, I have offered general and specific recommendations for drug policy consistent with our present scientific and medical knowledge. The central theme here again was that drug addiction should be regarded as primarily a brain disease and a public health problem, and addressed accordingly at all levels of government.

What You Can Do

Government actions are important in addressing the drug addiction problem, but they are not enough. In a democratic society, public involvement is also essential—to help bring about the needed statutory and regulatory changes through the political process, to create an environment supportive of those changes, and to promote the attitude that drug addiction is primarily a public health problem. I hope that concerned citizens, better informed after reading this book, will contribute in one way or another to making the "war on drugs" more effective by urging their elected officials to adopt more rational drug policies. A partial list:

Support organizations like Mothers Against Drunk Driving, which are influential in promoting the necessary tougher regulations on alcohol.

Make known to the media and the advertisers your outrage about the glamorization of alcoholic beverages, cigarettes, and other addictive drugs in motion pictures, television, radio, and print media.

Exert political pressure on Congress and the White House to reverse the absurd 70 to 30 funding ratio in favor of supply reduction over demand reduction in the "war on drugs," to abolish all forms of tobacco subsidy, and to stop the cynical export of our tobacco products to developing countries.

Demand that treatment be made readily available for all addicts who seek it, subsidized as required; and strengthen institutions like drug courts, which offer an alternative to incarceration.

Insist that we stop filling our jails and prisons with drug offenders who have not committed violent crimes; and restore judicial discretion by getting rid of the ill-advised mandatory sentencing laws for the "crime" of mere drug possession for personal use.

My recommendations for a more humane policy are not "soft on drugs." They are based on science and common sense and fiscal prudence. If you find merit in them, make yourself a crusader for change. Very likely, drug addictions will always be with us, but the harm they cause can be reduced considerably. The key strategy—through education as well as through laws that reinforce the social norm—is to change public attitudes, and thus to reduce demand. Addictive drugs affect us all. We can all help create a new climate of awareness and understanding of drug addiction.

Suggestions for Further Reading

This annotated list—in the same order as the chapters—contains a selection of both technical and popular books and articles that expand on some of the topics. Explanatory comments are omitted whenever a title speaks for itself. Included also here are references to a few original articles that describe experiments from the author's own laboratory, which are mentioned in the text.

Introduction (Chapter 1)

Biomedical journals devoted exclusively to addictive drugs and drug addiction:

Addiction (British Journal of Addiction, prior to 1993); *Addiction Research; Addictive Behavior; Addictive Diseases; Advances in Alcohol and Substance Abuse; Alcohol; Alcohol and Alcoholism; Alcohol and Drug Research; Alcoholism: Clinical and Experimental Research; American Journal of Drug and Alcohol Abuse; British Journal of Addiction; Chemical Dependencies; Drug and Alcohol Dependence; International Journal of the Addictions; Journal of Addictive Diseases; Journal of Drug Issues; Journal of Psychoactive Drugs; Journal of Studies on Alcohol; Journal of Substance Abuse Treatment; Recent Developments in Alcoholism*

The National Drug Control Strategy (Office of National Drug Control Policy, Washington, D.C.).

[Published annually and at other intervals, with numerous ancillary publications.]

National Institute on Drug Abuse (NIDA) Research Monograph Series, U.S. Department of Health and Human Services (DHHS), Rockville, MD, available from U.S. Government Printing Office, Washington, D.C. 20402.

NIDA NOTES. National Institute on Drug Abuse, National Clearinghouse for Alcohol and Drug Information, P O Box 2345, Rockville MD 20847–2345.

[Ongoing periodical, approximately monthly, with current information on numerous aspects of drug abuse.]

National Household Survey on Drug Abuse. U.S. Department of Health and Human Services, Public Health Service, Alcohol, Drug Abuse, and Mental Health Administration, Washington, D.C.

[Includes statistical source material for the prevalence data in chapter 1 and Figure 1.1. See also Web sites at samhsa.gov and health.org.]

Monitoring the Future: National Results on Adolescent Drug Use, Overview of the Key Findings. Also National Survey Results on Drug Use from the Monitoring the Future Study. L. D. Johnston et al., University of Michigan Institute for Social Research; National Institute on Drug Abuse, U.S. Department of Health and Human Services, Government Printing Office, Washington, D.C.

[These publications detail drug use by young people, with trends extending over more than 25 years.]

Diagnostic and Statistical Manual of Mental Disorders, DSM-IV, 4th Edition. American Psychiatric Association, Washington, D.C., 1994.

[Contains the official diagnostic terminology and descriptions of the psychoactive substance use disorders, especially on pages 175–272.]

M. D. Glantz, C. R. Hartel, eds. *Drug Abuse, Origins and Interventions.* Washington, D.C.: American Psychological Association, 2000.

Substance Abuse: The Nation's Number One Health Problem. Key Indicators for Policy Princton, New Jersey: The Robert Wood Johnson Foundation, 1993.

Substance Abuse in Young People Drug and Alcohol Dependence, special issue, I. B. Crome, ed. Vol. 55, No. 3, 1 July 1999.

Pathways of Addiction—Opportunities in Drug Abuse Research. Institute of Medicine, National Academy Press, Washington, D.C., 1996.

[Exhaustive summary of research needs, according to the various disciplines such as behavior, neuroscience, epidemiology, etiology, prevention, and treatment.]

H. Kalant and O. J. Kalant. *Drugs, Society and Personal Choice.* Ontario: Paper Jacks, General Publishing Co., 1971.

[Despite its early publication date, this little gem, directed primarily toward the intelligent lay reader, is still instructive and worthwhile.]

Part One: Drugs and the Brain (Chapters 2–7)

J. G. Hardman, L. E. Limbird et al., eds. *Goodman and Gilman's The Pharmacological Basis of Therapeutics.* 9th Ed. New York:McGraw-Hill, 1996.

[The definitive textbook of pharmacology. Includes major chapters on addictive drugs and on general aspects of drug metabolism.]

W. B. Pratt and P. Taylor, eds. *Principles of Drug Action—The Basis of Pharmacology.* 3rd Ed. New York: Churchill Livingstone, 1990.
[Detailed technical treatment of many pharmacological principles that are applicable to the addictive drugs.]

L. Stryer. *Biochemistry.* 3rd Ed. New York: W. H. Freeman, 1995.
[Beautifully presented, this is a widely used textbook of biochemistry, which covers in great detail receptors, gene action, membranes, enzymes, and fundamental mechanisms that underlie the actions of addictive drugs.]

J. R. Cooper, F. E. Bloom, and R. H. Roth. *The Biochemical Basis of Neuropharmacology.* 7th Ed. New York: Oxford University Press, 1996.
[A well-illustrated standard textbook on the chemistry of the brain, the neurotransmitters, the receptors, and the effects of psychotropic drugs.]

J. Frascella and R. M. Brown, eds. *Neurobiological Approaches to Brain-Behavior Interaction.* NIDA Research Monograph 124, DHHS Publication ADM92–1846, Rockville, MD, 1992.
[Technical articles with emphasis on modern techniques for studying reward pathways, self-administration, and mapping of sites in brain by PET scanning, microdialysis, and other techniques.]

G. F. Koob. Drugs of Abuse—Anatomy, Pharmacology and Function of Reward Pathways. *Trends in Pharmacological Research* 13: 177–184, 1992.
[A description of the reward systems on which addictive drugs act, with emphasis on their anatomic distribution in the brain.]

R. A. Wise. The Neurobiology of Craving—Implications for the Understanding and Treatment of Addiction. *Journal of Abnormal Psychology* 97: 118–132, 1988.
[Contains references to literature on the method of conditioned place preference and reviews the evidence for a dopaminergic reward system that underlies craving produced by opiates and cocaine.]

R. Restak. *The Brain.* New York: Bantam, 1984.
[The text for a widely praised TV series, with many outstanding figures in color.]

R. Bergland: *The Fabric of Mind.* New York: Viking Penguin, 1985.
[Historical insights into brain research, developing the theme that the brain is a hormonal organ with many of the same hormones as found in other parts of the body.]

A. Goldstein, ed. *Molecular and Cellular Aspects of the Drug Addictions.* New York/Berlin/Heidelberg: Springer-Verlag, 1989.
[The proceedings of a 1988 symposium, this volume contains eight tech-

nical contributions presenting recent basic research findings on the neurobiology of the drug addictions.]

A. Goldstein and E. J. Nestler, eds. *Neurobiology of Addiction.* Drug and Alcohol Dependence, special issue, Vol. 51, Nos 1, 2, June/July 1998.
[A multiauthor collection with up-to-date technical accounts of brain research on each drug family.]

C. P. O'Brien and J. H. Jaffe, eds. *Addictive States.* Vol. 70, Research Publications, Association for Research in Nervous and Mental Disease, New York: Raven Press, 1992.

A. Goldstein. Thrills in Response to Music and Other Stimuli. *Physiological Psychology* 8: 126–129, 1980.
[The full description of the music experiment described in chapter 5.]

M. M. Vanyukov and R. E. Tarter. *Genetics of Substance Abuse. Drug and Alcohol Dependence* 59: 101–123, 2000.

R. W. Pickens and D. S. Svikis, eds. *Biological Vulnerability to Drug Abuse.* NIDA Research Monograph 89, DHHS Publication ADM88–1590, Rockville, MD, 1988.

C. R. Cloninger and H. Begleiter, eds. *Genetics and Biology of Alcoholism.* Banbury Report 33, Cold Spring Harbor Laboratory Press, 1990.

Part Two: Drugs and the Addicts (Chapters 8–14)

Smoking and Health, Surgeon General's Report. (U.S. Department of Health, Education, and Welfare, PHS Publication No. 1103, U.S. Government Printing Office, Washington, D.C. 20402, 1964.)
[The original report documenting tobacco smoke as a health hazard. Further reports followed every few years (not listed here) on special aspects of smoking and health.]

The Health Consequences of Smoking: Nicotine Addiction. A Report of the Surgeon General, 1988. (U.S. Department of Health and Human Services, Rockville, MD 20857; U.S. Government Printing Office, Washington, D.C. 20402, 1988.)

J. Slade. The Tobacco Epidemic—Lessons from History. *Journal of Psychoactive Drugs* 21: 281–291, 1989.

NIAAA 25th Anniversary. (Alcohol Health and Research World. Vol. 19, No. 1, 1995, National Institute on Alcohol Abuse and Alcoholism, National Institutes of Health, NIH Publication no. 95–3466, Washington, D.C., 1995).
[Historical summaries of milestones in alcohol research and of NIAAA.]

D. B. Goldstein. *Pharmacology of Alcohol.* New York: Oxford University Press, 1983.

C. R. Cloninger, S. Sigvardsson and M. Bohman: Childhood Personality Predicts Alcohol Abuse in Young Adults. *Alcoholism, Clinical and Experimental Research* 12: 494–505, 1988.

F. E. Bloom. Neurobiology of Alcohol Action and Alcoholism. *Annual Review of Psychiatry* 8: 347–360, 1989.

N. K. Mello, J. H. Mendelson and S. K. Teoh: Neuroendocrine Consequences of Alcohol Abuse in Women. *Annals of the New York Academy of Sciences* 562: 211–240, 1989.

Alcoholics Anonymous. Alcoholics Anonymous World Series, Inc., New York, 1976.
[The official account of the principles and ideals on which the movement is based, with description of the first 12-step programs.]

D. L. Cheney and A. Goldstein. Tolerance to Opioid Narcotics. III. Time Course and Reversibility of Physical Dependence in Mice. *Nature* 232: 477–478, 1971.
[An experiment to determine the critical interval for development of dependence, as described in chapter 10.]

R. E. Meyer and S. M. Mirin. *The Heroin Stimulus—Implications for a Theory of Addiction.* New York: Plenum Medical Book Co., 1979.
[Reports of controlled experiments on heroin with volunteers in a closed ward.]

W. K. Bickel and L. Amass. Buprenorphine treatment of opioid dependence—A review. *Exp. Clin. Psychopharmacol.* 3: 477–490, 1995.
[Information on the early studies that led to approval of this partial agonist used as an alternative to methadone or LAAM maintenance.]

V. P. Dole. Implications of Methadone Maintenance for Theories of Narcotic Addiction. *Journal of the American Medical Association* 260: 3025–3029, 1988.

D. Latimer and J. Goldberg. *Flowers in the Blood—The Story of Opium.* New York: Franklin Watts, 1981.

J. Goldberg. *Anatomy of a Scientific Discovery.* New York: Bantam, 1988.
[A popularized account of the discovery of endogenous opioid peptides.]

I. Chein, D. L. Gerard, R. S. Lee and E. Rosenfeld. *The Road to H—Narcotics, Delinquency, and Social Policy.* New York: Basic Books, 1964.
[A classic sociological study of heroin addiction and heroin addicts.]

J. E. Zweben and J. T. Payte, eds. Opioid Dependence and Methadone Maintenance Treatment. *Journal of Psychoactive Drugs* 23, No. 2, 1991.
[Includes reprints of two classic articles from 1966 and 1973.

A. Herz, ed. Opioids I and II. *Handbook of Experimental Pharmacology,* Vol. 104 I/II, Springer-Verlag, Berlin/Heidelberg/New York, 1993.
[A definitive and detailed technical account of the biology, chemistry,

and behavioral aspects of the opioids. Nearly 1,700 pages in all, these two volumes will be the definitive source of information about opioids for years to come.]

Effective Medical Treatment of Opiate Addiction (NIH Consenus Statement, Nov. 17–19, 15(6):1–38,1997).

[Findings of an interdisciplinary panel, with selected references.]

A. Goldstein. Heroin Addiction—Sequential Treatment Employing Pharmacologic Supports. *Archives of General Psychiatry* 33: 353, 1976.

[A proposal by the author to bring heroin addicts into treatment by offering sterile pure heroin injections in a clinic, followed by obligatory progression to surrogate opiates, then to antagonists and eventually to a drug-free state.]

A. Goldstein. Heroin Maintenance—A Medical View. A Conversation Between a Physician and a Politician. *Journal of Drug Issues* 9: 341–347, 1979.

[A response to proposals made about 25 years ago that heroin should be legalized to solve the heroin addiction problem at that time. Of historical interest, reflecting how little the problems or the proposed solutions have changed over the years.]

D. T. Courtwright. Charles Terry, the Opium Problem, and American Narcotic Policy. *Journal of Drug Issues* 16: 42–434, 1986.

[A historian looks at the development of attitudes and policies toward narcotics in the early years of the twentieth century.]

F. Weiss et al. Control of cocaine-seeking behavior by drug-associated stimuli in rats: Effects on recovery of extinguished operant-responding and extracellular dopamine levels in amygdala and nucleus accumbens. *PNAS* 97:4321–4326, 2000.

A. R. Childress et al. Limbic activation during cue-induced cocaine craving. American Journal Psychiatry 156: 11–18, 1999.

C. Van Dyke and R. Byck. Cocaine. *Scientific American* 246: 128–141, March 1982.

[A history and pharmacology of coca and cocaine. Out-of-date biochemistry but interesting history. As the article was written early in the current epidemic of cocaine use, the authors tend to underrate the health hazards and addictiveness of this drug.]

G. Nahas. *Cocaine—The Great White Plague.* Middlebury, VT:Paul S. Eriksson, 1989.)

[A history of cocaine addiction, enlivened by personal accounts of this pharmacologist-physician's observations. The author's extreme antipathy toward the use of all the illicit psychoactive drugs is expressed throughout his book.]

F. H. Gawin. Cocaine Addiction—Psychology and Neurophysiology. *Science* 251: 1580–1586, 1991.

Cocaine—Scientific and Social Dimensions. Ciba Foundation Symposium 166, New York: John Wiley & Sons, 1992.

G. Le Dain et al. *Cannabis—A Report of the Commission of Inquiry into the Non-Medical Use of Drugs.* Ottawa: Information Canada, 1972.

[The widely quoted Canadian government examination of the problems associated with marijuana and hashish, and what to do about them. The commission's report led to changes in Canadian government policy, and the arguments for and against various recommendations make interesting reading even 20 years later.]

Marijuana and Health. Institute of Medicine, National Academy Press, 1982.

[Concise summaries of marijuana's effects on the various organ systems, with focus on the many gaps in our knowledge that call for further research. Contains a strong recommendation for increased federal research funding to a level commensurate with the widespread use of cannabis.]

E. W. Single. The Impact of Marijuana Decriminalization—An Update. *Journal of Public Health Policy* 10: 456–466, 1989.

[An examination of the effects of decriminalizing cannabis use in various U.S. states during the 1970s, with emphasis on the few controlled studies that were carried out at the time.]

J. E. Joy et al, Marijuana and Medicine—Assessing the Science Base. Washington, D. C.: Institute of Medicine, National Academy Press, 1999).

[An up-to-date analysis of the data that are relevant to the controversies over the therapeutic utility of marijuana.]

Herkenham et al. Cannabinoid Receptor Localization in Brain. Proceedings of the National Academy of Sciences USA 87: 1932–1936, 1990.

[Specific sites in the brain that bind a radiolabeled cannabinoid ligand.]

R. Seth and S. Sinha: Chemistry and Pharmacology of Cannabis. *Progress in Drug Research* 36: 71–115, 1991.

W. A. Devane et al. Isolation and Structure of a Brain Constituent that Binds to the Cannabinoid Receptor. *Science* 258: 1946–1949, 1992.

[Technical evidence that a natural brain lipid may be the endogenous ligand of the same receptor that responds to THC, the active principle of marijuana and hashish.]

H. Kalant et al., eds. *Health Effects of Cannabis.* Toronto: ARF Books, 1999.

P. A. Fried. The Ottawa Prenatal Prospective Study (OPPS): methodological issues and findings — it's easy to throw the baby out with the bath water. *Life Science* 56 :2159–2168, 1995.

L. L. Iversen. *The Science of Marijuana.* Oxford: Oxford University Press, 2000.

[This recent volume, by a leading neuropharmacologist, summarizes

cannabis history and neurobiology, with emphasis on potential therapeutic uses of marijuana.]

H. E. Jacob. *Coffee—The Epic of a Commodity.* New York: Viking Press, 1935.
[Although somewhat fictionalized to capture reader interest, this book
is a thorough history of coffee, coffeehouses, and coffee plantations, with
emphasis on the economics of the international coffee trade.]

R. S. Hattox. *Coffee and Coffeehouses—The Origins of a Social Beverage in the
Medieval Near East.* Seattle: University of Washington Press, 1985.
[A lively scholarly account of the origins of coffee in Ethiopia and
Yemen, and its sixteenth century spread through the institution of cof-
feehouses in Cairo, Damascus, and Constantinople.]

N. L. Benowitz. Clinical Pharmacology of Caffeine. *Annual Review of Medicine* 41: 277–288, 1990.
[A brief but thorough review of recent research on the health effects
and addictive potential of this most widely used drug.]

M. D. de Rios. *Hallucinogens—Cross-Cultural Perspectives.* Albuquerque: University of New Mexico Press, 1984.
[A study of 11 cultures worldwide—from Australia to Siberia, from Peru
to Equatorial Africa—in which hallucinogens are used in religious rituals
under the guidance of shamans.]

D. F. Aberle. *The Peyote Religion Among the Navaho.* 2nd Ed. Norman, OK:
University of Oklahoma Press, 1990.
[A scholarly text by a leading anthropologist, with descriptions and pho-
tographs of the peyote ceremonies, as well as a historical perspective on
the role of the peyote cult in Navaho society.]

Part Three: Drugs and Society (Chapters 15–20)

Single Convention on Narcotic Drugs, 1961, as Amended by the 1972 Protocol. United Nations, New York, 1977.
[Text of the international agreement covering opiates, coca, and
cannabis.]

D. R. Gerstein and H. J. Harwood, eds. *Treating Drug Problems.* Vol. 1. Washington, D. C.: Institute of Medicine, National Academy Press, 1990.
[An analysis by an expert committee of the multiplicity of health and
social problems associated with drug addiction in the United States.]

E. C. Senay. Drug Abuse and Public Health—A Global Perspective. *Drug
Safety* 6, Supplement 1: 1–65, 1991.
[A comprehensive worldwide survey, with several hundred references
and detailed tables.]

E. M. Brecher. *Licit and Illicit Drugs.* Boston: Little, Brown, 1972.
[This book, commissioned by Consumers Union, was a landmark first

attempt to treat all addictive drugs in an evenhanded manner. Although strongly biased in favor of decriminalizing possession of all drugs, it nevertheless remains an important source of information. Several of the specific recommendations for changes in drug policy are similar to those proposed here in chapter 20.]

D. F. Musto. *The American Disease—The Origins of Narcotics Control.* New Haven: Yale University Press, 1973. By the same author: Opium, Cocaine and Marijuana in American History. *Scientific American* 265: 40, July 1991.

Preventing Drug Use Among Children and Adolescents—A Research-Based Guide. National Institute on Drug Abuse, National Institutes of Health, NIH Publication No. 99–4212, 1999.

[Very useful explanation of the multiple prevention approaches that have been subjected, insofar as possible to outcome analysis. Includes discussion of risk and preventive factors, community programs, and specific prevention programs. An indispensable practical guide.]

Cost-Benefit/Cost-Effectiveness Research of Drug Abuse Prevention: Implications for Programming and Policy. W. L. Bukoski and R. I. Evans, eds. National Institute on Drug Abuse Research Monograph Series #176, 1998.

[M. A. Pentz and others present data on large-scale prevention programs, with interesting attempts to compute the dollar value of intervention programs.]

Principles of Drug Addiction Treatment: A Research-Based Guide. National Institute on Drug Abuse, National Institutes of Health, NIH Publication No. 99–4180, 1999.

[The most recent official summary of science-based treatments for each addiction, with emphasis on the practical aspects of therapy.]

J. Normand et al. eds., *Preventing HIV transmission—The Role of Sterile Needles and Bleach.* National Research Council and Institute of Medicine, Washington, D. C.: National Academy Press, 1995.

D. C. Des Jarlais et al. Declining seroprevalence in a very large HIV epidemic: Injecting drug users in New York City. *American Journal of Public Health* 88:1801–1806,1998.

G. Edwards. What Drives British Drug Policies? *British Journal of Addiction* 84: 219–226, 1989.

[An overview of historical developments that led to the present British policies on addictive drugs, by the "guru" of drug addiction research and policy in Britain.]

UK Action on Drug Misuse—The Government's Strategy. Home Office, UK, Central Office of Information, London, 1990.

[A summary of activities of the British government in relation to addictive drugs. Contains a list of 18 agencies, including the Standing Conference on Drug Abuse (SCODA, 1–4 Hatton Place, Hatton Garden,

London EC1N 8ND), which is the national coordinating body for non-governmental agencies in the field of drug abuse. Statistical bulletins may be obtained from Statistical Department, Home Office, Lunar House, Croydon, Surrey CR0 9YD.]

G. F. van de Wijngaart. The Dutch Approach—Normalization of Drug Problems. *Journal of Drug Issues* 20: 667–678, 1990.
[A clear exposition of the similarities and differences between drug policies in the Netherlands and in other countries, by a leading participant in their development.]

R. MacCoun and P. Reuter, Interpreting Dutch cannabis policy: reasoning by analogy in the legalization debate. *Science* 278, 47–52, 1997.

A. Uchtenhagen et al. Prescription of Narcotics for Heroin Addicts: Main Result of the Swiss National Cohort Study. Medical Prescription of Narcotics. Vol. 1. Karger, Basel, 1999.

Heroin Maintenance Treatment, Research Summary. New York: The Lindesmith Center, 1998.

G. Bammer et al. The heroin prescribing debate; Integrating science and politics. *Science* 284:1277–1278,1999.
[A summary by Australian, British, and Swiss clinicians of the studies in which they have been actively involved.]

G. Le Dain et al. Final Report of the Commission of Inquiry into the Non-Medical Use of Drugs. Ottawa: Information Canada, 1973.
[An exhaustive compilation (1,148 pages) of research summaries and policy recommendations for Canada, relevant also for the United States. See also separate report devoted exclusively to cannabis.]

A. Goldstein and H. Kalant: Drug Policy—Striking the Right Balance. *Science* 249: 1513–1521, 1990.

L. Cockburn. *Out of Control—The Story of the Reagan Administration's Secret War in Nicaragua, the Illegal Arms Pipeline, and the Contra Drug Connection.* New York: Atlantic Monthly Press, 1987.
[A well-documented account of how U.S. foreign policy affected the drug trade. Further revelations are found in the Kerry Committee Report, immediately below.]

Senate Committee on Foreign Relations, Subcommittee on Terrorism, Narcotics and International Operations: Drugs, Law Enforcement and Foreign Policy, Kerry Committee Report, U.S. Government Printing Office, Washington, D.C. 20402, 1989.
[An official report on how some aspects of U.S. foreign policy resulted in increased importation of illicit addictive drugs.]

A. W. McCoy. The Politics of Heroin—CIA Complicity in the Global Drug Trade. New York: Lawrence Hill Books, 1991.
[A revised and updated version of his classic, The Politics of Heroin in

Southeast Asia (1972), documenting the role of U.S. foreign policy in the illicit drug traffic during the Cold War. Includes references to findings of Senator John Kerry's subcommittee in the 1980s.]

E. A. Nadelmann Thinking Seriously about Alternatives to Drug Prohibition. *Daedalus* 121: 85–132, 1992. Also: Drug Prohibition in the United States—Costs, Consequences, and Alternatives." *Science* 245: 939–946, 1989.

[Arguments by a political scientist who is a leading advocate of legalizing some or all of the presently illicit drugs.]

M. Falco *The Making of a Drug-Free America—Programs That Work.* New York: Random House, 1993.

[A recipe for new drug policies, much along the lines laid out in this book, placing emphasis on reducing demand by expanding prevention and treatment programs. The author analyses the features of programs she judges to be effective.]

M. A. R. Kleiman. *Against Excess—Drug Policy for Results.* New York: Basic Books, 1993.

[Well-considered proposals for changes in our drug policies.]

D. D. Simpson and B. S. Brown, eds., *Treatment Process and Outcome Studies from DATOS.* Drug and Alcohol Dependence, special issue, Vol. 57, No. 2, 1 December 1999.

[Findings from structured studies on drug abuse outcome studies carried out at multiple sites under NIDA management.]

R. Bayer and G. M. Oppenheimer, eds. *Confronting Drug Policy—Illicit Drugs in a Free Society.* New York: Cambridge University Press, 1993.

[A dozen experts contribute thoughtful discussion concerning drugs and the law, with emphasis on decriminalization and legalization.]

D. R. Gerstein and L. W. Green, eds. *Preventing Drug Abuse—What do we know?* Washington D. C.: National Research Council, National Academy Press, 1993.

M. Massing. *The Fix.* New York: Simon and Schuster, 1998.

[Critical analysis of changes in national drug policies over the past 30 years.]

Index

abstinence syndrome. *See* withdrawal syndrome

acamprosate, 154, 259

accidents, highway, 139, 199

acetaldehyde, 85, 112, 144

acetaldehyde dehydrogenase, 112, 151

acetylcholine, 20, 23–24, 121

acetyl-homotaurine, 154

ACTH (pituitary hormone), 31–32

acupuncture, 79

addiction, 5, 12–13, 13, 20–21, 34–35; influences on, 61, 103

addicts, 4, 277; alcohol, 100; caffeine, 99–100; cocaine, 179; heroin, 158, 277, 322; nicotine, 102; street, 261, 262, 266, 282, 314

Addicts Index (Great Britain), 277

adenine, 44

adenosine, 25, 213

ADHD (attention deficit hyperactivity disorder), 187

adolescents, drug use by, 245

adrenaline, 20, 25

advertising, 327; of alcohol, 237–38, 320; anti-drug, 295, 317; cigarette, 103, 117–18, 237–38, 317–18

Advisory Council on Misuse of Drugs (Great Britain), 271, 278

Afghanistan, 299

AIDS: drug policy, 311–12; epidemic, 182, 272, 279; prevention, 267–68, 270–72, 283–84

Albuquerque (New Mexico), 174, 270

alcohol, 6, 86, 135–55; advertising of, 237–38, 320; behavioral effects of, 135–36, 137, 138; cravings for, 153; dosages of, 137–38; drug policy for, 319–21; effect on brain, 85, 137, 139–40, 142–44; health effects of, 10, 146–48, 310, 319; hedonic effects of, 138, 230; intoxication, 136, 137–40; and naltrexone, 152–53; societal impact of, 5, 10, 135, 138–39, 310, 319; tolerance, 89, 108, 137, 145; use of, 8–10, 12, 236, 245; withdrawal syndrome, 90, 91–92, 93, 144–45. *See also* benzodiazepines

alcohol addiction, 104–5, 144–45; genetic predisposition toward, 106–8, 112–13; treatment of, 148–54

alcohol dehydrogenase, 143, 151
Alcoholics Anonymous (AA), 130, 149–51, 251, 256
alcoholism. *See* alcohol addiction
Algren, Nelson, 159
alkaloids, 144
Amanita muscaria, 228
American Psychiatric Association (APA), 141
amino acids, 25, 30, 109; gluta- mate, 25, 109, 220, 227
amotivational syndrome, 202
amphetamines, 6–7, 179–80, 181; and dopamine hypothe- sis, 65; effect on brain, 186– 87; health effects of, 183, 184– 86; hedonic effects of, 182, 230; relapse into use of, 187– 88; withdrawal syndrome, 90, 185, 187. *See also* methamphetamines
amphetamines addiction, 296; treatment of, 187–90
amyl nitrite, 141. *See also* alcohol
anandamide, 26, 197
anesthetics, gaseous, 141, 142– 43. *See also* alcohol
angel dust. *See* PCP
Anslinger, Harry, 275
Antabuse, 151–52, 259
antidepressants, 132, 187, 252
antisocial personality disorder, 104
anxiety, 77, 159, 213, 241
arginine, 109
Armour Company (meat pack- ing firm), 32
arthritis, rheumatoid, 309
asthma, 128
atropine, 23

attention deficit hyperactivity disorder (ADHD), 187
Australia, 290
availability, drug, 298–99, 302
ayahuasca, 219. *See also* hallucinogens

bans, cigarette sales, 247, 317
barbiturates, 6, 87, 93, 140. *See also* alcohol
Basques, 112
beer, 136. *See also* alcohol
Beijing Medical University, 79
bell-shaped dose-response curve, 213
benzodiazepines, 6, 93, 140–41, 252, 321. *See also* alcohol
Bernard, Claude, 21
beta-endorphins, 30. *See also* peptides
Bill of Rights (U.S. Constitu- tion), 310
binging, 87, 183
biogenic amines, 24–25. *See also* neurotransmitters
black market, 318, 319
bleach, 271
bleeding, severe, 146
blood alcohol level, 319
brain, 83–97; and alcohol, 85, 137, 139–40, 142–44; and amphetamines, 186–87; and caffeine, 210, 213–14; and cannabis, 196–98, 201–2; ce- rebral cortex, 202, 220; chemical transmission within, 21–24; and cocaine, 186–87; and hallucinogens, 220–21; hippocampus, 201–2; locus coeruleus, 14, 220; mecha- nisms of adaptation, 94–96; neurotransmitters within, 33– 34; nucleus accumbens, 197,

220; and PCP, 227–28; receptors within, 41–42; seesaw model of, 83, 90
Breathalyzer, 137
breeding, selective, 105–6
bronchitis, 124–25, 126
buprenorphine, 6, 170–71, 189
bupropion, 132. *See also* antidepressants
buttons, 224

cactus, 7. *See also* hallucinogens; peyote cactus
caffeine, 7, 26, 86, 207–18; behavioral effects of, 208–9; drug policy for, 324–25; effect on brain, 210, 213–14; experiments, 207, 208–9, 210; genetic predisposition toward, 214, 217; health effects of, 209–12, 216–17; hedonic effects of, 209, 210, 212–13; tolerance, 89, 210–11, 213; use of, 8, 9, 237; withdrawal syndrome, 92, 93–94, 214–15
Canada, 204
cancer, 203; lung, 123–24, 125, 126, 201
cannabis, 7, 107, 195–206; appetite stimulation by, 198, 203; behavioral effects of, 198–200; drug policy for, 323–24; effect on brain, 196–98, 201–2; health effects of, 201–3; hedonic effects of, 198–99, 230; and law enforcement, 281–82; societal impact of, 204–5; use of, 9, 203–4, 236, 263, 274, 280–82, 324; withdrawal syndrome, 92, 197, 202
carbon monoxide, 126, 242
cardiovascular disease, 125–26

catalytic antibodies, 190, 259
cathinone, 181
cellular tolerance, 87–88
cerebellum, 202
cerebral cortex, 202, 220
Charles II (of England), 212
chemical transmission, 21–24
chemotherapy, 203
children: advertising to, 317–18; drug use by, 236–38, 244–45
China, 112–13, 295–96
chloroform, 141
Christianity, 136
chromatography, thin-layer, 167
cigarette smoking, 118, 246; by children, 236, 245; health effects of, 123–28
cilia, 124–25
Civil War (U.S.), 158
class, socioeconomic, 262
clonidine, 252
Coca-Cola, 181
cocaine, 5, 59, 65, 86, 107, 180–81, 214; administration routes of, 85–86, 182; chemical forms of, 6, 181–82; drug policy for, 322–23; effect on brain, 186–87; health effects of, 11, 183, 190–92; hedonic effects of, 180, 182, 230; relapse into use of, 187–88; tolerance, 89, 183; use of, 7, 9, 180, 181, 236–37, 244, 245; withdrawal syndrome, 90, 92, 184, 185, 187
cocaine addiction: treatment of, 171, 187–90
cocaine hydrochloride, 182
Cocaine Politics (Marshall and Scott), 299
coca leaf, 6, 180
codeine, 6. *See also* opiates

coffee, caffeinated, 210
coffeehouses, 212
cold turkey withdrawal, 90, 161, 252, 264, 296
Colombia, 299
comorbidity, 11–12, 104, 122, 252
complementary DNA (cDNA), 46
complementary pairing principle, 44
compliance problem, 4
conditioned association triggers, 129, 184, 187–88
conditioned place preference (CPP), 61–62
conditioned withdrawal, 257
condom distribution, 267, 268
Confessions of an English Opium-Eater (De Quincey), 159
contraception, compulsory, 313
controllability, 119–20
corruption, 299–300
cortisol, 45
Costa Rica, 112
counseling, 254
CPP (conditioned place reference), 61–62
crack. See cocaine
crank. See methamphetamines
crash, 183
cravings, 95–96, 153, 183, 188, 256–57, 258
CREB (protein), 186
crime, 261–64, 262, 314–15
critical interval, 88–89
cross-dependence, 145
crystal. See methamphetamines
curare, 21–22
cutoff effect, 144
cystic fibrosis, 111
cytosine, 44

DARE (Drug Abuse Resistance Education), 243–44
date rape drugs, 141
DAWN (Drug Abuse Warning Network), 11
Delancey Street Foundation, 252
delirium tremens. See alcohol, withdrawal syndrome
demand reduction, 294–95, 310, 327
dependence. See withdrawal syndrome
De Quincey, Thomas, 159
desensitization, 257–58
diabetes, 101
dimers, 51
disinhibition, 66
distillation, 136
disulfiram, 151–52, 259
DNA, 44; sequences, 108–9
Dole, Vincent, 164
dopamine, 25, 180, 214; hypothesis, 63–67
dosages, 86, 137–38, 168–69, 230
double-blind experimentation, 57, 168, 169, 211
Drug Abuse Resistance Education (DARE), 243–44
Drug Abuse Warning Network (DAWN), 11
Drug Action Teams, 278
drug administration: inhalation, 84–85, 118–20, 158, 182, 237; intravenous injection, 84–85, 119, 159, 182, 237
drug discrimination, 54–58
drug education, 238–40, 245–47
drug policy, 307–28; and AIDS epidemic, 311–12; for alco-

hol, 319–21; for caffeine, 324–25; for cannabis, 323–24; for cocaine, 322–23; and crime, 314–15; demand reduction, 310–11; for hallucinogens, 325; harm reduction, 308–9; and law enforcement, 313–14; for nicotine, 317–19; for opiates, 321–22; research funding, 315–16
drug problem, 293
drug reinforcement, 58, 61, 63
Drugs, Law Enforcement and Foreign Policy (Kerry Committee), 300
drunk driving, 320
drunkenness. *See* alcohol, intoxication
Durrell, Lawrence, 78–79
dynorphins, 30, 31–33, 67. *See also* peptides

ecstasy. *See* MDMA
Edinburgh (Scotland), 269
education: and cannabis, 199; complement to regulation, 313–14
Eighteenth Amendment (U.S. Constitution), 296
electron spin resonance (ESR) spectrometer, 168
EMIT (immunoassay), 168
emotions, suppression of, 79–81
emphysema, 123–24, 124–25, 126
endomorphins, 31. *See also* peptides
endorphins. *See* opioids, endogenous
England. *See* Great Britain
epena, 221, 229

epinephrine, 20, 25
erasing fluid. *See* inhalants
ergot, 221–22
ESR (electron spin resonance) spectrometer, 168
ether, 119, 141
ethical research, 54, 166
Ethiopia, 181
ethnicity, 262, 263, 285
ethnopharmacology, 229
expectation, 199
expression cloning, 45–47
extinction sessions, 188

FDA (Food and Drug Administration), 215, 322, 325
fermentation, 136
fetal alcohol syndrome, 146–47, 191, 312
fetal damage. *See* women, pregnant
Finland, 298
First Amendment (U.S. Constitution), 318
flashbacks, 224, 230
flunitrazepam, 141
fly agaric, 228
Food and Drug Administration (FDA), 215, 322, 325
fractionation, 32
France, 222, 298
free radical, 168
Freud, Sigmund, 180
functional magnetic resonance imaging (fMRI), 42

GABA (gamma-amino butyrate), 25, 49–50, 66, 139, 140, 228
gamma-hydroxybutyrate (GHB), 141, 277
gasoline. *See* inhalants

gateway drugs, 239–40, 262, 310
gay community, 270
gender, 107
gene: chip, 110; expression, 46; knockout, 48; technology, 108
genetic predisposition, 100, 104, 105–6, 107, 113; to alcohol, 106–8, 112–13; to caffeine, 214, 217; research on, 108–13, 113–14. See also vulnerability
genotype, 108; problem, 111–12
GHB (gamma-hydroxybutyrate), 141, 277
Glasgow (Scotland), 269
glaucoma, 203
glutamate, 25, 109, 220, 227
glycine, 25
gonadotropin (LH), 75
gonadotropin-releasing hormone (GnRH), 75
G-protein, 51, 95
Great Britain, 89–90, 136–37, 204, 212, 271; approach to drug addiction, 273–79
guanine, 44

half-way houses, 161–62
hallucinogens, 7, 9, 219–32; addiction to, 229–31; drug policy for, 325; effect on brain, 221–21; hedonic effects of, 222–23, 224–26, 227, 228; ritual use of, 219, 223, 224, 230, 270; therapeutic use of, 7, 231; types of, 221–28
halothane, 119
handedness, 39
happy hour, 319–20

hard drugs, 280
harm reduction, 130, 131, 255–56, 308–9; 302–304. See also needle park
Harrison Act (1914), 164, 181
hashish. See cannabis
health: and alcohol, 10, 146–48, 310, 319; and amphetamines, 183, 184–86; and cannabis, 201–3; and cigarette smoking, 123–28; and cocaine, 11, 183, 190–92; and heroin, 11, 174; and nicotine, 10, 123–28, 310, 317
hedonic effects: of alcohol, 138, 230; of amphetamines, 182, 230; of caffeine, 209, 210, 212; of cannabis, 198–99, 230; of cocaine, 180, 182, 230; of hallucinogens, 222–23, 224–26, 227, 228
hemoglobin, 109
hemp. See cannabis
hepatitis, 270
heroin, 6, 85, 86, 157, 160, 286; administration routes of, 6, 158; compared to methadone, 170; compared to morphine, 274; health effects of, 11, 174; relapse into use of, 161, 172; tolerance, 88–89; use in Vietnam War, 103, 168, 298; use of, 9, 236–37, 245; withdrawal syndrome, 160–61. See also opiates
heroin addiction, 158, 161, 252, 276; genetic predisposition toward, 107, 113; treatment of, 161–62, 255, 289–90
high, 83
Himmelsbach, C. K., 91
hippocampus, 201–2

hits, 183
HIV, 267–68, 270. *See also* AIDS
Home Office (Great Britain), 275
homology cloning, 47–48
Human Genome Project, 108, 316
hypothetical material receptive substance. *See* receptors

ice, 7. *See* methamphetamines
Iceland, 112
ICSS (intracranial self-stimulation), 62–63
illicit drug business, 299
immunoassay, 34, 167–68
incarceration, 253–54, 315, 327–28
Indian Hemp Commission (1894), 204
inhalants, 9, 321
inhalation, 84–85, 118–20, 158, 182; of secondhand smoke, 127–28
injection, intravenous, 84–85, 119, 159, 182, 237
in situ hybridization, 44–45
insomnia, 140
Institute for the Study of Drug Dependence, 278
Institute of Medicine of the National Academy of Sciences (Great Britain), 204, 271
insulin, 20, 101
intracranial self-stimulation (ICSS), 62–63
Italy, 112

Japan, 112–13, 180, 296
Joe Camel, 317
Judaism, 136

junkie. *See* Addicts, street
junkie union, 283
"Just say no!" slogan, 235, 310–11

Kalant, Harold, 307–8
Kerry Committee report (1989), 300
khat, 181. *See also* amphetamines
killer weed. *See* cannabis
Koop, C. Everett, 10
Kosterlitz, Hans W., 28–30

LAAM, 6, 169–70. *See also* methadone
La Guardia Commission (1944), 204
Langley, J. N., 22–23
laughing gas, 141, 142–43
law enforcement, 238, 295, 296–97, 314–15, 320; and cannabis, 281–82; corruption of, 300; and drug policy, 313–14; in Great Britain, 275–76; and opiate addiction, 163–64, 165–66
laws, drug, 204–5, 236, 247, 315, 328
legalization, drug, 4, 300–304
Leshner, Alan, 5
leucine, 30
leucine-enkaphalin, 30
Lewin, Louis, 179, 180–81
LH, 75
lidocaine, 181
ligand binding, 38–41, 40–41, 43
ligand-gated ion channel, 49
liquors, distilled, 136. *See also* alcohol
liver cirrhosis, 297–98

Livingstone, David, 77–78
locus coeruleus, 220
Loewi, Otto, 23
long-term potentiation (LTP), 43
low-threshold treatment programs, 321
LSD (lysergic acid diethylamide), 7, 40, 86, 221, 224, 230–31; hedonic effects of, 222–23. *See also* hallucinogens
LTP (long-term potentiation), 43
lung cancer, 123–24, 125, 126
lysergic acid, 221–22
lysergic acid diethylamide. *See* LSD
lysine, 109

McCaffrey, Barry, 14, 309–10
McCoy, A. W., 299
magic mushrooms, 7, 223–24. *See also* hallucinogens
magnetic resonance imaging (MRI), 42
Man with the Golden Arm, The (Algren), 159
marijuana. *See* cannabis
Marshall, J., 299
Mavrojannis, M., 27
MDMA, 7, 226, 277. *See also* hallucinogens
mecamylamine, 132
Mecca (Saudi Arabia), 212
media. *See* advertising
Medical Social Service for Heroin Users (Netherlands), 283
membrane fluidization, 142
memory loss, 199
mental illness, 111. *See also* comorbidity; schizophrenia
mescaline, 225. *See also* hallucinogens

mesolimbic dopaminergic pathway, 63
metabolic disease hypothesis, 171
metabolic tolerance, 87. *See also* tolerance
methadone, 6, 164, 168–69, 170, 255. *See also* LAAM
methadone buses, 284
methadone maintenance, 164–70, 264, 275, 276–77, 290; development of, 315–16; long-term results of, 171–76; programs, 165–69, 265–67, 272
methamphetamines, 5, 179. *See also* amphetamines
methionine-enkaphalin, 30
methylphenidate, 180, 187
Middle East, 212
Midwestern Prevention Project, 242–43
Monitoring the Future study (1999), 237, 244
morphine, 86, 157, 158; detection of, 166–69; pain suppression from, 72, 159, 162, 274; withdrawal syndrome, 90–91. *See also* opiates
Mothers Against Drunk Driving, 327
MRI (magnetic resonance imaging), 42
mRNA, 44
multiple sclerosis, 203
muscarine, 23
muscimol, 228. *See also* hallucinogens

naloxone, 29, 75–77, 79, 80, 88, 163, 241; medicinal use of, 28, 171; and withdrawal syndrome, 92–93 naltrexone, 57, 75, 152–53, 163, 189; and relapse prevention, 258–59

Narcan. *See* naloxone

National Health Service (Great Britain), 278

National Household Survey on Drug Abuse (NHSDA), 7–10, 244

National Institute of Mental Health (NIMH), 11–12

National Institute on Alcohol Abuse and Alcoholism (NIAAA), 146

National Institute on Drug Abuse (NIDA), 169, 237, 240, 250

National Institutes of Health, 203–4

Native American Church, 224, 325

needle exchange, 267–72, 311–12

needle park, 285–88. *See also* harm reduction

Netherlands, approach to drug addiction, 279–85

neurokinin, 72

neuromuscular junction, 22

neurons, opioidergic, 67

neurotransmitter release, measure of, 73–74

neurotransmitters, 19–35, 72, 220, 223; acetylcholine, 20, 23, 24; and addiction, 34–35; adenosine, 25, 213; anandamide, 26, 197; chemical transmission, 21–24; distribution within brain, 33–34; dynorphin, 31–33; endogenous opioids, 26–31; GABA (gamma-amino butyrate), 25, 66, 139; glutamate, 25, 109, 220, 227; identification of, 24–26; and receptors, 42–43, 45. *See also* peptides; receptors

New York City, 267, 270

New York Times, 117

nicotine, 22–23, 26, 60, 86, 89, 117–33, 121–22; administration routes of, 6, 118–20; advertising of, 103, 117–18, 237–38; behavioral effects of, 5, 122–23; drug policy for, 132, 294, 317–19; health effects of, 10, 123–28, 310, 317; relapse into use of, 129–30; use of, 8–10, 118, 313; withdrawal syndrome, 92, 94, 120–21, 132

nicotine addiction: environmental factors of, 102–3; genetic predisposition toward, 107, 113; treatment of, 128–32, 252, 255

nicotine chewing gum, 131

nicotine discrimination, 56–57

nicotine inhaler, 131, 256

nicotine skin patches, 131

nicotinic acetylcholine receptors, 48–49

NIMBY syndrome, 265–67

nitrites, inhaled, 141

nitrous oxide, 141, 142–43

NMDA receptors, 50, 227

nociceptin. *See* orphanin-FQ

noradrenaline, 220

norepinephrine, 25

Novacaine, 181

nucleotides, 44

nucleus accumbens, 197, 220

nutmeg, 225–26. *See also* hallucinogens

Nyswander, Marie, 164

Odyssey, The (Homer), 157
Office of the National Drug
    Control Policy (ONDCP),
    238, 278, 285, 295, 300, 309–
    10
operant behavior, 58
operant conditioning, 119
opiates, 6, 89, 157–77; and do-
    pamine hypothesis, 65–66;
    drug policy for, 321–22; pain
    suppression from, 159–62;
    withdrawal syndrome, 90, 91,
    93, 175. *See also* heroin;
    morphine
opiates addiction: and law en-
    forcement, 163–64, 165–66;
    treatment of, 163, 164–71
opioids, endogenous, 26–31,
    73, 79–81; pain suppression
    by, 72–74, 76–77; relation-
    ship to alcohol, 152–53
opium addiction, 295–96
Oriental flush, 112, 151
orphanin-FQ, 30, 48. *See also*
    peptides
Osler, William, 229

pain, relationship to pleasure,
    71–72
painkillers, 27, 158
pain suppression, 79, 209, 274;
    by endogenous opioids, 72–
    74, 76–77; from morphine,
    72, 159, 162, 274; from opi-
    ates, 159–62
paint thinner. *See* inhalants
panic attacks. *See* flashbacks
party drugs, 141, 277
Pauling, Linus, 109
PCP (phencyclidine), 7, 226–
    28. *See also* hallucinogens
PCR (polymerase chain reac-
    tion), 47

peer pressure, 102
peer support, 252
penicillin, 228
pentobarbital, 87. *See also*
    barbiturates
peptides, 25, 30–33, 67, 75. *See
    also* neurotransmitters
perceived risk, 245
Peru, 299
PET (positron emission tomog-
    raphy), 41–42
peyote cactus, 7, 224–25, 325.
    See also hallucinogens
pharmacology, 14
phencyclidine. *See* PCP
phenotype, 108; problem, 111
phenylalamine, 30
Phoenix House, 252
plasmid, 46
police. *See* law enforcement
Politics of Heroin, The (McCoy),
    299
polydrug abuse, 250
polymerase chain reaction
    (PCR), 47
polymorphisms, 108–9
Pont-Saint-Esprit (France), 222
popcorn jumping, 92–93
population isolates, 112
positron emission tomography
    (PET), 41–42
potency, drug, 40–41
prevention, 235; drug educa-
    tion, 238–40, 245–47; pro-
    grams for, 242–44; shaping
    behavior, 240–41
priming effect, 257. *See also*
    withdrawal syndrome
*Principles of Drug Addiction Treat-
    ment* (NIDA), 250–51
procaine, 181
Prohibition, 295–99
prostitution, 311

psilocybin, 223, 224
psychosis, 184–86, 200, 227
Purkinje, Johannes, 225–26

quarantine, 308

racism, 285. *See also* ethnicity
radioligand, 38
receptors, 37–52, 121, 162,
    213, 220; and addiction, 48–
    52; cloning by homology, 47–
    48; expression cloning, 45–
    47; GABA (gamma-amino
    butyrate), 49–50, 140, 228;
    ligand binding of, 38–41; lo-
    cation within brain, 41–42;
    and neurotransmitters, 42–
    43, 45; and nicotine, 22–23;
    NMDA, 50, 227; seven-helix,
    50–51, 196–97; structure of,
    43–45. *See also*
    neurotransmitters
regulation: complement to ed-
    ucation, 313–14
reinforcement, drug, 58, 61,
    63
relapse, 95–96; into ampheta-
    mine use, 187–88; into co-
    caine use, 187–88; into her-
    oin use, 161, 172; into
    nicotine use, 129–30; preven-
    tion of, 188, 256–60
restriction fragment length pol-
    ymorphisms (RFLPs), 110
reverse transcription, 46
rheumatoid arthritis, 309
risk factor, 215
Ritalin, 180, 187
rituals, 219, 223, 224, 230, 270
roadblocks, random, 320–21
Rohypnol (roofies), 141
runner's high, 73
rush, 159–60

St. Anthony's Fire, 222
saliva testing, 213, 242
Sandoz (pharmaceutical firm),
    221–22
San Pietro (Italy), 112
Saudi Arabia, 212, 296
scare tactics, 240
schizophrenia, 27, 111, 221,
    228. *See also* mental illness
scientific method, 211
Scotland, 269
Scott, P. D., 299
selective breeding, 105–6
self-efficacy, 241
self-report bias, 8, 147, 242,
    254
self-titration, 59–60
sensitivity. *See* tolerance
Sequential Treatment Employ-
    ing Pharmacologic Supports
    (STEPS), 256
serotonin, 220, 223. *See also*
    receptors
shooting galleries, 269
sickle-cell anemia, 109–10, 111
signal transduction, 43, 95
single nucleotide polymor-
    phism (SNP), 108–9, 110–11
sleep, 139, 209–12
sleeping pills, 87. *See also*
    barbiturates
sleep latency, 211, 212
smoke, secondhand, 127–28
snorting, 6, 237
SNP (single nucleotide poly-
    morphism), 108–9, 110–11
social acceptability, 102–3
social learning theory, 240, 241
soft drinks, 7, 181, 215, 237,
    324
soft drugs, 280
solvents, volatile, 141, 142–43.
    See also alcohol

Somalia, 181
Spain, 112
specificity, 34, 39
speed. *See* methamphetamines
spikes, 84
STEPS (Sequential Treatment
Employing Pharmacologic
Supports), 256
stop codon, 109
stress, 77, 159, 213, 241
subsidies, 319
substance abuse disorder, 12
supply reduction, 294–95, 299–
300, 310, 327
susceptibility, 12
Sweden, 104, 180, 320
Switzerland, 89–90, 256; approach to drug addiction,
285–90
Synanon, 264
synapses, 42

taxes, 247, 313, 318, 319
temperance movement, 296
testing, drug use, 137, 166–67,
213, 242, 254; vigilance, 207,
208–9, 212
tetrahydrocannibol. *See* THC
Thailand, 299
THC inhaler, 204
THC (tetrahydrocannibol),
196, 197. *See also* cannabis
thin-layer chromatography, 167
thiocyanate, 242
thrill, 80
thymine, 44
tobacco, 117–18; industry, 103,
237, 317
tolerance, 83, 86–90, 183, 199;
alcohol, 89, 108, 137, 145;
caffeine, 89, 210–11, 213
tranquilizers, 252. *See also*
benzodiazepines

transporters, 51–52
treatment, addiction, 163, 164–
71, 250–56, 279; for alcohol,
148–54; for amphetamines,
187–90; availability of, 311,
327; for cocaine, 171, 187–90;
for heroin, 161–62, 255, 289–
90; for nicotine, 128–32, 252,
255
Trexan. *See* naltrexone
trip, 231
tryptophan, 25
12-step program, 149–51
2-arachidonyl glycerol, 197
tyrosine, 25, 30

United Nations Single Convention on Narcotic Drugs,
274
U.S., approach to drug addiction, 275
U.S. Constitution: Bill of
Rights, 310; Eighteenth
Amendment, 296; First
Amendment, 318
U.S. Public Health Service hospital (Lexington, Kentucky),
91, 164
uracil, 44
urine testing, 166–67

valine, 109
Valium. *See* benzodiazepines
Vanderbilt University, 184
Vietnam War, 103, 168, 298
vigilance testing, 207, 208–9,
212
violence, 282
Volstead Act (1919), 296
vulnerability, 99–100, 172, 256.
See also genetic predisposition

"war on drugs," 13, 294, 299, 309

White House Panel on Narcotic and Drug Abuse (1962), 204

wines, 136. *See also* alcohol

withdrawal syndrome: of alcohol, 144–45; of amphetamines, 90, 185, 187; of barbiturates, 140; of caffeine, 92, 93–94, 214–15; of cannabis, 92, 197, 202; of cocaine, 90, 92, 184, 185, 187; of morphine, 90–91; and naloxone, 92–93; of nicotine, 92, 94, 120–21, 132; of opiates, 90, 91, 93, 160–61, 175; of PCP, 227. *See also* priming effect

women: and cigarette smoking, 118

women, pregnant, 302, 312–13; and alcohol, 146–48; and caffeine, 216–17; and cannabis, 202–3; and cocaine, 190–92; and nicotine, 126–27; and PCP, 227

xenon, 142–43

Yanomani, 221

Youth Anti-Drug Media Campaign, 317

Zyban, 132. *See also* antidepressants